Guide Medical Informatics, the Internet and Telemedicine

Guide to
Medical Informatics,
the Internet
and Telemedicine

Enrico Coiera

CHAPMAN & HALL MEDICAL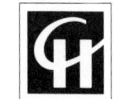
London · Weinheim · New York · Tokyo · Melbourne · Madras

Published by Chapman & Hall, 2–6 Boundary Row, London SE1 8HN, UK

Chapman & Hall, 2–6 Boundary Row, London SE1 8HN, UK

Chapman & Hall GmbH, Pappelallee 3, 69469 Weinheim, Germany

Chapman & Hall USA, Fourth Floor, 115 Fifth Avenue, New York, NY 10003, USA

Chapman & Hall Japan, ITP-Japan, Kyowa Building, 3F, 2-2-1 Hirakawacho, Chiyoda-ku, Tokyo 102, Japan

Chapman & Hall India, R. Seshadri, 32 Second Main Road, CIT East, Madras 600 035, India

First edition 1997

© 1997 Enrico Coiera

Printed in Great Britain at the Alden Press, Oxford

ISBN 0 412 75710 9

∞ Printed on acid free text paper, manufactured in accordance with ANSI/ NISO Z39.48-1992 and ANSI/NISO Z39.48-1984 (Permanence of Paper)

NOTE

Medicine is an ever-changing science. As new research and clinical experience broaden our knowledge, changes in treatment and drug therapy are required. The author and the publisher of this work have checked with sources believed to be reliable in their efforts to provide information that is complete and generally in accord with the standards accepted at the time of publication. However, in view of the possibility of human error or changes in medical sciences, neither the author nor the publisher nor any other party who has been involved in the preparation or publication of this work warrants that the information contained herein is in every respect accurate or complete, and they are not responsible for any errors or omissions or for the results obtained from the use of such information. Readers are encouraged to confirm the information contained herein with other sources.

Table of Contents

Preface

This book has been written for healthcare professionals who wish to understand the principles and applications of information and communication systems within healthcare. It is presented, I hope, in a way that will make it accessible to anyone, independent of their knowledge of technology. It should thus also be suitable as a component of undergraduate and postgraduate training.

It has not always been easy to explain to those outside the field what medical informatics is all about. Its terminology and concepts, and perhaps more than anything its focus on technology, have made it hard to bridge the gap to the concerns of those working day to day in clinical practice.

However, computing technology is now commonplace in healthcare, and the 'communications revolution' is transforming our daily lives through the likes of the Internet and mobile telephony. So now the technology gap does not seem so great. As importantly, clinicians are starting to understand that some of their biggest problems may only yield to the concerted application of information and communication technologies. Evidence-based clinical practice, for example, can only truly be possible within a clinical community that is set up to attack the mounds of clinical evidence, and then share the distillate through a richly woven communications web.

Yet, amidst all this change, it is often unclear what is fundamental and what is just the fleeting detail of ever-changing technology. Thus the very pace of change is both ally and enemy. It is one of the biggest barriers to informatics concepts and skills becoming a natural part of every healthcare worker's knowledge.

It is with this perspective that I have written this book. It is not so much about the details of the different information or communication technologies. Rapid technological change is a given, and it is impossible to track it all in a single text. More importantly, the finer details of different technologies are probably not relevant or even of interest to most healthcare workers. They want to drive the car, not know what goes on under the hood.

The book is also intended as an introductory text for those who wish to undertake a postgraduate career in informatics. For these readers, I have tried to include more advanced material where possible, along with a strong emphasis on basic principles throughout. Given the introductory nature of this book, I have intentionally avoided some more advanced or specialised areas that might properly be considered a part of informatics, such as formal decision analysis. The text also assumes that informatics students will be taught other more technological modules in parallel. Thus, this book intentionally does not explore subjects like statistics, the principles of programming computers, the basics of computer or communications hardware, computer networking, security or database design. There are many excellent texts available in these fields, and an informatics professional will need a solid grounding in these areas. A single text like the present one cannot, and should not, attempt to provide that. Nevertheless, I have included some introductory material on communications technologies and computer networks because this area is so rapidly changing that it may be difficult to obtain an appropriate text.

Finally, I have tried, however imperfectly, to do justice to history. It is a constant source of amazement to me when I read a mid-nineteenth century text like Oesterlen's *Medical Logic* to find a mind with a richer understanding of the nuances of informatics than many of us have today. It is easy to always look to those close to us in time, but we are richer if we can steal the wider view. It is harsh when it reminds us how little has changed, or how little further we have understood. It whispers encouragement too, because things do change and we do move forward. What would someone like Oesterlen have made of the World Wide Web, or of an expert system?

As enthusiastic as I am with the current shape of the book, I am very conscious that it will fall short of the mark in many places. It is my hope that readers will take the time to let me know where I have succeeded, and where I need to improve the text. I would like to see the book evolve over the next few years, to meet the changing needs of healthcare professionals, just as it needs to evolve because of the pace of technological change.

E.C.
ewc@pobox.com
http://www.pobox.com/~enrico.coiera

Bath, UK
March, 1997

Acknowledgements

I owe my continuing interest in medical informatics to a number of individuals, and I can think of no better place to thank them all than this book.

At the Royal North Shore Hospital in Sydney, Australia, Dr. David More took a young medical resident with a naïve interest in computers, and with much kindness, pointed me in the direction of informatics. Dr. Claude Sammut gently supervised me as I moved through a PhD in computer science, exploring the application of artificial intelligence in medicine. Professor Paul Compton warned me against the evils of Platonism, and was a never-ending source of good humour, ideas, and encouragement. My fellow doctoral students Tim Menzies, David Hume, Bill Kneipp, Ashwin Srinivasan and Ian Gibson were a bedrock, and taught me most of the computer science that I would otherwise had missed. It is a source of much sadness to me that Bill and Davey are already no longer with us.

After I left Australia to work in the UK, I had the good fortune to meet Professor John Fox. John not only gave me my first real informatics research job, but nurtured in me a self-belief without which I would not have dreamed of writing this book.

I also owe an enormous debt to my colleagues at the Hewlett-Packard Laboratories in Bristol. Over the last few years, I have been given the space and resources to explore my ideas in medical informatics, and to learn about new technologies in a way that I doubt I could have done anywhere else in the world. It is a unique privilege to work there. I thank Martin Merry, Ray Crispin and John Taylor for their support and encouragement to write this book. There are so many HP labbies that I should thank, that I am perhaps safer in not naming them all. However, Simon Lewis, an outstanding software engineer who has worked with me on many projects, deserves special mention for encouraging me to start this book. I am also indebted to Graham Higgins for introducing me to the perspectives of cognitive psychology, and the work of Elanor Rosch on basic level concepts, both of which have influenced my thinking greatly. Finally, Vanessa Tombs has worked side by side with me through most of my projects at the Labs, and her practicality, wisdom and insight into the clinical domain have been marvellous companions to me.

This book is much better for the detailed comments of Kate Berghaus, James Harrison, Helen van Horick, Michael Power and Stuart Stapleton who all read draft chapters for me. Andzerj Glowinski in particular deserves thanks for his insightful comments on the coding and classification chapters.

Finally, writing a book is a long and lonely marathon, and if I have finished, it is only because I have been sustained by the love of my parents and family, and most of all, Blair. I thank you.

Publisher's acknowledgements

Some material in the introduction, and in Chapters 9 and 18 has been adapted from *BMJ*, 310, 1381-7, (1995), and *BMJ*, 311, 2-4, (1996), with kind permission from the BMJ Publishing Group.

Figure 9.1 is taken from Fox et al. (1996) and appears with kind permission of the copyright holder John Fox.

Material form my papers in *Journal American Medical Informatics Association*,3,6, 363-366, (1966), and the *Proceedings of American Medical Informatics Association Autumn Symposium*, 17-21, (1996) has been adapted within Chapters 15 and 19, and appears with permission.

Figures 21.1, 21.2, 21.3, 21.5 and some material in Chapter 21 appear with permission of W. B. Saunders Company Ltd. London. They are adapted from my chapter on Automated Signal Interpretation, in P. Hutton, C. Prys-Roberts (eds.) *Monitoring in Anaesthesia and Intensive Care*, Bailliere Tindall Ltd., London, (1994).

Of what value, it may be urged, will be all the theorizing and speculation through which it would profess to guide us, when we come to practise at the bedside? Who has not heard so-called practical men say that medicine is a purely empirical science; that everything depends upon facts and correct experience; or, perhaps, that the power to cure is the main point? All arguments and theories, they say, do not enable the physician to treat his patients more correctly; in an art like medicine they rather do harm, or, at best, no positive good. It is there we are in need of experience - facts, and above all, remedies and their correct employment: all the rest is evil.

F. Oesterlen, *Medical Logic*, p. 8, (1855).

Introduction
to medical informatics

If physiology literally means 'the logic of life', and pathology is 'the logic of disease', then medical informatics is the logic of healthcare. It is the rational study of the way we think about patients, and the way that treatments are defined, selected and evolved. It is the study of how medical knowledge is created, shaped, shared and applied. Ultimately, it is the study of how we organise ourselves to create and run healthcare organisations. With such a pivotal role, it is likely that in the next century, the study of informatics will become as fundamental to the practice of medicine as anatomy has been to the last.

Medical informatics is thus as much about computers as cardiology is about stethoscopes. Rather than drugs, X-ray machines or surgical instruments, the tools of informatics are more likely to be clinical guidelines, formal medical languages, information systems, or communication systems like the Internet. These tools, however, are only a means to an end, which is the delivery of the best possible healthcare.

Although the name 'medical informatics' only came into use around 1973 (Protti, 1995), it is a study that is as old as medicine itself. It was born the day that a doctor first wrote down some impressions about a patient's illness, and used these to learn how to treat their next patient.

Informatics has grown considerably as a medical discipline in recent years fuelled, in part no doubt, by the advances in computer technology. What has fundamentally changed is our ability to describe and manipulate medical knowledge at a highly abstract level, as has our ability to build up rich communication systems to support the process of healthcare.

The rise of medical informatics

Perhaps the greatest change in medical thinking over the last two centuries has been the ascendancy of the scientific method. Since its acceptance, it has become the lens through which we see the world, and governs everything from the way we view disease, through to the way we battle it.

It is now hard to imagine just how controversial the introduction of theory and experimental method into medicine once was. Then, it was strongly opposed by the views of the empiricists, who believed that observation, rather than theoretical conjecture, was the only basis for the rational practice of medicine.

With this perspective, it is almost uncanny to hear again the old empiricists' argument that 'medicine is an art', and not a place for unnecessary speculation or formalisation. This time, the defenders are not fighting against those who wish to put our understanding of disease and treatment on a theoretical ground. Rather, it is against those who wish to develop formal theoretical methods to regulate the communal practice of medicine. Words like clinical audit, outcome measures, healthcare rationing and even evidence-based medicine now define the new intellectual battleground.

While the advance of the scientific method is pushing medical knowledge down to a fine grained molecular and genetic level, events at the other end of the scale are forcing the change. Firstly, the enterprise of medicine has become so large that it now consumes more national resources than any country is willing to bear. Despite sometimes heroic efforts to control this growth in consumption, the healthcare budget continues to expand. There is thus a social and economic imperative, coming from outside healthcare, that is intent on controlling its processes.

However, the structure of medical practice is also coming under pressure from within. The scientific method, long the backbone of medicine, is now under threat. The reason for this is not that experimental science is unable to answer the ever pressing questions about the nature of disease and its treatment. Rather, it is almost too good at its job. As medical research ploughs ahead in laboratories and clinics across the world, like some great theory machine, medical practitioners are being swamped by its results. So much research is now published each week that it can literally take decades for the results of clinical trials to translate into changes in clinical practice.

So, healthcare workers find themselves practising with ever restricting resources, and unable, even if they had the time, to keep abreast of the knowledge of best practice hidden in the literature. As a consequence, the scientific basis of clinical practice trails far behind that of clinical research.

Two hundred years ago, enlightened physicians understood that empiricism needed to be replaced by a more formal and testable way of characterising disease and its treatment. The tool they used then was the scientific method. Today we are in analogous situation. Now the demand is that we replace the organisational processes and structures that force the arbitrary selection amongst treatments with ones that can be formalised, tested, and applied rationally.

Modern medicine has moved away from seeing disease in isolation, to understanding that illness occurs at a complex system level. Infection is not simply the result of the invasion of a pathogenic organism, but the complex interaction of an individual's immune system, nutritional status, environmental and genetic endowments. By seeing things at a system level, we come ever closer to understanding what it really means to be diseased, and how that state, however defined, can be reversed.

We now need to make the same conceptual leap and begin to see the great systems of knowledge that enmesh the delivery of healthcare. These systems produce our knowledge, tools, languages and methods. Thus, a new treatment is never created and tested in intellectual isolation. It gains significance as part of a greater system of knowledge, since it occurs in the context of previous treatments and insights, as well as the context of a society's resources and needs. Further, the work does not finish when we scientifically prove a treatment works. We must try to communicate this new knowledge, and help others to understand, apply, and adapt it.

These then, are the challenges for medicine. Can we put together rational structures for the way clinical evidence is pooled, communicated, and applied to routine care? Can we develop organisational processes and structures that minimise the resources we use, and maximise the benefits delivered? And finally, what tools and methods need to be developed to help achieve these aims in a manner that is practicable, testable, and in keeping with the fundamental goal of healthcare - the relief from disease? The role of medical informatics is to help develop a rational basis to answer these questions, as well as to help create the tools to achieve these goals.

The scope of informatics is thus enormous. It finds application in the design of decision support systems for practitioners (e.g. Miller, 1994), in the development of computer tools for research (e.g. Hunter, 1993), and in the study of the very essence of medicine - its corpus of knowledge (e.g. Keravnou, 1992). Yet the modern discipline of medical informatics is still relatively young. Many different groups within healthcare are addressing the issues raised here, and not always in a co-ordinated fashion. Indeed, these groups are not always even aware that their efforts are connected, nor that their concerns are ones of informatics.

The first goal of this book is to present a unifying set of basic informatics principles, which influence everything from the delivery of care to an individual patient, through to the design of whole healthcare systems. Its next goal is to present the breadth of issues which concern informatics, show how they are related, and to encourage research into understanding the common principles that connect them.

Each area that is covered has been written with three criteria in mind - its **possibility**, its **practicability**, and its **desirability**. Possibility reflects the science of informatics - what in theory can be achieved? Practicability addresses the potential for successfully engineering a system or introducing a new process - what can actually be done given the constraints of the real world? Desirability looks at the fundamental motivation for using a given process or technology.

These criteria are suggested in part because we need to evolve a framework to judge the claims made for new technologies, and those who seek to profit from them. Just as there is a long-standing symbiosis between the pharmaceutical industry and medicine, there is a newer and consequently less examined relationship between medicine and the computing and telecommunication industries. Clinicians should try to judge the claims of these newcomers in the same cautious way that they would examine claims about a new drug (Wyatt, 1987). Perhaps more so, given that clinicians are far more knowledgeable about pharmacology than they are about informatics and telecommunications.

Overview of the book

The book is organised into a number of parts, all of which revolve around the two distinct strands of information and communication. The unique character of each strand is explored individually. There is also an emphasis on understanding the rich way in which they can interact and complement each other.

Part 1 - Basic Concepts in Informatics

Like medicine, informatics has both theoretical and applied aspects to its study. This first part of the book is focused on developing an intuitive understanding of the basic theoretical concepts needed to approach informatics practice in a principled way. Three fundamental ideas underpin the study of informatics - the notions of what constitutes a model, what one means by information, and what defines a system. Each of these three ideas is explored to develop an understanding of how one can develop complex information and communication systems.

A recurring theme in this part will be the need to understand the limitations imposed upon us whenever we create or use a model of the world. Understanding these limitations defines the ultimate limits of possibility for informatics, irrespective of whichever technology one may wish to apply in its service.

Part 2 - Information Systems in Healthcare

The chapters in this part explore the special character of information systems in healthcare. The electronic medical record (EMR) is discussed in many different guises throughout the book, and its role and scope are introduced here. Information systems like the EMR manage a wide variety of activities. Ultimately, the way that these activities are modelled, measured and then managed is determined by information system design.

Sometimes, leaving things unsaid or informal is more productive. Consequently, the important concept of system formality is also introduced here, since it is not always appropriate to build information systems. Indeed it can often be counterproductive. Understanding the role of formality helps informed decisions to be made before information systems are introduced.

The concept of formality also helps us to understand the different roles that communication and information systems play in healthcare. The final chapter in this part spends some time describing how one sets out to build such systems, and some of the design problems that bedevil that process.

Having laid down these foundational ideas in the first two parts of the book, the next two parts turn to focus on two information problems that are specific to healthcare - protocol-based care, and clinical coding.

Part 3 - Protocol-based Systems

Clinical guidelines or protocols have been in limited use for many years. The current emphasis on evidence-based medical practice has made it more likely that healthcare workers will use, and perhaps be involved in the design and maintenance of protocols.

In this part, the various forms and uses of protocols are introduced. Their characteristic advantages and limitations of are also discussed. These are then used to formulate a set of protocol design principles. Finally, the various roles that computer-based protocol systems can play in clinical practice are outlined. These cover both traditional 'passive' support where protocols are kept as a reference, and active systems in which the computer uses the protocol to assist in the delivery of care. For example, protocols incorporated into the EMR can generate clinical alerts or make treatment recommendations.

Part 4 - Language, Coding and Classification in Healthcare

If the data contained in electronic patient record systems is to be analysed, then it needs to be accessible in some regular way. This is usually thwarted by the variations in medical terminology used by different individuals, institutions and nations. To remedy the problem, large dictionaries of standardised medical terms have been created.

The chapters in this section introduce the basic ideas of concepts, terms, codes and classifications, and demonstrate their various uses. The inherent advantages and limitations of using terms and codes are discussed. The last chapter in particular looks at some more advanced issues in coding, describing the theoretical limitations to coding, and outlines practical approaches to managing these issues, as well as presenting open research questions.

Part 5 - Communication Systems in Healthcare

While interpersonal communication skills are fundamental to patient care, the process of communication has, for a long time, not been well supported technologically. Now, with the widespread availability of communication systems supporting mobility, voice mail, electronic mail and video-conferencing, new possibilities arise. The chapters in this section introduce the basic types of communication services and explain the different benefits of each.

Given that much of the technology is new for many, one chapter is devoted to describing the basics of the various different communication systems now available. The final chapter in this part examines the field of telemedicine, in the context of these new technologies. The potential of telemedical systems within different areas of healthcare is described, but the importance of carefully choosing the right set of technologies for a given problem is emphasised.

Part 6 - The Internet

Information systems are starting to become indistinguishable from communication ones, and this convergence is perhaps nowhere more apparent than with the Internet. This part explores in detail the phenomenal rise of the Internet and the World Wide Web, and examines why its technologies have proven to be so revolutionary. The complex way that the Web alters the balance of information publishing and access is explained, along with the consequences of these changes. The full impact of the Internet on healthcare has yet to be felt. Some of the many different ways that it will change healthcare are presented here, from the way communication occurs, through to the change it will have upon the doctor-patient relationship.

Part 7 - Intelligent Clinical Decision Support

The concluding chapters of the book look to some of the most complex computer systems created so far - those based upon the technologies of artificial intelligence (AI). The early promise of computer programs that could assist clinicians in the process of diagnosis have come to fruition, and they are now in routine use in many clinical situations. AI techniques also permit the creation of systems able to assist with therapy planning, information seeking, and the generation of alerts.

The final chapter in this part looks in detail at the way technologies like expert systems and neural networks can help interpret clinical signals. They find application in creating intelligent patient monitors, and potentially, autonomous therapeutic devices like self-adjusting patient ventilators.

Part
One

Basic Concepts in Informatics

*It is an established opinion amongst some men, that there are in understanding certain **innate principles**... stamped upon the mind of man which the soul receives in its very first being, and brings into the world with it. It would be sufficient to convince unprejudiced readers of the falseness of this supposition. If I could only show... how men, barely by the use of their natural faculties, may attain to all the knowledge they have, without the help of any innate impressions.*

John Locke, *An Essay Concerning Human Understanding*, Book 1, 1(1), (1689).

Man tries to make for himself in the way that suits him best a simplified and intelligible picture of the world and thus to overcome the world of experience, for which he tries to some extent to substitute this cosmos of his. This is what the painter, the poet, the speculative philosopher and the natural scientist do, each in his own fashion...
one might suppose that there were any number of possible systems ... all with an equal amount to be said for them; and this opinion is no doubt correct, theoretically. But evolution has shown that at any given moment out of all conceivable constructions one has always proved itself absolutely superior to all the rest.

A. Einstein, *The World as I See It*, (1935).

Chapter 1

Models

The study of medicine is based upon a few basic ideas like the cell or the concept of disease. Informatics, similarly, is built upon a few concepts like data, models, systems and information. Unlike medicine, where the core ideas are usually grounded in observations of the physical world, these informatics concepts are abstract ideas. As a consequence, they can be difficult to grasp, and for those used to the study of healthcare, often seem detached from the physical realities of the clinical workplace.

This is further complicated because we use the same words that describe these informatics concepts in everyday language. It is common to ask for more information about a patient, to question what data support a particular conclusion, or to read a textbook that describes a physiological model. In informatics, however, these intuitive ideas need to be much more precisely defined. Having mastered them, it is relatively easy to move on to the key issues facing informatics in medicine.

In this first chapter, we begin the study of informatics by exploring the central idea of models. As will soon become apparent, a deep understanding of what it means to create or apply a model underpins the way we interact with the world. Models define the way we learn about the world, interpret what we see, and apply our knowledge to effect change, whether that be through our own actions, or through the use of technology.

Whether diagnosing a patient's condition, or trying to deliver an efficient service to the public, we use models to direct our actions. Humans are naturally adept at developing mental models of the world, and manage to use them robustly, despite the inherent weaknesses of the models themselves. When these models are created within a technological system like a computer, the effects of modelling error can be amplified significantly (Box 1.1). This is largely because much of the knowledge used in creating the model is no longer available, and as a consequence, the technological system is unable to define the limits of its knowledge. One of the major ideas to be explored in this chapter is that the implicit and explicit assumptions we make at the time a model is created ultimately define the limits of its usefulness.

1.1   Models are abstractions of the real world

Models are commonplace in our everyday lives. People are familiar with the idea of building model aeroplanes, or looking at a small-scale model of a building to imagine what it will look like when built. In medicine, models are ubiquitous. They underlie all our clinical activities. For example, whenever we interact with patients, we use internalised models of disease to guide the process of diagnosis and treatment.

Models actually serve two quite distinct purposes, and both of these are of interest. The first use of a model is as some kind of copy of the world. The modelling process takes some aspect of the world, and creates a description of it. A simple example will make this clearer. Imagine a camera taking a photograph. The image that is captured upon the camera's film is a model of the observed world:

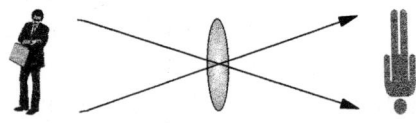

We can generalise from the way a camera lens and film record a physical object to describe the way that all models are created. The process of creating a model of the real world is one of abstraction:

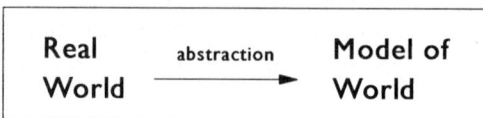

Box 1.1 - Therac-25

Between June 1985 and January 1987, Therac-25 linear accelerators operating in the USA and Canada delivered massive radiation overdoses to at least 6 patients, causing death or serious radiation injury. Patients received doses of up to 20,000 rads where a dose of 200 rads was a typical therapeutic dose, and a 500 rad whole-body dose will cause death in 50% of cases. These were arguably the worst radiation incidents associated with medical accelerators in the history of radiotherapy.

Medical linear accelerators operate by creating a high energy electron beam. The beam is focused onto a patient to destroy tumour tissue, and leaves healthy tissue outside the beam focus relatively unaffected. The high energy beam produced by these devices is focused through a tungsten shield. This 'flattens' the beam to therapeutic levels, and acts like a lens to focus the beam to a tissue depth appropriate for a given patient.

In the Therac-25 accidents, the tungsten shield was not in place when the radiation dose was delivered, resulting in patients receiving a full dose of the raw 25 MeV electron beam. There were a number of different causes of the various overdoses, but each essentially resulted from modelling errors in the system's software and hardware (Leveson and Turner, 1993).

One critical error resulted from the reuse of some of the software from a previous machine, the Therac-20. This software worked acceptably in the 20, but when reused in the 25 permitted an overdose to be given. This was because while the 20 had a physical backup safety system, this had been removed in the design of the 25. The Therac-20 software was thus reused in the 25 on the assumption that the change in machines would not affect the way the software operated. So, software modelled to one machine's environment, was used in a second context in which that model was not valid.

Another problem lay in the measurement system that reported the radiation dose given to patients. It was designed to work with doses in the therapeutic range, but when exposed to the full beam strength, became saturated and gave a low reading. As a result, several patients were overdosed repeatedly, because technicians believed the machine was delivering low doses. Thus, the measurement system was built upon an assumption that it would never have to detect high radiation levels.

All of these failures occurred because of the poor way models were used by the designers of the Therac-25. They did not understand that many of the assumptions that were left implicit in the specifications of the device would quickly become invalid in slightly changed circumstances, and would lead to catastrophic failure.

The effects of the abstraction process are directly analogous to the effects of using a camera. In particular, the image captured upon film has three important features which are characteristic of all models.

- Firstly, the image is simpler than the real thing. There are always more features in the real world than can be captured on film. One could, for example, always use a more powerful lens to capture ever finer detail. Equally, models are always less detailed than the real world from which they are drawn. A map for example, will not contain every feature of the city streets it records. Since models are always less detailed than the thing they describe, information is lost in the abstraction process.

- Secondly, the image is a distortion of the real world. Through the use of different light filters, lenses and films, very different images of the observed world are obtained. None of them is the 'true' image of the object. Indeed there is no such thing. The camera system just records a particular point of view on the world. Abstraction also imposes a point of view upon the real world, and inevitably the resulting model is distorted in some way. Thus a map looks very little like the terrain it models. Some land features are emphasised, and others de-emphasised or ignored. In physiology, the heart can be modelled as a mechanical pump. This model emphasises one particular aspect of the organ system, but it is clearly much more than this. It also has a complex set of functions to do with the regulation of blood pressure, blood volume, and organ perfusion.

- Thirdly, as a consequence of this process of distortion, there are many possible images that can be created of the same object. Different images might be taken for very different purposes, emphasising different aspects of the object. Similarly, since there are a variety of aspects that could be modelled of any physical object, and a variation in the level of detail captured, many models can be created. Indeed, the number of possible models is infinite. The mind for example, can be considered from a Freudian or Jungian perspective. It can also be likened to a computer, or be modelled as a collection of neurones (Figure 1.1).

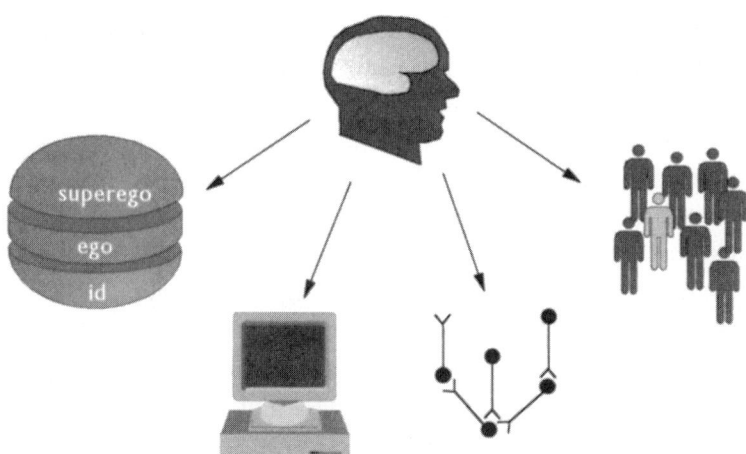

Figure 1.1: *Multiple models can highlight different aspects of the same object, to achieve different ends.*

Before a model is used, one therefore has to be clear about what has actually been modelled. This is because, when models are created, the circumstances at the time have a strong influence on the final value of the model. For example, before the work of the famous physician Galen, it was assumed that the arteries contained air. This was because arteries were observed to be empty after death (Schafer and Thane, 1891). The physicians making these observations had thought they had created a model of arterial function in living humans, but all they had created was a model valid in cadavers. So, the context in which a model is created affects its validity for any other context within which it might be used (see Box 1.1).

As a consequence of these characteristics of models, a final one now becomes evident. All models are built for a reason. When we create a model, we actively choose amongst the many possible models that could be created, to build one that suits our particular purposes. For example, the point of view captured in a map is determined by the way the map will be used. A driver's map emphasises streets and highways. A hiker's map emphasises terrain and altitude. Thus, one actively excludes or distorts aspects of the world to satisfy a particular purpose.

This last point is crucial to much of what will follow in later chapters. It leads on to a related idea, which has already been touched upon. Just as a camera cannot capture a 'true' image of an object, one cannot ever build a 'true' model of an object.

In philosophy, the argument against things ever being inherently correct is equivalent to arguing against the Platonic ideal. This is the idea that pure forms of physical objects exist outside the realms of the physical world. Thus, while a physical sphere may always have an imperfection, Plato believed there existed an 'ideal' mathematical spherical form. The arguments against Plato's ideas say that there is no such ideal or objective truth in the world. There can only be our subjective and local point of view, based upon the input of our senses.

And though the truth will not be discovered by such means - never can that stage be reached - yet they throw light on some of the profounder ramifications of falsehood.

Franz Kafka, *Investigations of a Dog.*

This philosophical argument continues into the present century, as the process of scientific enquiry has been debated, and the nature of experimental evidence defined. This is because a scientific hypothesis is nothing more than a model of some aspect of the world, which is to be tested by an experiment. However, if objective truth cannot be known, then our experiments can never actually prove anything to be true. We are never sure that we are right. The best that experiments can do is show us when our models of the world are wrong (Popper, 1976). What remain are theories that are in some way more or less useful than others in managing the world.

1.2   Models can be used as templates

So far, models have been described as copies or images of the world. There is a second sense to the word model that is equally commonplace. Some models, rather than being copies of real things, are the basis upon which a new thing will be created. An architect, for example, creates a set of drawings that will be translated into a building. Economists build mathematical models of a country's economy, and then use these models to predict the effects of changes in monetary policy. An emergency procedure is written down, and will come into effect if a hospital team is called to a major civil disaster.

Again, a simple example will make this second use of models clearer. If we take an image captured on a photographic slide, a lamp can be used to project a copy of the image onto a screen:

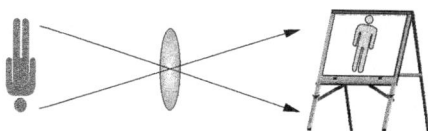

The image stored on the slide is a model of the real world. The projection process uses this model to create a second, slightly altered, image. We can generalise from this to understand how models can act as templates. The process begins with the creation of a model. This might be a design, perhaps recorded as a set of blueprints or specifications. This is followed by a process of construction that uses the model as a template. The result is a built artefact or process that exists in the physical world:

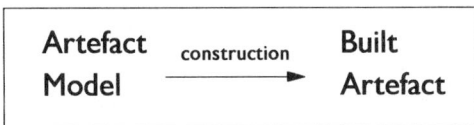

The value of the final image on the screen depends on how the original image was taken, and for what purpose it was taken. Similarly, decisions made at the time a model is created affect how the final product will function. These modelling decisions or **design assumptions** are based upon how the model was created, and its intended purpose.

Thus, the manner in which an image is taken determines the way in which it can be used. Slides are created with the assumption that they are to be used in a particular type of projector. Equally, the manner in which a model is created affects the final value of the artefact that is based on it. For example, different drug therapies are modelled upon knowledge of drug effectiveness. These models of different treatments are usually constructed from the results of clinical trials. However, the methodology adopted in a trial determines the quality of its results. A trial that does not use appropriate controls will have less value than one that is more rigorously designed. Consequently, a treatment based upon such a poor model will probably not be very effective.

Secondly, the success of a projected image in meeting a particular need depends in part on what was originally photographed. A chest

X-ray may be of less value than a CT scan of a skull when managing a head injury. Perhaps even more fundamentally, there is an assumption made at the time the image is taken that an image is the most appropriate way to represent objects. Instead of a coronary angiogram, one might obtain a better 'view' of a heart following an acute infarction through the eyes of a cardiogram or through serum enzyme levels.

When artefacts are created, they too assume that they are to be used for a particular purpose. If the purpose changes, then a design becomes less effective. Thus, the physical design of the waiting room and treatment areas for a general practice clinic will assume a certain number of patients need to be seen during a day, and that certain kinds of therapy will be given. If the clinic was bought by radiologists, they would have to remodel the clinic's design to incorporate imaging equipment, and to reflect a different throughput of patients.

Equally, we can consider a particular treatment of a disease written in a textbook to be a template for what should be done to any given patient. If that treatment was based upon assumptions about the incidence of diseases in a given population, then it may not work well if attempted in a different one. Treating infant diarrhoea in a developed nation is not the same task in underdeveloped nations where poorer resources, malnutrition, and different infecting organisms change the context of treatment.

A more general principle follows from these observations. It should

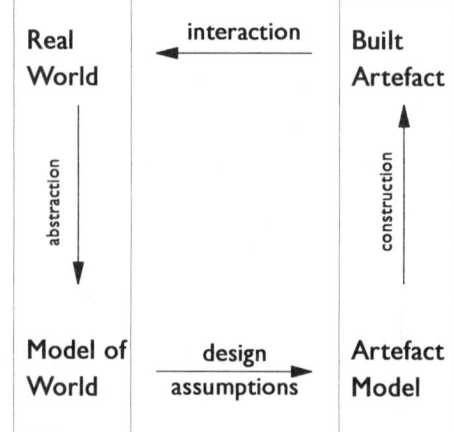

Figure 1.2: *Models of the world are used as a basis for creating template models which define how artefacts like devices or processes will be constructed.*

now be clear that there is no such thing as a general purpose design. All we can have are designs that are better or worse suited to our particular circumstances, and are better or worse at meeting the needs of the task at hand.

As we will see in later chapters, this means that there can be no 'correct' way to treat an illness, no 'right' way to describe a diagnosis, nor a 'right' way to build an information or communication system. There can thus never be an absolutely 'correct' design for a treatment protocol or information system, nor a 'pure' set of terms to describe activities in healthcare. This principle explains why clinical protocols will always have varying effectiveness based upon local conditions, and why medical languages can never be truly general purpose. What we do have are protocols, languages, information and communication systems that are better or worse suited to our purpose than others.

1.3 The way we model the world influences the way we affect the world

In the previous sections we saw how models acted either as copies of the world, or as templates upon which new things are created. These two aspects of modelling are deeply interrelated. In the photography example, decisions at the moment an image is made influence the way it can ultimately be used.

More generally, any designed artefact, whether it be a car, a drug or

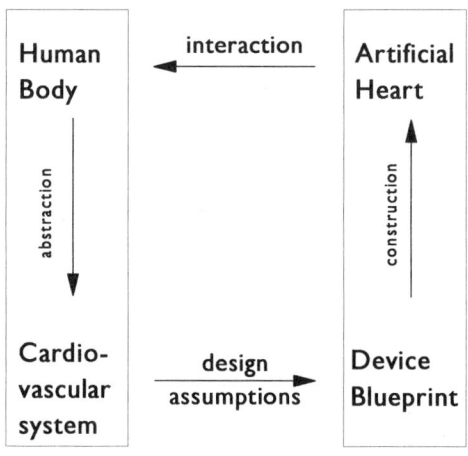

Figure 1.3: An artificial heart is based upon two kinds of model. Firstly, the cardiovascular system has to be modelled, and secondly, a mechanical blueprint is used to model the way the heart will be constructed.

a computer system, has to be designed with the world it will operate within in mind. In other words, it has to contain in its design a model of the environment within which it will be used. These specifications constitute its design assumptions. Thus there is a connection between the process of model creation, the construction of artefacts based upon such models, and their eventual effectiveness in satisfying some purpose (Figure 1.2).

A few examples should make the cycle of model abstraction and construction clearer. Firstly, consider an artefact like a car. The design blueprints of the car reflect both the purpose of the car, as well as the environment within which it will operate. The car's engine is built based upon the not unreasonable assumption that it will operate in an atmosphere with oxygen. The wheels and suspension are designed with the assumption that they will operate on a highway or local street. The car thus carries within its construction a kind of implicit model of the world within which it is designed to work. If the car was put into another physical environment like the lunar surface, it probably would not work very well. Sometimes such design assumptions are left implicit, and only become obvious when a device is used in a way in which it was not intended, sometimes with catastrophic results (Box 1.1).

The human body also makes assumptions about its environment. The haemopoietic system calibrates the number of red blood cells needed for normal function based upon the available oxygen in the atmosphere. As a consequence, individuals living at sea level have calibrated their oxygen carrying system differently to those living in high altitudes. An athlete training at sea level will not perform well if moved quickly to a high altitude because these 'working assumptions' are no longer met.

Finally, consider an artificial heart (Figure 1.3). Such a device must model the heart in some way, since it will replace it within the cardiovascular system. The artificial heart thus is based upon a model of the heart as a mechanical pump, and is designed with the assumption that supporting the pump mechanisms will be beneficial. It is also designed on the assumption that it will need to be implanted, and as a consequence is crafted to survive the corrosive nature of that environment, and to minimise any immune reaction that could be mounted against it.

1.4   Conclusions

In this chapter, the basic concept of a model has been explored in some detail. Models underpin the way we understand the world we live in, and as a consequence guide the way we interact with the world. In the next chapter, a second basic concept of information will be introduced. These two ideas will then be brought together, as we begin to see that knowledge is a special kind of model, and is subject to the same principles and limitations that afflict all other models.

Chapter summary

1. Models are the basis of the way we learn about, and interact with, the physical world.
2. Models can act either as copies of the world like maps, or as templates that serve as the blueprints for constructing physical objects, or processes.
3. Models that copy the world are abstractions of the real world.
   - Models are always less detailed than the real world they are drawn from.
   - Models are abstractions of the real world, ignoring aspects that are not considered essential. This abstraction imposes a point of view upon the observed world
   - Many models can be created of any given physical object, depending upon the level of detail and point of view selected.
   - The point of view used to build a model is based upon the use the model will be put.
   - There is no such thing as the most 'correct' model. Models are simply better or worse suited to accomplishing a particular task.
4. Models that act as templates are used to create objects or processes that are used in the world.
   - When models are created they assume a context of use. When objects or processes are built from a model, this context forms a set of design assumptions.
   - When models are created, they assume that they are to accomplish a particular purpose.
   - As a consequence, there is no such thing as a general purpose design. All we can have are designs that are better or worse suited to our particular circumstances and task.
5. The assumptions used in a model's creation, whether implicit or explicit, define the limits of a model's usefulness.

Chapter 2

Information

Whether delivered in conversation, captured in a set of hand-written notes, or stored in the memory of a computer, the same basic principles govern the way information is structured and used in decision making.

In this chapter, a basic framework will be presented that defines what is formally meant by information. The ideas presented here will build upon the work on models presented in the previous chapter. The simple way that models, data and information interrelate will then be unfolded. At this point it should become apparent that these ideas about models and information underpin not just the specialised study of informatics, but every aspect of medicine and the delivery of healthcare.

2.1 Information is constructed from data and knowledge

One might informally say that we have received information when what we know has changed (Gregory, 1987). In some sense this information must be measurable, since intuitively some sources of information are better than others. Some newspapers are generally more informative than others. A summary of a patient case history might be full of facts but contain little new information.

One can actually develop statistical measurements for the amount of 'information' communicated from a source, with information theory being the classic example (see Box 2.2). However, such measurements do not help us much when it comes to understanding information in the way we commonly understand the concept.

Despite the central importance of information, the words we use to describe what we know about the world often become entangled. Terms like data, information and knowledge are often used interchangeably in common speech. Each of these terms however, has a quite precise and distinct definition in the information sciences. A simple way to conceptualise the difference between these terms is to think of a hierarchy of meaning. The hierarchy starts with raw data at the bottom, moves up through information, and ends at the top with knowledge. Each of the layers builds upon the one below so that meaning increases moving up the hierarchy:

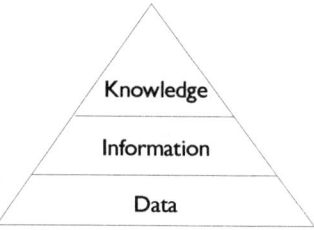

The way data, information and knowledge build upon each other starts to become apparent as we define each more precisely.

Data sit at the bottom of the hierarchy, and consist of facts. For example, 'today is Tuesday' or 'the patient's blood pressure is 125/70 mmHg'.

Information is usually taken to be data that gains significance in a certain context. Thus, the fact that 'the patient's blood pressure is 125/70 mmHg' becomes information when it is added to the context of managing a patient's high blood pressure. For example, the data may inform a clinician that a patient's blood pressure is under control.

Knowledge is at the top of the meaning hierarchy. It defines general relationships between different kinds of data. The rule 'if a patient's blood pressure is greater than 135/95 mmHg on three separate occasions then the patient has high blood pressure' is an example of a piece of knowledge.

One can now start to see how each of these three concepts is related. Using a piece of knowledge, in a given context, data are interpreted to produce information. Since these ideas are at the very foundation of informatics, we will need to understand their interrelationships in

Information is constructed by people in a process of perception; it is not selected, noticed, detected, chosen or filtered from a set of given, static, pre-existing things. Each perception is a new generalization, a new construction.

Clancey, p229, in Steels and Brookes, (1995).

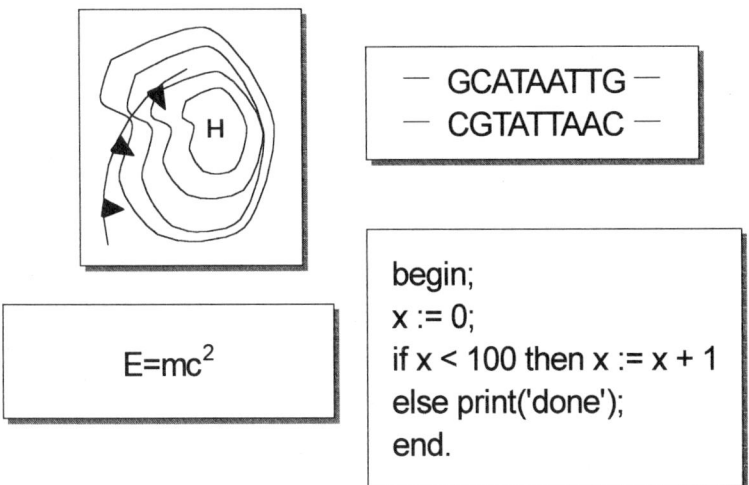

Figure 2.1: *Symbolic models cannot be understood unless the symbol language, and the possible relationships amongst the symbols, are also understood.*

even more depth. To this end, the concepts of models developed in the previous section will be of assistance.

2.2   Some models are built from symbols

Knowledge can now be recognised to be the set of models we have built up to understand and interact with the world. Often that knowledge is stored in the heads of individuals. With the development of language and writing, it has become possible for these models to be transferred from being purely mental constructions, to something we can examine and manipulate in the physical world.

Sometimes these models are physical analogues of the real thing. For example, a scale model of a township captures in miniature some physical aspects of the real town. An image captured on film is a direct physical abstraction of the object that has been photographed. Other models bear no physical resemblance to the things they model. A weather map, for example, tries to capture processes that do not look anything like their diagrammatic representation. If we move into the realms of science and mathematics, it is common to create models in the form of diagrams, or equations. These models are all created from a set of symbols, where the symbol is some form of marking that is understood to represent something else. When people talk about formal knowledge, they are usually referring to this kind

Figure 2.2: Data remain uninterpretable in the absence of a language that defines what each datum represents.

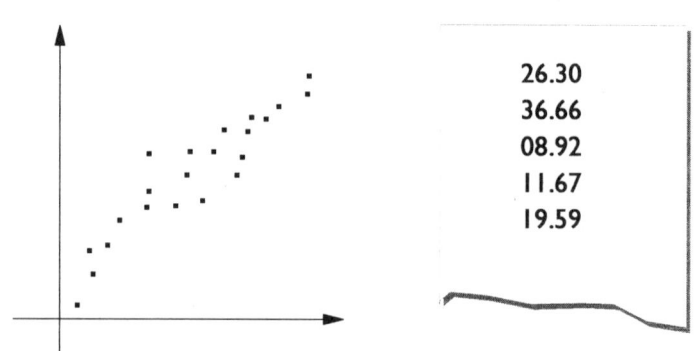

26.30
36.66
08.92
11.67
19.59

of symbolic model, and that is the sense in which knowledge will be used here.

A fundamental characteristic of all symbolic models is that, on their own, they have no intrinsic meaning. If a child was to be shown the equation $e = mc^2$, it would be meaningless unless each of the letters in the equation was named, and the concepts they stood for understood. It would also be meaningless if the child did not understand the mathematical operations that related each of the concepts. A weather map could be equally mysterious.

Symbolic models thus require a **language** and a **set of relationships** to be defined before they can be understood (Figure 2.1). In the information sciences, the languages that are used to create models are usually based upon logic or mathematics.

2.3 Inferences are drawn when data are interpreted according to a model

Healthcare is an information and knowledge intensive activity. Data are constantly being gathered, and their meaning evaluated against a set of models. Whether these interpretations and decisions are made based upon direct observations of a patient or complex measurements from sophisticated diagnostic equipment, the process is the same.

The process of interpretation begins when a set of data is obtained. The data are simply a collection of symbols, for example a series for numbers, and as should now be apparent, they have no meaning on their own. For example, in medicine, it is common for experimental

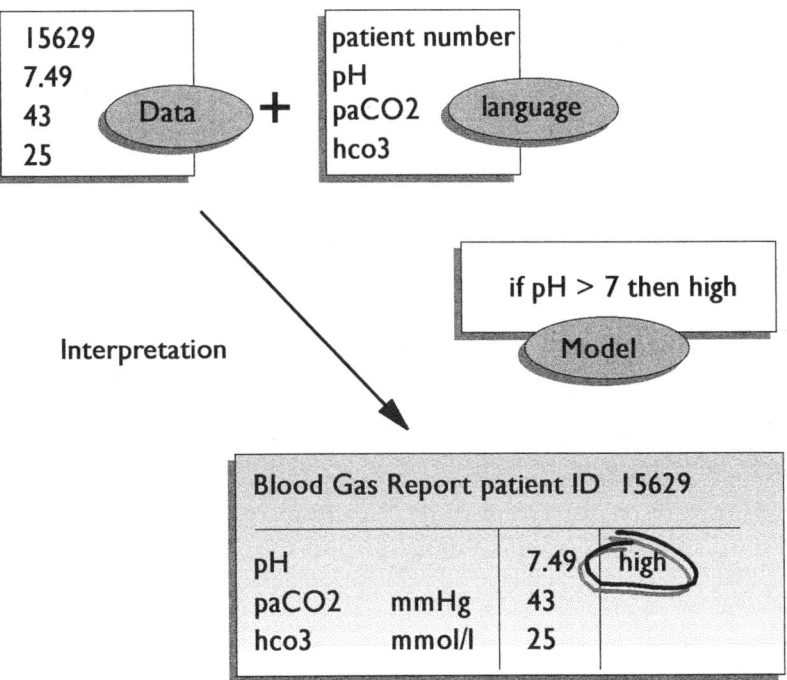

Figure 2.3: Data are interpreted with reference to a model and a modelling language.

data to be plotted on a graph. If one does not know what each of the axes of the graph represents then there is no way that the plotted data can be interpreted (Figure 2.2).

Another example may make this even clearer. Imagine that you are being spoken to by someone in a language that you do not understand. You might have received a large amount of data during that conversation, but since you do not understand the language, it is meaningless to you. You cannot say that you have received any information.

The context that allows data to be interpreted is provided by two things. Firstly, a language is required to give meaning to the symbols contained in the data. This language is called the **data model** in an information system. Secondly, a model that contains knowledge about the way concepts are related is needed to draw inferences based upon the data.

For example, one might have a laboratory test result for a patient (Figure 2.3). Without a language, the results are simply a collection of numbers. With a language, one is able to define what the meanings of each of the symbols on the result record are. They

*Model languages provide the grammar or **syntax** which defines relationships between data. Knowledge models are then used to interpret the meaning or **semantics** of the data.*

might be numbers corresponding to particular tests or a patient identification number.

Next, the model must provide knowledge that will allow the test result to be interpreted. A rule like 'if the pH is greater than 7 then it is abnormally high' would be part of a clinician's model of acid-base physiology.

The model in this case also may contain a patient-specific component. Thus the blood gas test results shown in Figure 2.3 would change their meaning depending on the context in which they were taken. The interpretation would change for example, depending upon which patient the tests were taken from, what treatment the patient was been given, and where in a sequence of tests this particular result lay.

In general, the more a model tells us about the source and content of the data, the richer is the potential for interpretation.

2.4　Assumptions in a model define the limits to knowledge

In the previous chapter, we saw that the assumptions made at the time a model is created affect the way it is used. The way a model is constructed, the context within it is defined, what is included in it, and the purpose for which is intended, all affect its ultimate usefulness.

This is also the case for the models that define our knowledge of the world. The implication then, is that the inferences we are able to draw from a model are strongly influenced by the assumptions made when the knowledge in the model was first created.

For example, it is now common for clinical protocols to be used to define a standard way in which a particular illness is to be treated. Such a protocol is a kind of template model, that drives the actual treatment delivered to a patient.

When the protocol is created, the designers have to make many assumptions, not all of which are necessarily obvious to them at the time. For example, the protocol designers might make an implicit assumption that the drugs or equipment they include in the protocol will actually be available.

What they are actually doing when they make such an assumption is to model the environment within which they expect the protocol to operate. This is usually their own local environment, and it is only when a designer is forced to check with others in very different circumstances that such implicit environmental assumptions are unearthed. This is because a protocol becomes less useful in a

---

Box 2.1 - DNA is just data

Conceptualising an information system into model, data and interpretation components has a certain universality. In biology, in particular, there is a strong information paradigm arising out of our understanding of the role of DNA.

Since its structure and function began to be unfolded, DNA has been seen as some form of master molecule, dictating the development of individual organisms. The doctrine of DNA has perhaps reached its most extreme position in the notion of the selfish gene (Dawkins, 1982). Here, DNA is characterised as clothing itself in cells, which allow the DNA to survive and reproduce from generation to generation. DNA, in this view of the world, creates and dictates the development and activity of organisms. The organism phenotype is merely the survival machine used by the genetic sequence.

There is another view which sees DNA as part of a far more complex system. DNA is amongst the most non-reactive and chemically inert molecules in biology. It thus is perfectly designed for its role, which is to store instructions, much like the memory in a computer. DNA is a kind of database, nothing more.

Thus, while DNA stores the models used to create proteins, it is of itself incapable of making anything. It is actually the cellular machinery that determines which proteins are to be made. While it is often said that DNA produces proteins, in fact proteins produce DNA (Lewontin, 1993). The symbolic language of DNA, and thus the ability to interpret DNA, resides in the surrounding cellular structures. Without these molecules, there would be no way that we could decode the symbolic meaning of DNA - the data stored in the DNA would be uninterpretable. In other words, an organism's DNA has no meaning outside the context of the cellular structures that contain it.

We can thus regard a complex organism as being the result of a cell's interpretation of the models stored in the DNA database, using a language encoded within its proteins, and within the context of the data provided by the intra and extracellular environment.

Figure 2.4:
Knowledge is acquired through the construction of models, and these models are then applied to data, to draw interpretations of the meaning of the data.

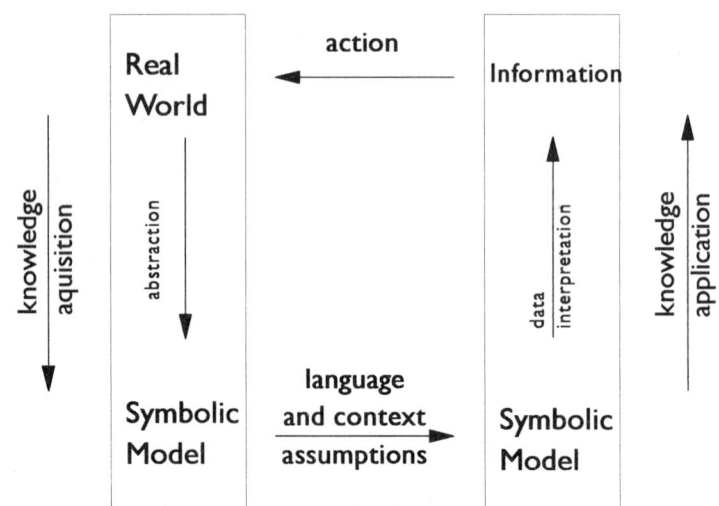

context in which some of its implicit assumptions are not valid.

Thus, a protocol created for a well-equipped modern hospital is unlikely to be useful in a poor village in an under-developed nation. Equally, a protocol might be created with the assumption that a patient has no other significant illnesses. In the case of an individual patient, this implicit assumption might be exposed when the treatment advised by the protocol cannot be used because it interacts with the patient's other medications.

Similarly, a set of rules and procedures might be developed in one hospital, and be spectacularly successful at improving the way it handles its cases. One would have to be very cautious, given that these procedures implicitly model many aspects of that particular institution, before one imposed those procedures on other hospitals. Very small differences, for example in the level of resources, type of patients seen, or experience of the staff, may make what was successful in one context, unhelpful in another.

With these examples in mind, we can cast the creation and application of knowledge into the same form as the cycle of model creation and application developed in the last chapter (Figure 2.4). Firstly, the process of model abstraction is equivalent to the knowledge acquisition process. Observations made of the world are generalised into a model that describes how different parts of the world interrelate. Recall from the last chapter that such models are always limited, and that they emphasise certain observations and omit others.

Next, the knowledge model is applied to data. We can view this process as the construction of an inference, based upon a template model which represent our knowledge, and a set of data. As we have just seen, design assumptions made at the time that the model is created affect how it can be used.

One special set of design assumptions associated with symbolic models are its language. Just as a photographic slide cannot be used unless the right projector is present, a symbolic model cannot be used unless the language and modelling relationships used are also available. In other words, the modelling language becomes a design assumption, which needs to be explicitly catered for when the model is used.

2.5 Computational models permit the automation of data interpretation

If the model and data components of an information problem can be written down, then it can also in principle be solved using a computer. In most cases, the actual work of data interpretation for a given problem is shared between human and computer. For example, the computer may organise and consolidate data into a graphical presentation, and the human then examines the processed data to make a final interpretation.

The amount to which models are resident in the computer or exist as mental models in the head of a human determines where the interpretation takes place. Computer systems thus form a spectrum, from those that have minimal ability to assist in the interpretation of data, to those that are able to carry out a complete interpretation, within the bounds of a given task (Figure 2.5).

Computers can act as data stores

If a computer is used solely as a repository for data, it acts as a database. The data is organised according to a data model, so that

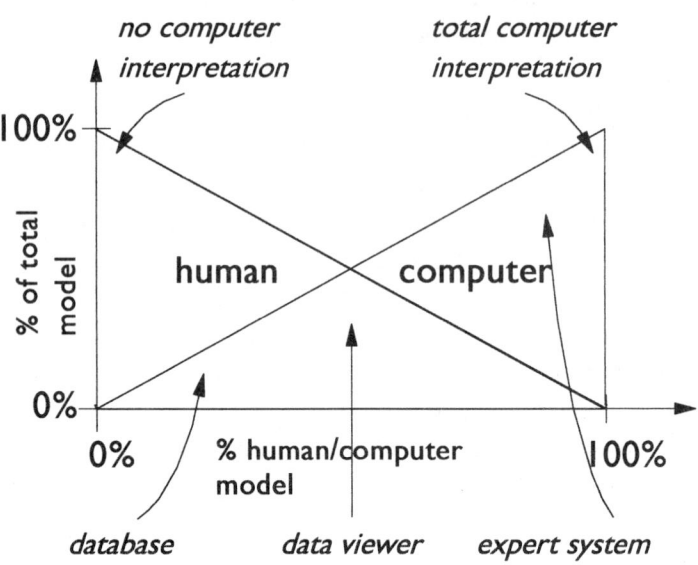

Figure 2.5: *Humans and computers can share the burden of data interpretation. The amount of interpretation delegated to the computer depends upon the how much of the interpretative model is shared.*

the origin of each datum is recognisable. Medical data often consists of images or physiological signals taken from monitoring devices, and may occupy a vast amount of storage space. As a consequence, the databases that store complex patient data can be huge.

Designers of database systems are concerned with issues like the efficient use of computer memory, the design of filing systems that permit the rapid retrieval of data from massive stores, and methods for ensuring the safety and security of the stored data.

Computerised models can generate views that assist interpretation

In contrast to passive databases, a computer can attempt some degree of interpretation by generating a view into a body of data. In this case, given some large data set, the computer system only shows a user that portion of data that is of immediate interest, and in a way that is best suited to the task at hand.

Consider a database that holds publication data and abstracts of articles from medical journals. Given the thousands of papers published weekly, there would be little value in a researcher simply inspecting each record in the database. It would be practically impossible to locate an article within it. What is required is a way of viewing a relevant subset of the data that matches the researcher's interests.

For a computer system to provide such 'views' of stored data, a model of the user's needs has to be conveyed to the computer. At its most rudimentary, this communication between the database and the human might be provided by what is known as a **query language**. This is a method commonly used to search library catalogues. Using special words like 'and', 'or' and 'not', the user constructs a question for the query system about the things that should be displayed. Since it recognises these special words and their meaning, the query system is able to retrieve those records from the database that match the terms provided by the user.

A patient monitor is also kind of viewer. If a clinician was to look at the raw data stream, he or she would be confronted with streams of rapidly changing digits that would be completely unusable in a clinical setting. It is the monitor's role to prepare sensor data in such a way that it can be viewed sensibly. In this case, the view might show data as a set of waveforms like the ECG, or numeric values like the blood pressure. To do this, the computer must have models of the signals, the kinds of noise and artefact that may corrupt the signals. It also needs a model of the preferred ways of displaying the signals to allow humans to carry out the interpretation.

The same process occurs with computer generated images. Computerised tomography (CT) and magnetic resonance imagery (MRI) for example, are both dependent on complex models that reconstruct raw data into images that can be interpreted by clinicians. By varying the models applied to the data, the imaging systems can produce different views, or 'slices' through the raw image data.

In general, the division of responsibilities for data interpretation between human and computer may occur for a number of reasons. It may be that it is inherently difficult to formalise all the knowledge used in the interpretation of data, or it may simply be that the effort involved in modelling is greater than the reward. This is often the case when problems are highly variable. In such cases, it is not the case that a model does not exist, but it may be simply be poorly formed or difficult to articulate. Recent developments in computer science, for example in areas like case-based reasoning, fuzzy logic, and qualitative reasoning have helped us understand how such poorly formed models can still be captured in a way that they can be amenable to computer interpretation.

Computers can be responsible for all data interpretation

As the understanding of how knowledge could be represented in a computer developed, it became clear that computers could be used to perform quite powerful forms of reasoning on their own.

Such computer interpretation can occur in real-time. For example, a pacemaker may analyse a cardiogram looking for the development of an arrhythmia. Interpretation by computer can also occur in a more exploratory fashion on data archived in a database. In this case, a variety of different models can be used on the data. It may be useful, for example, to create a number of financial projections using historical data, based on different modelling assumptions about the likely ways a health service might evolve.

Computers are now often used as backup on reasoning tasks that are performed by humans. For example, in safety-critical situations like the operation of a nuclear power plant, the human benefits from a computer watching over the complex system with a second pair of fail-safe 'eyes' looking over the operator's shoulder. Computers are also used to interpret data when the task is routine, but occurs with high enough frequency that automation would help. The automated interpretation of laboratory test results is a common example of this use of computers.

In all these cases, the interpreting computer does not just possess data and the knowledge that will be used to interpret the data. It also needs a third thing - a model of the way the computer will 'think' about the problem. More precisely, the computer needs a representation of the way the knowledge is applied to the data. For example, the reasoning system may use rules of formal logic - most **expert systems** are built in this way. Sometimes the systems reason with rules of mathematics, probabilities or other more modern techniques like fuzzy reasoning or neural networks. These fascinating ideas will be returned to in greater detail in Chapter 20.

2.6   Conclusions

In this chapter, we have used the idea of a model to help develop an understanding of what it means to have information. In reaching more precise definitions of data, information and knowledge, it has been possible to look at how they interact, and arrive at a rich understanding of everything from the way people draw conclusions to the role that DNA plays in the cell.

These last two chapters have been a prelude to introducing a third fundamental informatics concept - the notion of a system. In the following chapter, the discussion will introduce the concept of systems, and lead on to an exploration of what it means to create an information system. In this way, one can begin to understand the ways in which information systems can be forces for good, as well as understand some of their inherent limitations.

Box 2.2 - Information theory

Claude Shannon developed the mathematical basis for information theory while working at Bell Laboratories during the 1940s (Slepian, 1974). Motivated by problems in communication engineering, Shannon developed a method to measure the amount of 'information' that could be passed along a communication channel between a source and a destination.

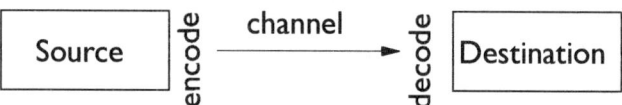

Shannon was concerned with the process of communicating using radio, and for him the transmitter, ionosphere and receiver were all examples of communication **channels**. Such channels had a limited capacity and were noisy. Shannon developed definitions of channel capacity, noise and signal in terms of a precise measure of what he called 'information'.

He began by recognising that before a message could enter a channel it had to be **encoded** in some way. For example, a piece of music needs to be transformed through a microphone into electronic signals before it can be transmitted. Equally, a signal would then need to be decoded at the destination before it can be reconstructed into the original signal. A hi-fi speaker thus needs to decode an electronic signal before it can be converted back into sound.

Shannon was principally interested in studying the problem of maximising the reliability of transmission of a signal, and minimising the cost of that transmission. Encoding a signal was the mechanism for reducing the cost of transmission through **signal compression**, as well as combating corruption of the signal through **channel noise**.

The rules governing the operation of an encoder and a decoder constitute a **code**. The code described by Shannon corresponds to a model and its language. A code achieves reliable transmission if the source message is reproduced at the destination within prescribed limits. After Shannon, the problem for a communication engineer was the find an encoding scheme that made the best use of a channel while minimising transmission noise.

Although Shannon saw his theory helping us understand human communication, it remains an essentially statistical analysis over populations of messages, and says little about individual acts of communication.

Chapter summary

1. Information is based upon data and knowledge.
   - Data are collections of facts.
   - Data interpreted in a context provide information.
   - Context is supplied by our knowledge of the world.
2. Knowledge can be thought of as a set of models describing our understanding of the world.
   - These models are composed of symbols.
   - A symbolic model is created using a language that defines the meaning of different symbols, and their possible relationships amongst each other.
3. Inferences are drawn when data are interpreted according to a model.
   - Data on their own have no intrinsic meaning.
   - A language identifies concepts within the data.
   - Next, the knowledge stored in a model can be used to draw an inference from the labelled data.
4. Assumptions in the knowledge model affect the quality of the inferences draw from it.
   - Assumptions may implicitly model the context within which the model was created.
   - These design assumptions include the language used if the model is symbolic.
5. Knowledge acquisition and application are an example of the cycle of model abstraction and template-based construction.
6. Once a model and data have been sufficiently formalised, the interpretation can be automated using a computer.
   - Computers can store data according to data models.
   - Computers can provide views onto data according to user models.
   - Computers can interpret data when they are provided with models of knowledge, and models of the method of inference.

One doesn't add a computer or buy or design one where there is no system. The success of a project does not stem from the computer but from the existence of a system. The computer makes it possible to integrate the system and thus assure its success.

C. Caceres, in Dickson and Brown, (1969), p207.

Chapter 3

Systems

Systems pervade medicine, and there are countless examples of them. In physiology, one talks of the endocrine system or the respiratory system. In clinical practice, we develop systems for questioning and examining our patients. Indeed, the whole of healthcare itself is often described as a system. In essence, all these different systems are just models, and as such, they can operate either as descriptions of the world or templates to action.

As descriptions of the observed world, systems are vital to human reason because they take us beyond simple cause and effect, and allow us to look at complex interrelationships. Indeed, when we first encounter new system behaviours in the world, they are often surprising or even counter-intuitive. Imagine for example, the shock of a physician trying to understand how Jenner's inoculation of humans with living cowpox actually led to protection from smallpox infection. In Jenner's time, simple cause and effect predicted that inoculation would produce disease. It needed the development of a complex model of the immune system to eventually explain what was occurring.

In common usage, a system is often understood to be some kind of routine or regular way of working. One can have a system for betting on a horse race, or a filing system for storing and retrieving documents. These systems can be seen as models providing templates to action in the world. Knowledge and data can also be used in such a systematic way. When the same kinds of decision are made on a regular basis, they will require access to the same kind of data and use the same knowledge. In these circumstances, one can develop a regular decision process or **information system** to accomplish the task. An information system could thus be anything from the routine way in which a clinician records patient details in a pocket notebook, the way a triage nurse assesses patients on arrival in an emergency department, through to a complex computer-based system that regulates payments for healthcare services.

In this chapter, we will introduce the topic of systems by first providing a general definition of systems, and identifying a few of their key characteristics. This will be a prelude to the main focus of the chapter, which is the introduction of what is formally meant by an information system, and a discussion of how information systems are used to control the way decisions are made.

3.1 Systems are models

At its most abstract, a system is a special kind of model within which we have identified a set of interacting or connected components. As we have seen, systems can either be abstractions of the world, or can act as templates for the things we wish to accomplish.

As abstractions, like all models, systems help compartmentalise a portion of the world in a way that makes it more understandable. For example, a collection of anatomical structures whose function is closely related might constitute a system. Thus we may speak of the nervous system, and collect within its definition organs like the peripheral nerves, the spinal cord, and the brain.

The collecting together of such elements into a system can be a particularly powerful way of enhancing our understanding of the way things work. For example, when Harvey first proposed the notion of a system of circulation for blood through the body in 1628, he essentially constructed a model that connected together for the first time the arteries, veins and heart into a functioning whole. So powerful was this model that it was adopted despite its inadequacies at that time. It was for example, not until 1661 that Malpighi finally demonstrated that it was the capillaries that connected the arterial and venous systems together (Schafer and Thane, 1891).

As templates, systems are also a common feature of modern technology. Cars have fuel systems and brake systems. Patients are connected to ventilator systems. Societies have health or educational systems. All these systems describe complex, interconnected structures that have been designed to achieve a particular purpose, based upon a system blueprint.

There are three basic features of any system that distinguish them from other kinds of model. Firstly a system must have a definable **structure,** and it must have a **behaviour**. As a consequence, a system also has a **function**. Further, like all models, systems are arbitrary, purposive, and embedded in an environment. Each of these points will be examined in turn, and they will echo what we have already learned in the earlier discussion on models.

Systems have behaviour

For a system to be distinguishable from its environment, it should exhibit some characteristic behaviours. Thus, a weather system might be a set of related pressure bands, whose collective behaviour stands out and demands attention. One of the behaviours of the vascular system is that it can be observed to contain flowing blood within certain pressure bands. This behaviour distinguishes the vascular system, from say, the nervous system. It is this identification with a particular behaviour that helps conceptually separate a system from other parts of its environment.

Critically, a system's behaviour cannot usually be predicted by an examination of its individual components, but emerges out of the way that the components interact with each other. Thus the behaviour of social groups, communication networks, roads, neural processes and so forth are all emergent properties of their components (Box 3.1).

Systems are embedded in an environment

From an informatics perspective, the emergence of system behaviour means that the effect of anything we build is not directly predictable, irrespective of how well we understand it. This holds for everything from clinical guidelines, information systems, through to medical devices. It is because these things exist within an environment, and it is a system's interaction with its environment that produces the overall behaviour.

Box 3.1 - Braess' paradox

Simple cause and effect predicts that putting more resource towards achieving a goal should improve performance, but this is not always the case. The creation of new roads can lead to greater traffic congestion. The installation of new telephone or computer network elements can lead to degraded system performance. Introducing new workers to a team may actually result in a decrease in the team's performance.

To understand these apparently paradoxical results, one needs to examine events from a system view. Studying the effects of new roads upon traffic, Dietrich Braess discovered that if a new road is built in a congested system, everyone's journey unexpectedly lengthens (Bean, 1996). He explained this result by examining the behaviour of drivers, who made individual decisions about their journey, and the emergent effects of all these individual decisions upon the whole system. Consider a journey from A to D that can follow several routes like ABD or ACD:

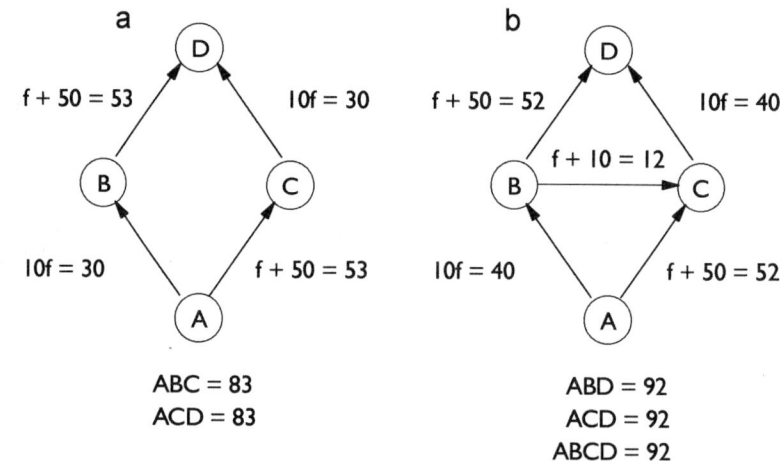

The delay on any link is a function of f, which is the number of cars on that link. In case a, there are two equidistant path choices. With 6 cars in the system, they will tend to distribute equally, with 3 cars on each path ABD and ACD. If they did not distribute equally, the congestion on one link would over time cause drivers to choose the less congested path. The expected delay is thus 83 on both routes. In case b, a new link BC is added, creating a new path ABCD. Assuming previous path costs, drivers think ABCD is now the quickest route. Users take the new path to try and minimise their journey (Glance et al., 1994), but the choice hurts the whole system. Equilibrium eventually occurs when 2 cars choose each of the paths ABD, ACD and ABCD. This puts 4 cars on the link AB. Now, the new road has increased the expected delay for everyone to 92.

The environment in some sense becomes part of the system. For practical purposes, we usually restrict the description of a system to including a limited set of elements of the environment that are of immediate interest (see Box 3.2). Thus, one cannot divorce a system from the environment within which it exists because, by doing so, the very context for the system's existence disappears. This is as true if our system is a description of a part of the real world we are interested in, or is a man-made artefact.

Systems have internal structure

If a system's overall behaviour arises out of the behaviour of its parts, then it has some internal structure. It is the way in which the components of that structure interact that generates the system behaviour. The behaviour of a mechanical clock is thus determined by its internal structure of springs and cogs. The cardiovascular system's behaviour arises out of its constituent pump and conduits.

As with all models, the amount of internal detail that can be described within a system is probably limitless. The description of the cardiovascular system could descend to the cellular level, or even the molecular level and beyond. The amount of detail one includes in a system is usually determined by the purpose of the description, which is usually to describe its function.

Systems have function

The usual sense in which a system's function is understood is that it is an explanation of the behaviour of the system, based upon the workings of its internal structure. Thus one of the vascular system's functions is to maintain the pressure of circulating blood within a certain range. Another function is to transport blood.

Systems are arbitrary

We create descriptions of systems to help us understand the observable world. So, by their very nature, systems are completely arbitrary human creations. There can thus never be something called 'the correct' definition of a system, whether one is talking about a description of something in the world or a design to accomplish some function.

Box 3.2 - Penicillinase and the closed-world assumption

The introduction of antibiotics in the second half of the 20th Century heralded a period of optimism. Infectious diseases were soon to be a thing of the past, and every year saw the discovery of new drugs that attacked an ever wider spectrum of bacteria. Then, as time went on, the tide started to turn the other way, as individual organisms like penicillinase producing bacteria developed resistance to specific drugs. Through a process of natural selection, the drugs that were created to kill bacteria were actually selecting individual organisms that were immune to their effects, allowing them to survive and dominate the gene pool. Some organisms now have such widespread resistance that their detection can shut down large sections of a hospital.

Modern medical science is often challenged by critics who cite examples like the development of antibiotic resistance as proof that its methods ultimately do more harm than good. It is the case that this 'fight-back' of natural systems following the introduction of technology is not a phenomenon confined to medicine, but potentially affects every technological intervention made by man (Tenner, 1996).

From a systems viewpoint, whenever a technology is introduced, the 'fight-back' effect is not so much a fault of the technology as it is an inevitable consequence of the way that we understand systems. When we model the world, we intentionally simplify or exclude whole sections of reality to create a point-of-view. When a technology is applied, it is aimed at solving a particular problem with a system, with the assumption that its effects are predictable 'everything else being equal'. This clearly is never completely possible.

The assumption that everything that can be known **is** known is called the **closed-world assumption** in logic (Genesereth and Nilsson, 1988). Its function is to allow reasoning to proceed, even if our knowledge is incomplete. It serves a similar role when a technology is introduced into a system, because without it, we would never be sure we understood all the possible consequences of its actions.

So, rather than being a specific consequence of technology, unexpected outcomes are a result of the imperfect way we in which we understand the world. Our only way around it is to assume, at some stage, that we know enough to try things out. The alternative is to do nothing.

There are many possible ways in which one might choose to create a system, and it is often only a matter of convention and practicality that one set of descriptions is chosen over another. Equally, it should come as no surprise that two system descriptions might overlap, and have common elements. Are the pulmonary arteries more properly part of the cardiovascular system, or are they part of the respiratory system? It depends entirely upon one's point of view.

Systems are purposive

This brings us to a key point. Descriptions of a system are constructed with a purpose in mind. They are goal directed, or teleological. The reason people developed the modern descriptions of different physiological system was with the intent of treating illness. The reason that one particular system begins to gain common acceptance over another is that it is seen to be inherently more useful for that purpose. Thus phrenology, the study of bumps on the skull, was replaced by a system of thought we now call neurology, as this newer viewpoint proved itself to be a more useful approach to the treatment of illness. So, over time whole systems of thought gradually fall into disuse as newer and more valuable ones appear.

People also tend to develop systematic routines because they find themselves doing the same task again and again. They thus pick out some elements of their actions that recur, and give them some objective existence by calling them a routine. So, with a purpose in mind, a part of the world is labelled, and a system is born.

3.2 Information systems contain data and models

An information system is distinguished from more general systems by its components, which include data and models (Fenton and Hill, 1993). A patient record system is a prime example. Its purpose is to provide a way to record data about particular patients in some formalised fashion that allows the data to be used in ongoing management. The patient record system is thus composed of patient data, and template models of the way that data should be organised, based upon models of the way clinicians use data in their decision making process. For completeness, the system definition might also include the medical language used in the records, the way that the records are accessed and filed, and possibly even the individuals

During the French revolution, a method was devised to create logarithm tables en masse. *Individuals called* computers *each carried out a small calculation, and as a result the team of individuals was able to carry out a large number of complex calculations. In his seminal treatise* On the Economy of Manufacture *(1833), Charles Babbage reasoned that, since such complex calculations could all in principle be broken down into simple steps of addition or subtraction, then these could be carried out by machine. This inspired him to devise his difference engine, which was the first proposal for a general purpose calculating machine.*

who use the records. All these elements together constitute the whole of a system which has been created to capture and re-use information about patients to facilitate treatment.

Information systems can be created for a number of reasons. In the main, it is because an information process is very common, very complex, or it is in some way critical. In the first case, the goal of introducing an information system is to reduce the effort of decision making by streamlining the process. In the case of complex or critical decisions, the information system's role is either to reduce complexity, or to minimise the likelihood of error.

Information systems share all of the characteristics of systems described earlier. We pick out decisions, data and models that are in some way consistent as a group, that are of interest for some purpose, and then look upon them as a system. Each information system exists within an environment, and is usually purpose built to interact with the environment. In other words, we want to manage specific activities within that environment, and want to influence their outcomes in a certain way.

3.3 Information systems are designed to manage activities

The main reason an information system is developed is to manage a set of activities. This is true whether one is talking about clinical activities like the delivery of therapy, or more administrative tasks like deciding staffing levels for a hospital unit. In every case, information is used to indicate the state of the activity, and decisions are made about that activity based upon that information.

For example, consider the case in which we are treating a patient for an acid-base disorder. The **goal** of management is to maintain the patient's acid-base status in a range that is consistent with good health. Measurements are taken to provide data about acid-base state, like pH and serum bicarbonate. The model used in this case is physiological. It might include rules that state the relationship between the measured acid-base parameters in health and in disease. Based upon this knowledge of acid-base disease, one can interpret the measurement data for a given patient (Figure 2.3). Associated with each interpretation, there usually exists a set of **management**

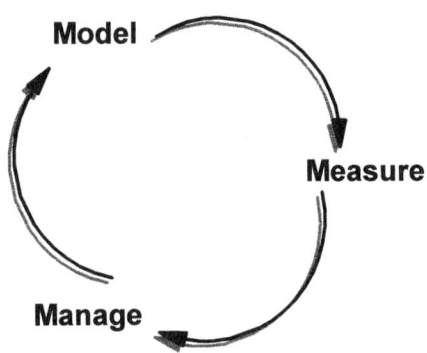

*Figure 3.1: The
model, measure,
manage cycle.
When the outcome
of a management
decision is fed
back into another
cycle, a feedback
control loop is
formed*

actions that can be taken. In this case, the management actions are a set of therapeutic interventions.

In general, the process of activity management consists of the following steps.

- Define a set of management goals.
- Construct a model of the system.
- Gather measurement data.
- Assess the state of the thing being managed, by interpreting measurements in relation to the model.
- Take actions to alter that state, based upon the management goals.

Usually, once an action has been taken, a check then needs to be made to assess the outcome of that decision. For example, if a treatment is given, measurements are subsequently taken of the patient to see if the treatment has been effective. If the outcome is not exactly as hoped for, further action may need to be taken. In this way the result of the first decision feeds back into the next decision-making round, creating a feedback control loop. Depending on the task at hand, the decision making loop can cycle through its steps many times.

This decision control loop within the information system can be characterised as the **model, measure, manage cycle** (Figure 3.1). It is at the heart of nearly every information system designed to control an activity. 'If you can't measure it', goes an old engineering saying, 'then you can't manage it'. The model, measure, manage cycle defines the function of most information systems. As will become apparent in later chapters, it is the basic way in which computer-based information systems function in healthcare, whether they are concerned with the delivery of clinical care, the administration of services and organisations, or clinical research. Indeed, the relatively complex model abstraction and application cycle that was introduced in Chapter 1 (Figure 1.2) can be mapped directly onto simple model, measure and manage cycle in Figure 3.1.

3.4   Conclusions

We have thus now reached a point where we can look at an information system in a fairly complex and rich way, based upon an understanding of the basic principles of models, information structures, and systems. Through a variety of examples, we have seen how information systems are used to manage activities. Whenever a decision is important enough, or is made often enough, then an information system is built to manage the process. With this background, it is now possible to move on and look at the healthcare system as a whole. In the next section of the book, we will see how healthcare is structured from an informational viewpoint, and see how information systems reflect and contribute to that structure.

Chapter summary

1. A system is a model that conceptually connects together smaller elements into a functioning whole.
2. System models can act either as abstractions of the world which explain its behaviour, or act as templates for the design of structures that have a specific purpose.
3. A system has a definable structure, a behaviour, and as a consequence, a system also has a function.
4. Like all models, systems are arbitrary, purposive, and embedded in an environment.
5. An information system is characterised from more general systems by its components, which include data, models, and the means to use them to draw conclusions.
6. An information system is developed to manage a set of activities, and its functioning can be characterised as repeated cycles of modelling, measurement and management.

Part Two

Information Systems in Healthcare

It appears to me a most excellent thing for the physician to cultivate Prognosis; for by foreseeing and foretelling, in the presence of the sick, the present, the past, and the future, and explaining the omissions which patients have been guilty of, he will be the more readily believed to be acquainted with the circumstances of the sick; so that men will have confidence to entrust themselves to such a physician. And he will manage the cure best who has foreseen what is to happen from the present state of matters.

Hippocrates, *The Book of Prognostics.*

Chapter 4

Information cycles and formality

In a complex environment like healthcare, there are many activities that need to be managed, and countless decisions to be made. The manner in which the model-measure-manage cycle can drive such activities was introduced in Chapter 3. In this chapter we will specifically explore the way that this cycle operates within healthcare.

Information flows through healthcare organisations in an often bewildering fashion, as a multitude of separate information management cycles interlace. These cycles occur in many guises and can be identified at all levels of the healthcare system. They govern everything from the day to day management of clinical decisions, all the way through to decision making about the operation of the healthcare system as whole.

This chapter will introduce two key concepts. Firstly, it will show that information management cycles have three quite distinct, but interlocking roles, and most of what occurs in healthcare can be described by this model. Secondly, it will be shown that it is not always necessary or indeed appropriate to completely formalise an information management system in all its details. To do so may introduce excessive bureaucracy and can be counterproductive, especially when flexibility in decision making is needed. Consequently, we will see that many information systems are left in an informal state, and as a consequence, are more likely to be supported by communication processes.

4.1 There are three distinct information management loops

As information moves through an information system, it can be used in several quite distinct ways. In particular, it is useful to distinguish three distinct information cycles or loops which reflect different roles for the model-measure-manage cycle. These loops are responsible for the direct **application**, **selection**, and **refinement** of knowledge. Indeed, these information loops exist in some form in most large enterprises, not just in healthcare. Together, they form the **three loop model,** which describes the main ways that information is used within an organisation, or indeed within many other systems requiring informed control (Figure 4.1).

The three-loop model was originally developed to describe computer network management (Phaal, 1994). The work of a team of Hewlett-Packard engineers, it describes measurement, operational and strategic loops that manage the way network policies are applied, selected and redefined over time.

The essence of the three loop model is to recognise that there is a life cycle for information as it percolates through any complex system. We start by assuming that there is a set of models of the system we want to manage. In the case of clinical medicine, these models correspond to medical knowledge. If we are talking about administering an organisation like a hospital, then the models will capture our understanding of economics, organisational dynamics and so on. The knowledge contained in these models might exist in books and journals, in the programs of information systems, or be in the heads of people.

In the first loop, information is used to directly manage a specific activity, like the selection of a diagnostic test for a patient. Secondly, as checks are made on the progress of an individual task, changes might need to be made to the models used to manage the task. For example, the model of treatment might need to be changed if a patient does not make appropriate progress. Thirdly, over time the data and models used in one task can be pooled with similar ones to make broader assessments about the quality of decisions. For example, decisions about the cost-effectiveness of a particular test might be made based upon the evidence of its use with a large number of patients. Such longer term decisions can then be used to refine the way tests are selected, and consequently feed back into the original clinical decision process.

Each loop thus has a different role. Each involves different information sources, and different operations on that information. As

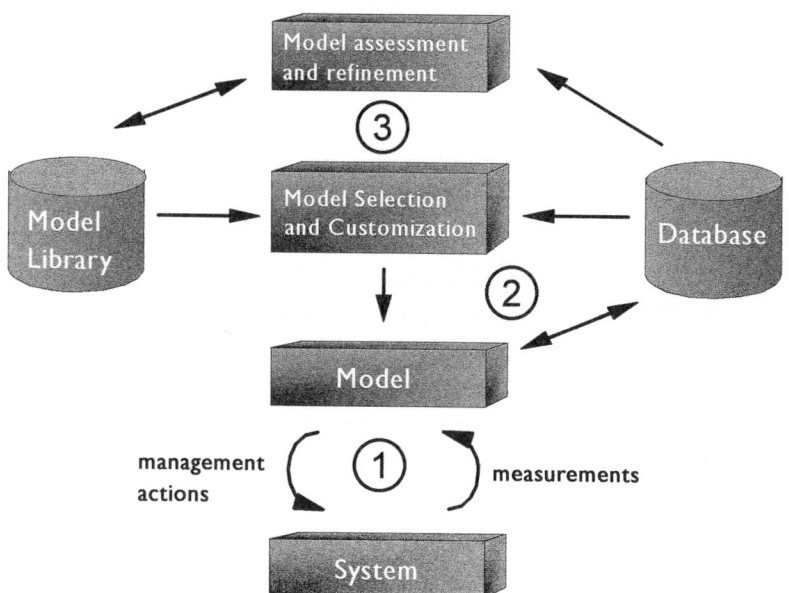

Figure 4.1: *The three loop model. Three separate information systems interact in the health system. The first and second select and apply models to the management of specific systems. The third information system tries to assess the effectiveness of these decisions and improve the models accordingly.*

a result, each cycle has quite different requirements for the kind of information or communication system needed to support them. We can now examine each loop in some more detail.

Loop 1 defines the direct application of a model to a task

The first loop is all about the application of knowledge to achieve a particular task. Using the knowledge contained in a model, and based upon some measurements, actions are taken in a way prescribed by the model. This is the model-measure-manage cycle described in Chapter 4 in its simplest form.

For example, a clinician may choose an insulin treatment regime for a diabetic patient. Having chosen that regime, the clinician applies it to the management of the patient's condition. Measurements of the patient's blood sugar levels will be taken, and the dosage of insulin will be varied based upon the rules contained in the regime.

Similarly, in a hospital, there might be a set way of determining the number of nurses required to staff a ward adequately. This might be based upon the number of patients in a ward, and the level of dependency of its patients. For any given day, based upon measurements of patient numbers and an assessment of their level of dependency, the nurse manager uses the model to decide upon staffing levels for different wards.

Loop 2 defines the way models are selected and customised

In most cases there are a number of different ways in which a task could be completed. This is because there are many possible ways that the world can be modelled, and many ways in which that model can be translated into a prescription for action. One can think of loop 2 as the ongoing process of deciding which models and measurements are most appropriate for a task. Thus, before a loop 1 management cycle can be set up, there has to be a decision which selects the most appropriate manner to complete the task.

In the example of the diabetic patient, the clinician must decide which insulin regime is the most appropriate one for the patient. This could be based, for example, upon an assessment of the patient's disease, the patient's ability to test their own blood sugar and to self-administer the insulin. It may be the case that the regime prescribed will vary many times over the period in which the clinician manages the patient. When the patient is ill, the clinician may prescribe so called 'sick-day' rules that alter the doses of insulin that can be given. These rules constitute a different model of the way the insulin dose is determined.

In the example of the hospital ward, a nurse manager may find that the rules for deciding staffing levels will need to be re-examined depending on the type of ward being considered. A different set of rules might be applied to an Intensive Care Unit, which has different requirements for staff skills, and different levels of patient dependency to a general surgical ward.

It may not always be the case that there are a complete set of models to help with a task. Patients have many individual variations in their circumstances that may require the normal treatment to be customised to suit an individual's specific needs. A particularly 'brittle' diabetic may need to be closely monitored and treatment varied because of the unpredictability of their disease. Nursing staff on a ward in a teaching hospital may need to vary the balance of their daily activities if they are expected to train students as well as carry out clinical duties. Sometimes these variations in approach reflect very particular circumstances, and are not frequent enough to be turned into general policy. It is also the case that if a model does not fit circumstances regularly, then it is the model that needs changing. This is the role of loop 3.

Loop 3 is responsible for model creation and refinement based upon the results of application over time

All our knowledge is constantly being re-examined. As a consequence our understanding of the world evolves with time. In loop 3, the knowledge that was used to complete a task is itself examined against the outcome of its application. To make such an assessment, the results from repeated attempts at a particular approach are pooled. When several different approaches have been tried out, this historical data is examined, and over time the most successful approach is adopted.

Loop 3 is thus the place where the scientific examination of existing theories leads to the creation of new ones. The models selected in loop 2 are all regarded as hypotheses about the best way to approach a task. These hypotheses are then examined based upon the 'tests' that occur every time they are applied in loop 1.

Thus the many different treatment regimes used in the management of diabetes have all hopefully been tested in trials across large numbers of patients. As the outcomes of the treatments are examined, decisions are made about which regimes should be retained, which should be modified, and under which conditions particular regimes should best be applied.

Equally, over time, the way in which hospital units are staffed will be modified when measurements like patient outcomes, staff retention and satisfaction levels are examined. Those hospitals that perform best on these measurements will be used as role models by hospitals that want to improve in a similar fashion.

4.2 Formal and informal information systems

Just because it is possible to define an information system, it does not follow that it is always reasonable to do so. If that was the case, then our lives would be regulated in minute detail. What happens in reality is that most organisations, whether they are small groups of individuals or large institutions, try to find a balance between creating formal processes and allowing individuals to behave freely and informally. That balance shifts, depending on the group, and realises a different set of costs and benefits. Large organisations gain stability through formal processes, but are often criticised for being overly bureaucratic. Smaller ones, whilst being flexible and able to respond rapidly to change, are often chaotic to work in as a result. The difference between these two extremes lies in the organisation's view of the need to formalise its internal systems.

So, while there are clear advantages to structuring processes, including improved reliability, efficiency and consistency, it does not come without cost. There are actually several different costs that need to be considered before a system is formalised.

- Firstly, the creation of a process, by definition, limits flexibility of response. Recall from the discussion on models in Chapter 1 that all models are just views of the world, and a formal process is a kind of model. Consequently, a particular view of how things should be done is captured within the rules, regulations and procedures of any formal process. Alternative views exist, and in some circumstances they would produce better results. The trade-off in adhering to a single view is the hope that the number of times the process produces a good result outweighs the cost of those times when an alternate approach would have been better.

- Secondly, formalising the information elements that contribute to a process usually requires considerable effort. An explicit model of the process needs to be created, which includes definitions of the data that needs to be collected. In some situations it is too costly to engage in this formalisation process, given the likely return.

- Finally, it may just not make sense to contemplate formalisation if the situations being dealt with are highly variable. If situations are unlikely to recur, then it would probably be better to come up with a way of handling them from 'first principle' each time, rather than looking to a formal cook-book of solutions.

In the first section of this chapter we saw that there are different cycles of information through healthcare. The way such information cycles can in principle be codified into an information system was

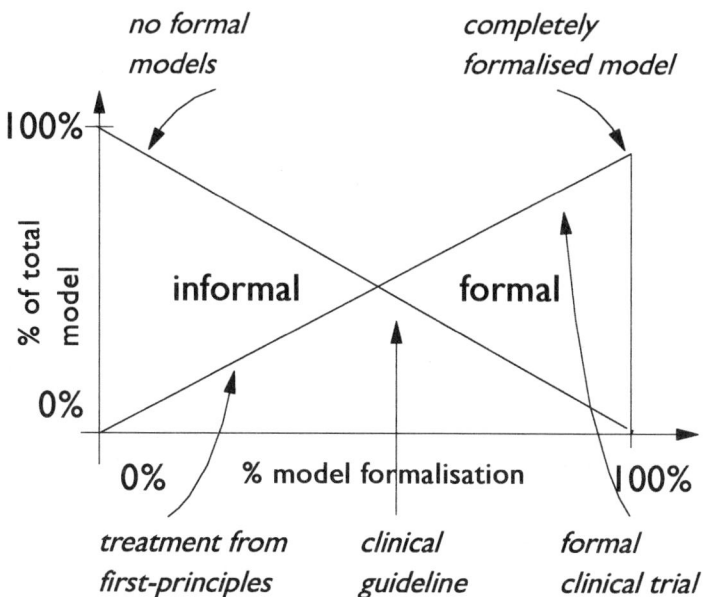

Figure 4.2: There is a
continuum of possible
formalisation of
information systems.
Formal and informal
models combine
together to cover the
total modelling needs
of a given problem.
The degree of
formalisation depends
on the type of
problem being
addressed.

demonstrated in Chapter 3. What should now be apparent is that, before a formal information system is created to manage a process, there needs to be an explicit choice made based on a cost-benefit analysis. In many circumstances, the result of that analysis may be that it is preferable to not build the system.

In Chapter 2 we saw that there is a continuum of possible model localisation between humans and computer (Figure 2.5). One can imagine a similar continuum stretching between those situations in which everything needs to be formalised, and those where a process can be left completely informal. In between these two extremes, depending upon specific needs, one can formally define some parts of a system, and leave the remaining interactions undefined (Figure 4.2). The proportion that is formalised will depend on the specific needs of a given situation.

Thus while a hospital will have many formally defined procedures for managing different activities, most activity in the organisation will be left informal. Similarly, the way patients are managed falls along this continuum of formality. Patients enrolled in a clinical trial have their management completely regimented, to maximise the scientific significance of any results. Patients with common conditions may be treated according to well-defined guidelines, but will have some aspects of their treatment modified informally to match individual needs. At the other end of the spectrum, a patient's problems may be approached in a non-standard way, perhaps because of the uniqueness of circumstances. While there may be a few general guidelines on how to approach such patients, most of what occurs has to be created 'from scratch'. This does not mean that such a treatment, if it is repeated over time, cannot slowly become part of the formal treatment of similar patients.

In the remainder of this section, we will explore the trade-off that exists between creating explicit models that permit formal information systems to be created, and leaving the system in an informal state, with minimally defined models and data.

Not all data need to made available for computer interpretation

Since not all processes need to be formalised, it follows that just because data is available, it may not necessarily benefit from being analysed. There clearly are many examples within healthcare when data is collected so that it can be analysed in depth. Data from clinical trials for example, are all defined in precise detail, so that the value of different treatments can be analysed.

Sometimes data is only of short-lived value and does not warrant the construction of formal a model to interpret it. Consider for example, a recorded voice message that is left by a member of a healthcare team for a colleague, containing an update on a patient's progress. The message is likely to be loosely structured, and cover a number of topics that would not normally be predictable in advance. It is also likely that the message will be of most interest only to the individuals who recorded and listened to the message.

Nevertheless the recorded message constitutes data that is stored, perhaps even on a computer system, and clinical decisions may be altered based upon the content of the message. Unlike the data that might be written into a patient record, or collected on a hospital information system and used by many people over an extended period, the data in such cases are of interest to a very few individuals and have a limited life-span.

As a consequence, the message data is treated in a very different way to data that might be formally recorded in a patient record. In such cases, it is unlikely that anyone would want to develop a model that allowed a computer to analyse the message. There is no formal agreement in advance on the content of the message or the ways in which it will be used. Such agreements are at the heart of traditional computer-based information systems, where data formats are specified in advance of system construction.

It thus follows that the model and the interpretation of the data are owned by the recorder and listener of the message. The machine that stores and transmits the data takes on a more passive role. It is used as a data repository, or as a channel between the communicating parties, rather than for any active interpretation it might make.

In general, one can make a distinction between information systems in which data is explicitly modelled and those in which data which is left unmodelled.

A **formal information system** contains an agreed model for the interpretation of data, and data within the system is structured in accordance with that model.

An **informal information system** is neutral to the interpretation of data, containing no model, and thus imposes minimal structure on any data that is contained within the system. Further, we can say that the model and the act of interpreting the data contained within an informal system are external to that system.

Thus an informal system does not imply the absence of a model or the inability to interpret data in the light a model. With an informal information system, the model exists externally to it. In practice these models are often kept in the heads of those who create or access the informally stored data (Figure 2.5).

There is thus no sense in which the data in an informal system is less valuable than formally structured data. It is used in fundamentally different ways, and in different situations. In general, we can say that informal information systems are used when data is only of temporary value, of interest to a very few people, is complex or its content is not predictable in advance.

Communication systems frequently support informal exchanges

We have already seen that when examining the information processes in an organisation, a distinction should be made between those that are worth supporting formally, perhaps with a computer-based information system, and those which are best left informal. This does not mean, however, that informal tasks cannot be supported by tools. Some tasks, like storing and retrieving phone numbers lend themselves to being formally organised. Other, like writing quick notes, are impaired by such structured methods. Thus, people often use simple tools like pen and paper to manage a variety of unstructured tasks. The key requirements for any tool used to support informal tasks is that it provides a means of managing information that is flexible, and can be used in a variety of ways.

One of the commonest ways of supporting informal processes is to use a communication system to channel data between people. This is because these systems are usually designed to be very informal about the content of the data they transfer. Thus, although usually thought of as a communication system, a telephone is a good example of an informal information system. The models for interpreting the data transmitted across the telephone are in the heads of the parties conversing, and not in the machinery responsible for mediating that conversation.

In fact, communication systems are commonly used to support informal information processes, because they are so flexible. When examining the flows of information through an organisation, it would be a mistake to only look at the formal processes in place, since this would give a very skewed picture of what really is going on. There is a complementary, and probably significantly larger, body of information coursing through the informal channels of the organisation's communication infrastructure.

An example will make the contrasting roles of communication and information systems in managing information clearer. Consider the information that might pass between a primary care physician and a cardiologist when a patient requires specialist assessment by the cardiologist. While the patient is still with him, the physician could transmit an ECG by fax to the cardiologist for an immediate opinion. In contrast, a more complex system could be set up to capture the

ECG signal directly from the cardiograph. Such a system would store the ECG data on a local computer, and the transmit the signal as a data file across the phone line to a computer used by the cardiologist.

Faxing an ECG. In the fax case, the ECG is printed out by the cardiograph and is then sent across the telephone system. The fax system is not configured in any special way to recognise that it is transmitting an ECG. It just as well could be sending text or a photograph. Thus the fax system is informal with respect to the content of the data. The model for the interpretation of the ECG is possessed by the cardiologist who reads the fax image.

The advantage of using a fax is that it is relatively cheap, easy to use, and widely available. The physician could be at a patient's home with a portable cardiograph, and use the patient's own fax machine, for example. Further it does not need to be in any way dedicated to a particular task like ECG transmission, since no model will be associated with the data it transmits. These are generally the characteristics of most informal communication systems like the telephone or paper. The disadvantage of using this system is that it requires someone with expertise on the receiving end of the fax to provide the model and interpretation.

Transmitting the ECG signal. If a patient's cardiogram is transmitted directly from a cardiograph to a remote computer in the cardiologist's office, the remote computer can take the original waveform signal and reconstruct the cardiogram. This is because the data is specifically structured according to a data model that allows it to be recognised as an ECG by the second computer system.

The advantages here are largely the inverse of the case with the faxed image. Having data that is structured according to a model permits flexible manipulation of the data. One could choose to display only some portions of the signal, at different resolutions. Equally, the signal could be automatically interpreted by an expert system, since the waveform data arrives in a highly structured form that is amenable to computer interpretation. The disadvantages of this system are that one requires a dedicated system at the sending and receiving ends to encode and decode the signal.

It is usually the case that there are many more general purpose systems available than there are complex and specialised ones. Thus at present there are more fax machines in the world than computer systems connected up to an ECG machine. A primary care practitioner who rarely has the need to transmit an ECG would find the cost of purchasing such a dedicated system unjustifiable. A cardiologist, for whom this was a common occurrence would find the case easier to make.

So, in summary, the fax system is able to be used on many different tasks, but will perform each of them less effectively than a system that has been formally designed for the task. Like most communication systems, the fax is relatively informal about what data is transmitted. When tasks are infrequent, it is more cost-effective to use an informal solution. In contrast, as a task starts to require formalisation because of its frequency or importance, more expensive and specific tools can be brought in to support it.

Chapter summary

1. Three quite separate information loops exist which reflect different instances of the information management cycle. Loop 1 defines the direct application of a model to a task. Loop 2 defines the way models are selected and are customised. Loop 3 is responsible for model creation and refinement based upon the results of application over time.

2. There are considerable advantages to structuring information processes, including improved reliability, efficiency and consistency. There are also costs associated with formalisation, including lack of flexibility to varying circumstances, and the effort involved in defining the system.

3. Not all data need to made available for computer interpretation. There is a trade-off that exists between creating explicit models that permit formal information systems to be created, and leaving the system in an informal state, with minimally defined models and data.

4. A formal information system contains an agreed model for the interpretation of data, and data within the system is structured in accordance with that model.

5. An informal information system is neutral to the interpretation of data, containing no model, and thus imposes minimal structure on any data that is contained within the system. The model and interpretation for data contained within an informal system is external to that system.

6. Communication systems are frequently used to support informal exchanges. Information flows through an organisation occur both through formal processes as well as through the informal channels of the organisation's communication infrastructure.

7. Informal information systems are used when data is of temporary value, of interest to very few people, is complex or its content is not predictable in advance. When tasks are infrequent, it is more cost-effective to use an informal solution. However, if a task requires formalisation because of its frequency or importance, more expensive and specific tools can be brought in to support it.

The problems of medical practice and hospital functioning are rapidly approaching crisis proportions, in terms of cost, limited personnel resources, and growing demands. The application of computer technology offers hope, but the realization of this hope in the near future will require a much greater commitment than is presently true of ...the medical academic community, and the health services community.

G. Octo Barnett, H. J. Sukenik, in Dickson and Brown (1969), p268.

Chapter 5

The electronic medical record

In the previous chapter, we saw that three distinct information cycles govern the operation of the healthcare system. The content of the information coursing within these cycles ranges from staff salaries, through to details about the care of patients. The last chapter also explained how some of that information is captured formally, but that a large part of it was left informal and communicated without necessarily ever being recorded. The formal aspects of clinical information are largely contained within the patient record, which serves as the single point of deposition and access for nearly all archival clinical data. The patient record is thus one of the primary mechanisms supporting the three information loops.

The medical record is so pivotal a topic in informatics that it makes sense to begin our detailed discussion of healthcare information systems here. Consequently, the remainder of this chapter will attempt to look at the benefits and limitations of existing paper-based systems, and the major functions that could in principle be replaced or enhanced by the electronic medical record.

Since the functional scope of the electronic record is so broad, the survey will inevitably widen to touch upon information and communication aspects of healthcare that extend beyond the pure record of care. In particular, the need to support communication amongst healthcare workers, protocol-based care, and the need for controlled medical terminologies will all be introduced here. However, given the importance and complexity of each of these topics, they will be returned to individually in greater detail in later sections of this book.

5.1 The electronic medical record is not a simple replacement of the paper record

The medical record has traditionally had a number of distinct functions, both formal and informal, and not all of these are always immediately recognised.

- The patient record provides a means of communicating between staff who are actively managing a patient. Notes left by staff assist those who work in different shifts, or who are unable to meet up during the working day.
- During the period of active management of a patient's illness, the record strives to be the single data access point for workers managing a patient. All test results, observations and so forth should be accessible through it. The record thus provides a 'view' onto data about a patient's illness.
- More subtly, the record offers an informal 'working space' to record the ideas and impressions that help build up a consensus view, over the period of care, of what is going on with a patient. One can view the evolution of such a consensus as storytelling or the development of a narrative about the patient (Kay and Purves, 1996). In this narrative, healthcare workers assemble data into a story that can then be communicated to others. This amounts to the imposition of an interpretation upon the patient data, and explains why the patient record is never the patient's own story, but rather the story as told by those who care for the patient.
- Once an episode of care has been completed, the record ultimately forms the single point at which all clinical data are archived, for longer term use. This might be to assist in later treatment for the same patient, or to be pooled with other data to assist in research.

The amount of patient data stored around the world in this record system is bewilderingly large, complex, and far flung. Every primary care practitioner's office contains patient records. Every hospital has dedicated professional staff whose main focus is to act as custodian and guide through its record store.

For today, this information exists in a multitude of forms, sometimes unintelligible except to those who created the record, and usually not accessible to anyone except those who are caring for individual patients. Oftentimes, it is not even available to these individuals as

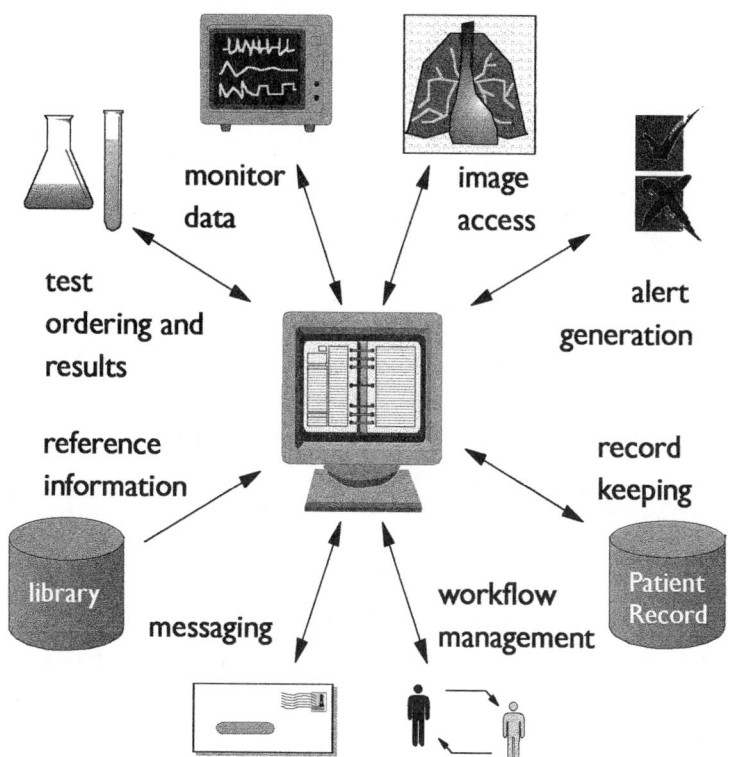

monitor data

image access

test ordering and results

alert generation

reference information

record keeping

library

messaging

workflow management

Patient Record

Figure 5.1: *The electronic medical record has a variety of potential functions that it can fulfil, requiring different degrees of investment and technological sophistication to implement them.*

records are misplaced, lost, or being used by someone else. It is also the case that one of the purposes of information is to help the growth of knowledge. With the medical record in such a form, it can only be a poor participant in this wider process.

With drawbacks both at the point of care and outcomes assessment, many have turned away from paper systems to computer-based ones in the hope that they will more closely meet the information needs of healthcare. The computer-based systems that are intended to deal with this formal information are known variously as the electronic medical record (EMR), computer-based patient record (CPR), or the electronic patient record (EPR).

Without doubt, over the last three decades there has been an enormous amount of controversy, confusion and distress associated with the development clinical computer record systems. At the core of much of this difficulty lie the very different views individuals have held over the role and importance of the electronic medical record.

For some, the EMR is simply the computer replacement for existing paper medical record systems. The computer provides mechanisms for capturing information during the clinical encounter, stores it in some secure fashion, and permits retrieval of that information by those with a clinical need.

The advantages that are often cited for moving to such a computer record system include a reduction in storage space, the possibility of simultaneous access to the records by many individuals, and the possibility of using data for a variety of clinical research activities. Individual clinicians, for example, could do rapid searches through their practice records for audit purposes. Data pooled from many patients in a region could be used to study local aspects of the epidemiology of disease, and so forth.

At the other extreme, for many the EMR represents the totality of information and communication systems that could be made available in the support of clinical activities. The label 'record' in the name 'electronic medical record' starts to become increasingly inappropriate as the functionality expected of the EMR broadens far beyond the computerised duplication of a paper record system. Everything from systems for ordering tests and investigations, digital image archiving and retrieval, the exchange of messages between different workers in the healthcare system, through to the automated coding of patient data for administrative purposes might be included as components of the extended EMR's function.

Indeed in 1991, when the Institute of Medicine (IOM) in the United States issued a highly influential committee report on the computer-based patient record, it intentionally used a broad and inclusive definition of the EMR (Dick and Steen, 1991). The EMR was defined as 'an electronic patient record that resides in a system specifically designed to support users by providing accessibility to complete and accurate data, alerts, reminders, clinical decision support systems, links to medical knowledge, and other aids.'

With such a wide variation in the functions that could be expected from an EMR, it is probably unwise to try to define the EMR in any formal way. It is more fruitful to observe that there are a range of clinical activities that use and communicate information, and that some of these can be supported through the introduction of technology (Figure 5.1). The extent to which that is actually done in any one locality depends entirely on the resources, needs and expertise of those concerned. We saw in the previous chapter, for example, that it is not always appropriate to introduce a formal computer system when a more informal solution might be more effective.

The main recommendation of the 1991 IOM report on the computer-based patient record was that health care professionals and organisations should adopt the EMR as the standard method for recording all records related to patient-care (Dick and Steen, 1991). The justification for such a recommendation rests as much on people's aspirations for transforming clinical practice as it does on the limitations ascribed to paper-based methods of recording clinical information, for which there much evidence.

5.2 The paper-based medical record

In one form or another, the method of recording patient data on paper has served medical practice successfully for centuries. However, while the physical nature of the paper record has remained relatively unchanged, the formal structure of the information contained within the record has undergone much change in the last fifty years. The patient record has moved from being an unstructured chronological record of events, to being problem or task oriented, and structured according to the expertise and role of those creating the record (Tange, 1996).

There are thus two quite separate aspects to the paper record that need to be considered. The first is the physical way individuals interact with paper. The second is the structure and content of the information that is recorded upon it. It is important to make such a distinction, because it is easy to confuse criticisms of existing record systems with criticisms of paper as a recording medium. In many cases, the reason a paper record system is poor has much to do with the processes in place to support it and the effort people choose to make when creating a record.

Physical aspects of the paper record

The way paper lends itself to being handled, marked upon, and stored are often taken for granted, but have some remarkably rich implications. As a physical system, the paper record thus has many positive attributes.

- Paper is portable, and access is self-contained. Apart from needing a light source, there is nothing preventing notes being worked on in most places. A computer system requires power to be supplied to it, and may require connection to a computer network.

- Paper and pen are a highly familiar method of recording information, and require no special training of medical staff. The educational process has occurred well before individuals come to interact with the paper medical record. In contrast, for many existing health professionals, use of a computer system may require specific training in the workplace.

- Access to data written on paper can feel very direct. Browsing through a reasonable sized volume of notes permits a form of rapid scanning of what is recorded there.

There are also some drawbacks associated with the physical characteristics of any paper system, some of which only become apparent when record systems become quite large.

- A paper record can only be used for one task at a time. If two people wanted to look at a patient's notes, then one would have to wait for the other to finish with it. Thus, a patient's records may be unavailable during a consultation because they are being cared for by a number of different workers. Notes might be lying in a different clinic, in a physician's office or home, or elsewhere. Several studies have found that records are unavailable up to 30% of the time in larger institutions (Dick and Steen, 1991). It is also sadly the case that records can be lost, with the percentage varying according to the record processing and tracking procedures of different institutions. Even if they are available, the time required for notes to be requested and delivered can be unacceptable, and the process of retrieval may require substantial expenditure of human resource.

- Paper records consume space when large amounts of data are recorded. There are methods of reducing this, for example creating copies on microfiche, but these require additional effort and expense, as well as imposing new barriers to easy retrieval.
- Large records for individual patients can be physically cumbersome, heavy, and difficult to search through for specific information. Patients whose chronic illness span a number of years of care can generate particularly unwieldy records.
- Paper is fragile, susceptible to damage, and unless well cared for, will degrade over time.
- The production of paper has environmental consequences, related for example to the bleaching processes and forest management.

Informational aspects of the paper record

Somewhat independent of the physical nature of paper is the choice of the structure and content of the information that is recorded upon it. It is thus not necessarily the case that a record is poor simply because it is captured on paper. The quality of a record might have more to do with the quality of data written upon it, or the way the data are structured.

Information entry. One of the great advantages of paper relates to how little structuring it demands. The way that data can be recorded on paper is quite unconstrained in both its form and content. A paper entry might capture a terse set of laboratory results, a record of physical examination with hand-drawn diagrams, or a long and detailed narrative containing subjective assessments of a patient's mental state. In the terms of the previous chapter, paper is a relatively informal medium, since it imposes few models on the data that is captured. The models that interpret the data captured on paper are contained within the head of the reader. This means that paper is a quite general purpose means for capturing data. Everything from the most personal scribbled note, to highly standardised forms can be captured on the same medium. Unfortunately, this freedom of structuring that comes with the use of paper is not without its drawbacks.

- Since the structuring used to create a paper record may be very personal, it may be difficult for someone other than the writer to understand what is recorded there. In model terms, the reader may not possess the model used when the data was captured, making interpretation difficult. This may simply mean that what is recorded is illegible, or that the words are clear, but their intended meaning is not.

- In the absence of any formal structure to guide record creation, there is increased opportunity for errors to occur, for example the omission of relevant data. There has been much study of the quality of patient records over the years, focusing on the amount of missing or inaccurate data. Many of the causes of these record defects are due to the manner in which examinations are conducted, and their results recorded, and have little to do with the fact that records are made on paper. The imposition of a formal structure for data capture such as pre-printed forms can certainly improve this situation, at the cost of making the process very directed. It seems fair to say then, that many difficulties with the content of existing record systems are largely due to the processes in place for data capture. In principle, it is possible for a well-designed set of paper forms to be far more effective in improving the quality of a medical record than a poorly designed computer-based one.

Information retrieval. A very different, but equally important aspect of the structuring of information relates to the way one is able to search within a given record, or across a body of records, for specific data. Clinicians use a wide variety of information sources during decision making, and patient specific data stored in the record is a major component of that (R. Smith, 1996b).

There is now clear evidence that clinical workers routinely fail to find pieces of information that they need during a patient consultation from the paper medical record. Tang et al. (1994) studied 168 outpatient consultations and found that data was searched for but not found in 81% of cases. In 95% of these cases, the medical record was available during the consultation. The categories of missing information were laboratory tests and procedures (36%), medications and treatments (23%), history (31%), and other (10%). It is not clear from this study what the effect of the failure to locate data had on the delivery of care or patient outcomes. Nevertheless, the physicians in the study expended additional effort pursuing the data they needed. These included searching alternate data sources, making decisions despite the missing data, or relying on the report of patients or their relatives. In another, earlier study, the consequence of missing laboratory data was that 11% of tests in a hospital setting were duplicated (Tufo and Speidel, 1971).

A different type of problem with data retrieval arises when data need to be extracted from a subset of records from within a larger number of records. All substantial record systems, in whatever form they exist, require some form of indexing to allow individual records to be retrieved. Libraries have the Dewey system for the classification and retrieval of books. Medical records are similarly accessed via an indexing system, at a minimum allowing a record to be found according to patient name or identification number.

It is a feature of large paper systems that fixed indexes need to be created before such searches can occur. For example, it would not be possible to walk into a paper record office and obtain the notes from every patient admitted with a particular disease over the last two years, unless a disease-based index had already been created. The only solution in this case would be to read each record individually to check if it contained the diagnosis in question. This is such a time-consuming process that it not frequently done.

Despite such a large set of shortcomings, the perceived advantages of the paper-based medical record are sufficient to make its continued use attractive in some circumstances. Indeed, there are data that suggest that at least some medical practitioners are quite happy to stick to the paper record for their everyday clinical activities (Tange, 1995).

5.3 The electronic medical record

With so many difficulties associated with the paper record, there has been a growing drive to replace it with a computer-based one for most of the last half-century (e.g. Barnett and Sukenik, 1969). This has resulted in the design and implementation of many different systems, with varying functionality, and variable success. In 1990, one of the most successful implementations of the EMR reported that only about 25% of all patient data in the hospital were available electronically, the remainder residing in the paper system (Kuperman and Gardner, 1990).

Consequently, despite such significant investments in information technology, some today still feel that it is difficult to quantify the explicit benefits of doing so. In several recent reviews of the literature on hospital information systems, the evidence for their cost-benefit was found to still be inconclusive (van der Loo et al., 1995; Lock, 1996). This is partly due to the inherent difficult associated with the evaluation of complex systems, but it may also reflect the lack of clear objective measurements in many studies. It is also the case that for many, the case for the introduction of computer-based systems is 'obvious', and so the need for detailed assessment is not apparent to them.

It is clear that this situation is changing rapidly, as medical informatics develops a more scientific basis. Thus, today it is at least possible to make a comprehensive qualitative assessment of the value of replacing paper with computer, and individual studies that demonstrate specific advantages are increasingly becoming available. Nevertheless, there is still a great need for the development and application of robust formal methods for the evaluation of information technology in health care (Friedman and Wyatt, 1997).

In the next sections, some of the advantages and disadvantages of a computer-based medical record compared to paper-based systems will be discussed. With a constant stream of technological innovation, and changes in the cost of information technologies, many of the traditional drawbacks associated with computer systems are disappearing. It is likely that soon the most profound difficulties will reside in the design of these information systems, and not their technological implementation.

Physical aspects of the computer-based record

Computer-based systems have a number of powerful physical attributes that make them ideal data capture and storage systems.
- Perhaps first amongst these, and now taken for granted, is the enormous quantity of data that can be stored in a small physical space once data are in electronic form. With continual advances in

the technologies of optical storage, and in magnetic particle systems, this capability will continue to deliver ever greater storage capacity for some considerable time to come.

- A second physical implication is the ability to easily create duplicate copies of data, either to allow sharing of data, but more importantly to act as back-up copies for security reasons. The costs and efforts involved in transferring paper records to microfiche, or in scanning them into electronic form, make them much less attractive in this respect. In the worst case, paper records are never duplicated and remain susceptible to physical damage and even loss through disasters like fire or flooding.

- One of the traditional advantages of paper is its informality. If needed it can support a wide variety of data. In contrast, computer systems have traditionally demanded far more formal data models, and as a consequence, imposed these on their users during data entry (Figure 4.2). It is common to hear comments about the rigidity of the way data have to be entered into a computer, and how much simpler it would be to use paper. Fortunately, this situation is changing for a number of reasons.

  ○ Firstly, the interaction technologies that define the way data are entered into a computer are becoming less constraining. Rather than forcing individuals to use a keyboard, it is now possible for data to be captured in a number of alternate ways. Thus, raw data can be entered as a dictated voice recording, or as hand-written notes and diagrams using a pen-based computer system (e.g. MacNeill and Huang, 1996). Such data can be stored and left uninterpreted, still permitting subsequent retrieval when the data can be viewed or listened to in their original form. Further, using advanced pattern recognition methods, voice and handwriting data can be converted by the computer system into text. These interpretation methods are variable in their success, depending upon the situation in which interpretation occurs, but can usually achieve recognition levels greater than 90% accuracy. Ultimately, recognition systems are limited by the way that the meaning of spoken or written language is based upon an understanding of the context within which a word is used (see Chapter 12). This ability to fully interpret natural language requires a computer to posses some degree of artificial intelligence in a computer system, and remains an open research problem in computer science.

○ Secondly, as more system designers realise the value in capturing spontaneous and unstructured data as part of the computer-based medical record, they will design features that allow this type of data to be entered. Thus, even without advanced interpretation systems, it is now physically easier to enter unstructured data into computer systems. This move to more familiar methods of data entry will also reduce the discomfort some individuals who have not grown up with computer systems experience.

• It was stated earlier that an advantage of the paper record is its portability, as if to imply that this was not an attribute of a computer-based one. This may have been the case in the past, when a computer system consisted of heavy fixed terminals connected to wired hospital computer networks. This no longer need be the case. It is now possible to provide wireless connections to lightweight portable computer systems, allowing workers to roam within a campus like a hospital, or even widely across much larger regions using cellular radio and satellite technologies (see Chapter 14). As a consequence, data can be accessed or retrieved in a wide variety of circumstances.

• The situation in which records are missing, lost or unavailable because they are elsewhere in an organisation does not arise with an electronic system. Database technologies permit multiple individuals to read a record simultaneously, and network technologies permit these individuals to be geographically separated. Thus it no longer should be the case that if data exist on file that they should not be immediately available to those with permission to access that data.

• Finally, physical access to the computer record can be protected by a variety of different security measures. These are designed to prevent unauthorised individuals accessing the clinical record. Complex schemes involving restricting access to different components of the record based on an individual's role and need to know can also be devised. Associated with such advantages are a different set of security risks (Anderson, 1995; Barrows and Clayton, 1996). It is often possible for knowledgeable and determined individuals to 'hack' into computer networks, despite security barriers like password entry systems. This type of risk can be reduced through the use of data encryption methods that make data unintelligible in the event that it is accessed by unauthorised individuals. Further discussion of security on computer networks is presented in Section 17.7.

Informational aspects of the computer-based record

Many of the advantages of an EMR become apparent when there are a large number of patient records, or when information tasks are complex. One of the most immediate benefits of having data available electronically is that the speed of searching for data is significantly improved. While a computer has searched through thousands of records for specific items, a human could still be leafing through one paper record.

Perhaps even more importantly, the types of search that can be performed are complex. A primary care physician should be able to search through the records of the practice, and extract files for patients with specific attributes, such as age or diagnosis and conduct a local audit of care, or search for patients that are similar to a current case. A researcher should be able to conduct retrospective studies of the epidemiology of specific diseases by accessing the records in a region that match specific study criteria. The ability of a computer database to search according to a number of different attributes means that each record is 'indexed' in a large number of different ways - certainly far more than could easily be accomplished by hand generated indexes. It is possible to move completely away from the notion of creating fixed index structures. In principle every word in a document can act as an index, permitting what is known as full text retrieval to be performed.

The EMR can actively participate in clinical care

Up until now, the EMR has been considered as if it were simply a repository of clinical data, which is either added to or looked at, as

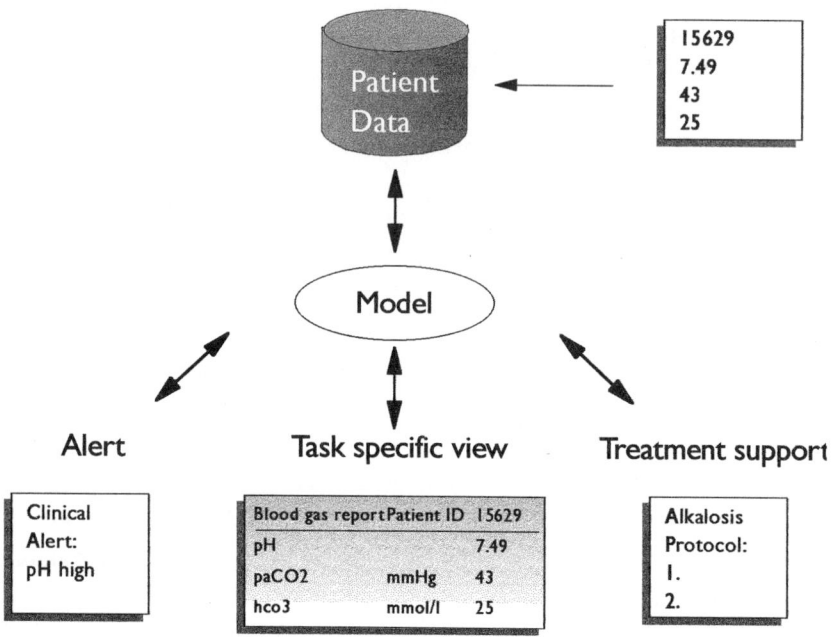

Figure 5.2: Using models of clinical tasks, the EMR can actively participate in clinical care, for example by generating specific views of clinical data, by sending alerts or by invoking models of treatment protocols.

the situation demands. One might characterise the EMR's role in this case to be a passive supporter of clinical activity. This is the traditional way in which the record has been used during care. Perhaps the greatest advantage of the EMR will ultimately be that it can be used in a more active way, by contributing more directly in the process of clinical care. An active EMR might suggest what patient information needs to be collected, or it might assemble clinical data in a way that assists a clinician in the visualisation of a patient's clinical condition.

For the EMR to become more active in clinical care, there must be some mechanism by which the computer system is able to 'understand' what is needed of it. More precisely, the EMR must possess some model of the clinical process which allows it to interpret data in a way that is clinically useful. At present, most research into active aspects of the EMR is focused on the generation of clinical alerts and reminders, the construction of task specific views of data, and the structuring of care around protocols or guidelines (Figure 5.2).

Alerts and reminders. It is commonplace to flag test results that fall outside the normal range, directing clinicians to results that might be particularly worth considering. This represents an interpretation of data based upon statistical models of normality. It is also possible to capture other types of model, representing different forms of clinical knowledge. For example, simple 'rules of thumb' or heuristics can be used by a computer to look at patterns in clinical data, and generate prompts for clinicians.

Even simple alerts and reminders can have a positive impact on care. Computer-generated reminders of the appropriate length of stay for a particular diagnosis have been show to reduce the median length of stay in hospital (Shea, et al., 1995). In a meta-analysis of 16 randomised controlled trials of computer generated reminders in ambulatory care, there was clear evidence that they improved preventative practices. Clinicians were found to perform better with the reminders on tasks like breast and colorectal cancer screening, cardiovascular risk reduction, and vaccination (Shea, DuMouchel et al., 1996). Much more complex reminders can be generated, based upon data contained within the EMR, including laboratory results and current medications. The methods used to accomplish this type of interpretation can be quite complex, and this advanced topic will be explored in much more detail in Chapters 20 and 21.

Task specific views of data. One of the basic roles of the medical record is to provide a 'view' onto all the known patient data, so that it can be used to make clinical decisions. As records grow in size, searching for data relevant to a specific decision becomes increasingly difficult. This problem is not specific to health care, but is common to many professions in which large quantities of data need to be searched before a decision can be made. Airline pilots are surrounded by a variety of instruments and manuals in their cockpits, and nuclear power plant operators are similarly beset with data. Research into the psychology of engineering systems suggests that the creation of task-specific data displays can assist in decision making by presenting views of only the data which are directly relevant to a decision (Wickens, 1992). Such displays both reduce the effort expended in collating data, as well as focusing the attention on important data that might otherwise be ignored.

Figure 5.3:
Using models of clinical decisions, different views of patient data can be constructed to support distinct tasks. Here data relevant to determining fluid balance during surgery is collected together on one screen as part of an anaesthetic EMR. © Hewlett-Packard, 1992.

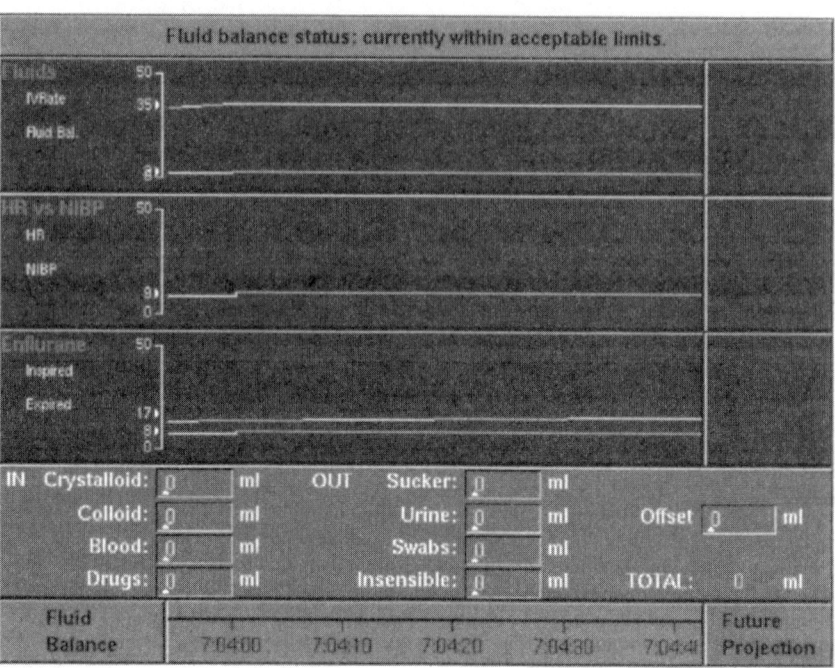

The creation of task-specific views is also supported by research into clinical behaviour, which suggests that the creation of data displays specific to particular clinical contexts can be of value (Fafchamps et al., 1991). The creation of such task specific data views requires some model of what the different tasks might be, as well as what data are 'relevant' for that particular task. Such models can be created by system designers, or be specifically designed by the staff who will use the system (Gierl et al., 1995). Most commonly, task-specific views are created around measured data, which might be obtained from laboratory tests or instruments (Figure 5.3). With appropriate structuring of record entries in an EMR, it should also be possible to view segments of unstructured text that relate to any given problem (Tange, 1996).

Protocol-guided care: The notion of a problem-oriented medical record is based upon the assumption that care can be best delivered when the record focuses on the management of specific problems. With the EMR, this notion of record structuring around problems can become more active when the EMR has models of the management of different problems. Clinical protocols or guidelines can provide such models, and if integrated into the EMR, could support a rich variety of new functions. Guidelines can be used to ensure that specific data are gathered, to suggest tests that need to be ordered or treatments that could be contemplated.

Clinical audit and outcomes assessment. Patient records contribute not just to the immediate care of individual patients, but can be pooled to assess the efficacy of particular treatments, determine cost-benefits, or to audit the performance of individual care centres. To do this, data often need to be condensed. It may, for example, only be necessary to record a patient's ultimate diagnosis for some purposes.

Much of this data condensation is done through the process of coding. Here, the treatments and diagnoses of a specific patient are assigned a code out of a predetermined list. For example, the World Health Organisation (WHO) has a set of epidemiological codes called the International Classification of Diseases (ICD), which are used to track broad global health patterns. Most countries return data to WHO based upon their local records. This has for a long time been a manual process, but the data stored in the EMR could be used to partially or completely create such codes.

5.4 Conclusions

This chapter has presented a broad survey of the rationale for and potential roles of the EMR. It should now be clear that the role of a computer-based information system in healthcare extends significantly beyond the simple storage and retrieval of patient data. Many of the aspects of the EMR introduced here will be returned to in subsequent sections. In particular, protocol-based care, clinical coding and classification, and the support of communication in a clinical setting will all be examined in much greater detail.

The final chapter in this section looks at the way all such information systems are designed. Within the constraints of these design principles, we can understand better how information and communication systems fit into the clinical workplace, and work more comfortably with some of their inherent limitations.

Chapter summary

1. At its simplest, the EMR is the computer replacement for existing paper medical record systems. It provides mechanisms for capturing information during the clinical encounter, stores it in a secure fashion, and permits retrieval of that information by those with a clinical need.

2. For many, the EMR represents the totality of information and communication systems that could be made available in the support of clinical activities. Systems for ordering tests and investigations, digital image archiving and retrieval, the exchange of messages between different workers in the healthcare system, through to the automated coding of patient data for administrative purposes may be components of the EMR's function.

3. There are two quite separate aspects to record systems. The first is the physical nature of the way individuals interact with it. The second is the way information is structured when entered into or retrieved from the system.

4. Advantages of the paper-based medical record include its portability, its support of informal and formal data capture, and its familiarity and ease of use.

5. Disadvantages of the paper-based medical record include its poor use of space, its fragility, its limitation to a single user at any one time, the ease with which records can be misplaced or lost, and the effort required in searching for information either in large single records, or from collections of records.

6. The computer-based medical record can be used passively as a repository of data, or actively by assisting with the shaping of care. Active use requires the EMR to contain models of care, permitting some degree of interpretation of the data contained in the record.

7. Active uses of the computer-based medical record include the generation of clinical alerts and reminders, task specific views onto clinical data, protocol-guided data entry and action suggestion, and generation of codes for the classification of the contents of the record.

Chapter 6

Designing and building information systems

Given that there are limits to resources in healthcare, just because something is possible, it may not be desirable, or indeed affordable. This certainly is the case with information technologies, and the last few decades are littered with examples of healthcare information systems that were ill-considered in their design, or in the resources they consumed. Equally, there are many examples of well conceived projects that have delivered considerable benefit. The difference between success and failure often comes down to the approach taken by the creators of a system.

There are essentially two ways in which a technology can be applied to solve a problem. The first approach is **technology driven**. Here one asks 'What problems will best be solved by using this new technology?' Inevitably, whatever the problem, the answer will always be that the technology is the solution. This approach is often useful when trying to demonstrate the potential of a particular technological innovation.

The second approach to the application of technological is **problem driven,** and asks the question 'What is the best way to solve this particular problem?'. In this approach, all kinds of solutions are explored, from changes in clinical process to the introduction of a new technology. Consequently, sometimes the answer to the problem may be that new technology is not the best solution.

Informatics, when it is focused on building healthcare systems that will be routinely used, should fundamentally be problem driven. It should first and foremost be concerned with understanding the nature of information and communication problems in healthcare. Only then should informatics try to identify if it is appropriate for technology to solve these problems and, if necessary, develop and apply these technologies.

Sadly however, this is not always the case. It is not uncommon for information system developers to put most of their effort into the technology, leaving problem definition scarcely addressed. One thus sometimes finds clinical information systems that are designed in a way that does not address the needs of the clinicians who will use them. Equally, sometimes informatics research explores exotic technologies that solve problems that could be more easily solved with simpler existing technology, or indeed in non-technological ways.

So, how does one choose which clinical problems are good candidates for a technological solution? Further, how should one design an information system in a way that maximises the likelihood that it will actually solve the problem it is intended to? These are complex questions, with many technical ramifications. This chapter will simply try to examine the problem selection and system design processes from a general perspective. In particular, the focus will be on understanding what is theoretically possible, what is technically practicable, and in the context of limited resources, what is desirable.

The chapter is divide into three sections. In the first section, methods of arriving at good problem-driven formulations will be examined. Next, some key issues that limit what is possible in the design of systems will be outlined, in particular looking at the life cycle of an information system. The final section will look, in a relatively systematic way, at how one arrives at a well engineered specification of an information system.

6.1 Defining clinical needs

There is an initial stage in the life of any information system in which its role, costs and benefits are debated. Eventually, this leads on to the creation of a system design that reflects the trade-offs that inevitably will be made at this point. The clarification of the role that a system will play is perhaps the most critical aspect of this process, since it influences everything that will follow.

How does one gain an understanding of the needs of clinical practice, and then convert these into a set of specifications for an information system? There are many approaches, each of which is aimed at understanding what people need. They can be roughly grouped into the following four categories.

Anecdotal or individual experience. At the most superficial level one can draw upon individual experience, or rely on anecdotal evidence from other colleagues, to help pinpoint the tasks with which clinicians need help. This method usually operates within a framework of the existing assumptions about user needs. In other words, it is unlikely that novel needs will be uncovered to challenge the prevailing wisdom.

Asking clinicians. If one wants to be a little more methodical, a survey can be conducted, and ask clinicians about their way of working and their needs. While this may seem attractive, it has its problems. The biggest is that it is unlikely that clinicians really know what they want or need. 'Although users are expert at what they do, they have difficulty predicting what they would like' (Fafchamps et al., 1991).

More specifically, both the anecdotal and survey approaches suffer from a number of methodological difficulties. The problem of attitudinal bias has long been understood in the social psychology literature - people's actions differ from their verbalised responses (Wicker, 1976). We don't necessarily do as we say. Secondly, these methods require a degree of self-reporting. When asked why they made a certain judgement, or how they solved a particular problem, people are capable of providing apparently plausible reports of their mental events. However, asking people to introspect about their behaviour is a contentious investigative method in psychology because verbal reports of influences on behaviour may not be valid. Since there is no method of independently checking the validity of self reports, the details of cognition remain private to the individual (Nisbett and Wilson, 1977).

Non-participatory observation. The next set of methods do not ask clinicians what they want, but study the way they work in the field. There are many approaches that one could take, including techniques derived from ethnography (Fafchamps et al., 1991), as well as the more traditional software design methods of data-flow and task analysis. Here researchers try to understand the demands made upon individuals through detailed observations of them engaged in routine tasks. By making such observations, one is in a position to identify needs that may not be apparent to the individuals being studied.

Formal psychological experiments. Finally, at the most detailed and scientifically rigorous level, one might have a set of hypotheses about specific aspects of behaviour, and set up controlled studies to test them out. In this way, the impact of different changes to a decision process can be robustly assessed in a controlled situation. Some of the classic work in clinical decision making has been of this type (e.g. Elstein et al., 1978).

While it may seem that the ideal method of proceeding is to invest in formal psychological studies of clinical decision making, this is not necessarily the case. Laboratory experiments run the risk of treating decision making as an abstract process, independent of the vagaries and interrupts of working life. By their nature, such studies are conducted in laboratory conditions which factor out the interruptions and pressures of the real clinical workplace. In the real world, time pressures mean that short cuts are taken, and that people and events interrupt clinical activities.

What is usually needed is a characterisation of clinical decision processes as much as possible in the way they really occur, as opposed to the way they **should** occur. This will give us the best chance of designing systems for use in working environments, as opposed to designing what would be needed if everything else was ideal. It may be the case for example, that in an ideal consultation a doctor may want to consult a computer to help with the diagnostic process. However, with the pressures of the real workplace, the bottlenecks to increased performance may be much more mundane and less glamorous. They may, for example, be more closely associated with easy and timely access to information, or better communications between professionals, or even simply reducing the amount of paperwork in the clinical workplace.

This argument strongly favours pursuing non-participatory methods in the field, such as the ethnographic approach. Such qualitative research methods are sufficiently formal to allow robust statements to be made about results, and have the advantage of being grounded in the realities of the clinical workplace (Mays and Pope, 1996). Formal experiments will only answer narrow questions and are relatively expensive to conduct. One must therefore have a broad understanding of the domain to make a value judgement about the most likely avenues for investigation prior to making the investment in experimentation. This does not mean that there should not be a more formal psychological basis to defining clinical need, but simply that when defining the functions of individual systems, other approaches are more appropriate.

It is nonetheless valuable to have an appreciation of the rich literature connecting cognitive psychology and systems engineering (e.g. Wickens, 1992). Sadly, there seems to have been little connection between the design of many clinical decision support systems, and the work on the cognitive aspects of clinical decision making. Thus, much of the work done in information system development has paid lip service to the notion of task understanding, and has operated on a set of largely untested assumptions about clinical need.

For example, there is a strong belief that providing health care workers with diagnostic assistance is of great value. The working model proposed might be that, during a clinical encounter, a health care worker turns to a computer system that suggests possible diagnoses. This model was possibly motivated by early research in decision analysis that suggested that human judgements were prone to decision biases (Kahneman et al., 1982). The implication of this work was that such flawed judgements could be normalised by relying on sounder, more formally based, diagnostic systems.

There is now growing evidence that questions such an assessment. Based upon studies of individuals in the field rather than in controlled laboratory situations, evidence now suggests that the primary effort for decision makers is not at the moment of choice, but rather in situation assessment (Klein and Calderwood, 1991). In other words, it may well be the case that the majority of clinicians do not have difficulty in making a diagnosis. Rather, they encounter problems in establishing a clear picture of the state of the world, and clarifying their goals and assumptions, prior to attempting to make a diagnosis. If situation assessment is the key bottleneck in decision making, this has implications for the design of decision support tools for monitoring and control. Systems that assist clinicians in making an assessment of data through clear presentation may be of more utility than systems that attempt to manufacture a diagnosis.

In summary, the design of individual information systems should be preceded by a period of investigation, relying on qualitative research methods, which help define the needs of individuals in the workplace. Wherever possible, this work should be shaped by our best understanding of cognitive processes and their implications for systems engineering.

6.2 Designing for change

Understanding user needs helps determine what a system should do, based upon the constraints of environment in which it will work. The working environment also affects how the system should be constructed. Indeed, we saw earlier that the construction of any object, device or system begins with set of assumptions about the environment in which it will operate (Figure 2.4). Of these assumptions, the intended lifetime of the system is perhaps one of the most fundamental, since it affects the choice of materials and quality of design. Something that is meant to be temporary is engineered in a very different way to something that is intended to stand for many years.

One of the greatest challenges for any designer is arriving at ways of coping with change during a system's lifetime. As the world changes, the design assumptions with which systems are built become outdated. As the effects of these changes accumulate over time, a system becomes increasingly out of tune with the environment for which it was built. There are countless examples of this process of system 'decay' (Hogarth,1986). Political systems arise out of the needs of a society, only to become increasingly inappropriate as the nature of society changes underneath them. Antibiotics become increasingly ineffective as the bacteria they are intended to attack change their pattern of drug resistance.

The rate of obsolescence of a human artefact is thus directly related to the rate at which its design assumptions decay. Since building an artefact like a hospital or an information system is often an expensive affair, coping with the process obsolescence is often critical. This is especially so if the costs of building need to be recouped over an extended period. If the system becomes obsolete before it has paid back the investment in it, then it may fail financially. Consequently, its builders may not be in a position to design and build the next generation of system to replace it.

Time cycles for information systems

An information system is particularly susceptible to the effects of change. We can think of an information system experiencing the effects of change at several different time scales, corresponding to different aspects of its design and construction:

- the user needs that define the role of the system,
- the model of user needs, and subsequent system design,
- the technology used to construct the system,
- organisational resources, including finance and staff availability.

A change in any one of these will effect the performance of the system as a whole. For example, if the original need for a system changes, irrespective of how advanced the technology is, the system as a whole has become obsolete. Equally, technology can change rapidly, and a well designed system may become obsolete because newer technologies make it seem slow compared to newer ones introduced at a later date.

The time scales over which each of these different aspects of a system age are different, making it very difficult to get any synchronisation in replacement cycles. Thus, once it has been built, an information system is probably already obsolete either in its modelling of user needs, its definition of organisational structure, or the computer technology used to implement it.

Informal systems are much less susceptible to this sort of obsolescence, since they avoid modelling specific attributes of an organisation, and consequently are much more permissive about the information that is being stored or transmitted within them. Consider, for example, how the telephone system in an institution like a hospital may undergo little change, whilst its information systems may go through several revisions or complete change. Indeed, informal systems are often used increasingly during the period that a

Figure 6.1: *The time scales over which user needs, information models, and computer technologies change, and over which financial replacement cycles extend may all be different. This results in an differential rate of obsolescence for these different aspects of an information system.*

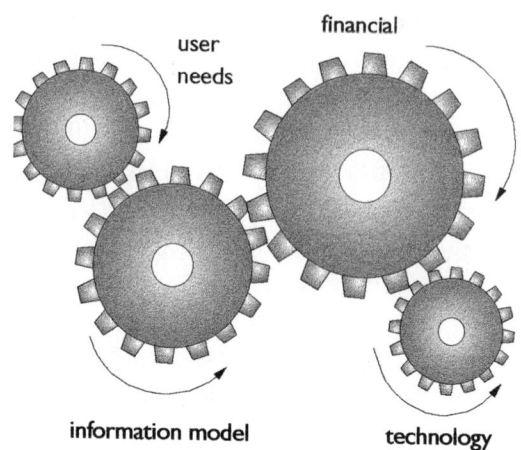

formal information system becomes out of date, bridging the gap between the deficiencies of the formal system and actual situation.

Withholding design

One solution to this problem of managing replacement cycles in the face of differential ageing, is to hold back the introduction of a new design, even through it is appropriate to retire an existing one. This is often the solution chosen when there is a mismatch between the period needed to pay for a system, and the period over which it becomes obsolete.

For example, as healthcare becomes increasingly expensive and the nature of medical practice evolves, the burden of care is being shifted from institutions like hospitals to smaller entities in the community. It is implicit in this change that much of the hospital system as it exists is becoming increasingly obsolete. However, given the huge investment in the hospital system, from the buildings through to the people whose skills are needed to make it work, it is impossible to make the change overnight. The investment in the existing system is too big, and the cost of creating a new one enormous.

As a result, larger hospitals are slowly closed down or change their function, and staff slowly trickle out to community-based institutions. At the same time, the cost of ramping up the new community-based care system is so large that it also takes time.

Change is expensive. The consequence of these costs is that obsolete systems are kept in use well beyond the point at which they could in principle be replaced.

Design modularity

Part of the solution to the problem of designing for a changing world is to construct a system, built upon the assumption that parts of its design will be altered over its working lifetime.

At the heart of designing for change is the concept of design modularity. The designer creates a system in such a way that it's different components, or sub-systems, are cleanly separated. In a car for example, the braking system is designed to be a separate set of components to the suspension. When change demands that a component be redesigned, the effects are contained within that component module. It is redesigned and replaced, while the remainder of the system is left unaffected.

The most useful way of creating modules is to consider the different purposes for which parts of the device's inner structure are intended. Each separate purpose, or function, is then contained within a module. There is a hidden catch to this simple idea. Recall from Chapter 3 that the definition of a system is ultimately arbitrary. In other words, when a designer looks at a system, the decision to separate it into sub-components could be made in many ways. Consequently, there can never be a guarantee that a particular way of compartmentalising a design will always insulate it from change. What it does achieve is that it decreases the likelihood that changes will affect the whole system - on average using design modularity allows a system's design to gracefully degrade over time.

6.3 Designing the information management cycle

Once a set of user needs has been determined, and constraints of the working environment understood, the next step in the construction of an information system is the formal specification of its design. This specification is used as a blueprint to drive the actual building process.

There are many different methodologies for designing information systems, their popularity changing with time. DeMarco's (1982) influential approach to the software engineering process is a classic example. In this, final section, rather than exploring the technical details of any specific design method, the design process will be looked at from first principles. Whether the goal of an information system is to manage the operation of a nursing unit, reduce infection rates, or conduct research into basic medical science, the principles determining the successful design of its management cycle should be the same.

The first section of this book examined the general process of creating a model of the world, and of designing artefacts based upon that model. The specific interaction of information systems with the world was characterised through the model, measure and manage cycle, containing the following steps.

- defining a set of management goals,
- constructing a model of the system,
- gathering measurement data from a system,
- interpreting the meaning of the measurements,
- taking actions based upon the interpretation.

For each step, we will now look at the principle issues that affect the design process.

Designing a goal

Goals are the outcomes that a management system tries to achieve. If we are trying to control a patient's cardiovascular system, for example, our goal might be to obtain a blood pressure in the normal range. If we are managing a hospital unit, the goal might be to treat a certain number of patients over a year within a given budget, and with a specified clinical outcome.

Having worked through the first chapters, the prerequisites for a goal to be achievable should come as no surprise.

- The goal should be measurable. If it is not, then there is no way of knowing when it has been achieved. Consider the difference between the goals 'I want to be successful' and 'I want to be a qualified neurosurgeon by the age of 35'.

- The measurements should be interpretable. We should have a model of the system we are trying to influence, and should be able to determine the meaning of the measurements we take in relation to our goal. Thus, for example, we should be able to say whether an action has resulted in a move towards or away from a goal.
- The interpretations should be manageable. We should know what actions to take given a specific interpretation, or at least have a way of finding out what actions to take.

Feedback control systems are a very special kind of information management system. Here the goal is called an equilibrium state (Klir and Valach, 1967). If the system being controlled is deflected from that equilibrium state, then a controller takes actions to try and reach a new equilibrium state. For example, an IV pump containing drugs that alter blood pressure could be coupled to a blood pressure measurement system. Based upon deviations in the blood pressure from some defined value, the IV pump would change the dosing rate of the medications, always attempting to keep the patient's pressure within some target range.

Designing the model

We already know that for a management goal to be achievable, a model must exist to allow any measurements to be interpretable. For a model to actually fulfil this requirement, there are several things that need to be in place.

- The model must be sufficiently accurate. Irrespective of how well we understand any given system, our knowledge of it and the environment within which it exists will never be complete. This means that any management system operating in the real world will never be able to completely guarantee an outcome. As our models of the systems we wish to control improve, so too do our chances of success in managing them. Inevitably, there will always be unforeseen problems that are not included in our models, and for which we will not have developed a plan of management.
- A model must be sufficiently detailed for the task at hand. The more closely that model approximates the system in question, the more fine-grained will be our prediction of its response to actions

performed upon it. However, it is not always the case that one should use the most detailed model available. Creating and using models consumes resources (Coiera, 1992b). Time, for example, may be limited. If a model is too detailed then it may take too long to work out what is going on, and consequently urgently needed control measures will be delayed. In this case, simple 'rules of thumb' may be sufficient to control a system within a roughly acceptable range. This is often the philosophy taken, for example, in the immediate management of critically ill patients. Rapid assessment and management by simple principles are followed later by a more painstaking assessment, once a patient has been stabilised. Then, when there is more time available, the patient's status can be assessed according to more complex models and the management can be fine-tuned.

- The model must be timely. As we saw in the first part of the chapter, systems in the real world change. Consequently, what has been a good model may over time become less useful - as the system has changed, the model has remained static. It is thus a good rule of thumb that over time a model becomes increasingly inaccurate - models decay (Hogarth, 1986). The consequences for system control are significant. The system seems to become increasingly unmanageable using the old model. Control actions that once worked are no longer as effective as they once were.

- The model must be the right one. A model of the pathophysiology of pneumonia and its treatment will not help to treat cardiogenic heart failure. In effect, a model is a hypothesis about how a system operates, and if the hypothesis is wrong, then it is unlikely that the system can be well managed. If, for example, the treatment goal is incorrect, then so too will be the specific knowledge that is brought to bear in achieving the goal.

Designing the measurements

Measurements provide the data with which we drive our inferences, and represent samples we take from the system we want to control. For example, we examine a patient to obtain physical measurements. These will then be mapped, through a diagnostic process, onto a disease state. In more general terms, we want to map measurement data onto a state description of the system being managed.

For a measurement system to produce data that will be useful to the interpretation process, the following conditions should exist.

- The measurements chosen must accurately reflect the system being observed. Is a patient's core temperature most accurately measured by their axillary temperature or their sublingual temperature? Clearly, the choice of measurement is influenced by the management goals. There is little value, for example, in making a highly expensive and very accurate measurement when a more approximate and cheaper one will do. Further, it is not just the case that some measurements are more accurate versions of others, but some measures may not correspond closely to the elements that are being modelled. Do the number of sick days taken by staff in a nursing unit measure the incidence of illness among the staff population, or do they measure staff morale? When multiple factors affect the value of a measurement, like total number of sick days, then interpreting the measurement becomes more problematic. Before the interpretation has taken place, we would have to be sure that all the confounding factors affecting its value have been taken into account

- Next, the values of measurements must themselves be accurate. Errors in the determination of the value of a measurement can translate into errors in the management of the system. Errors can occur in several places. They might arise from within the measurement system itself. For example, a thermometer may not be reading correctly, or a CVP transducer might not be placed at the right height. Secondly the error might arise from the way the measurement system is applied. For example, an incorrect reading of arterial oxygen saturation might be given because of poor positioning of a finger probe.

- If we are measuring a process over time, then we need to measure it frequently enough not to miss any important events. For example, if we are trying to measure the number of days a bed is occupied, then we need to visit the bed with a rate that is more frequent than it is possible to discharge patients. If it is possible for a unit to have two short stay patients occupy the one bed during a day, then visiting it once per day will miss periods in which the bed is either occupied or unoccupied. In signal processing terms, this problem of missing events because of measurement undersampling is called **aliasing**.

Designing the interpretation

It usually the case that it is hard to separate the details about the reasoning process used to manage a system from the details of the model being used. Knowledge and inference are inextricably interdependent.

We have already seen that a model should only be as detailed as necessary for the task at hand. There is no point in using a very detailed model when the details of the results do not matter. Similarly, an interpretation should be as simple as possible given the task at hand. Carrying out complex calculations and deriving an answer to several decimal places of precision is inappropriate if the possible control actions do not have such fine precision.

There are several basic forms of reasoning that are possible with a model. One can try to draw a conclusion about the world based upon a measurement of the world. One can try to draw a conclusion about whether the current model is the right one to be using. Finally, one can try to alter the model as new things are learnt about the world. These three types of reasoning correspond to the three-loop model of information use. We shall return to examine these very important reasoning processes in greater detail in Chapters 19 and 20.

Designing the management actions

Management actions should be chosen to maximally effect the system being controlled, and to minimally affect other systems. In the same way that a measurement may not always accurately reflect the system being modelled, some actions may more directly affect the component of the system being controlled than others. Drugs for example, are favoured if they treat a condition without side-effects. Some drugs have an effect closer to the causative mechanism of disease, while others are more indirect, treating downstream consequences of a primary cause. For example, in the case of gastric ulceration, the H2 antagonist class of drugs reduce gastric acidity. However, the control action that is most direct in controlling the disease process is the elimination of the infection with *H. Pylori* that probably triggered the increase in gastric acidity in the first place.

Chapter summary

1. Technology can be applied to a problem in a **technology** or a **problem** driven manner. Information systems should be created in a problem driven way, starting with an understanding of user information problems. Only then is it appropriate to identify if and how technology should be used.
2. There are many methods available to capture user needs, and they can be grouped into four categories: anecdotal or individual experience, asking clinicians, non-participatory observation and formal experiments.
3. While formal experiments will only answer narrow questions and are relatively expensive to conduct, qualitative research methods relying on non-participatory methods are formal enough to allow robust statements to be made. They also have the advantage of being grounded in the realities of the clinical workplace.
4. An information system is susceptible to the effects of change over time at several levels: the user needs that define the role of the system, the model of user needs and system design, the technology used to construct the system, and organisational resources, including finance and staff availability. A change in any one of these will effect the performance of the system as a whole. Aiming for modularity in design will help minimise these effects.
5. Many specific methodologies are available for designing information systems. In general, they are all focused on defining the different elements of the **model, measure, manage cycle,** i.e. defining a set of management goals, constructing a model of the system, defining measurement data for a system, interpreting the meaning of the measurements, and defining appropriate actions based upon the interpretation.

Part Three

Protocol-based Systems

But printed flow charts should not be regarded as a problem-solving panacea! They ... serve as recipes for a mindless cook. They are difficult to write, rigid, may inhibit independent thinking, and are often so intricate as to require a road map and a compass. Perhaps their greatest use lies in teaching. The good physician generates his own flow chart every time he sees a patient and solves a problem. He should not need to follow printed pathways.

(Cutler, 1979, p53)

Shortly thereafter, I had the last of the 'insights' to be recorded here: a clinician performs an experiment every time he treats a patient. The experiment has purposes different from those of laboratory work, but the sequence, and intellectual construction are the same: a plan, an execution, and an appraisal. Yet ... Honest, dedicated clinicians today disagree on the treatment for almost every disease from the common cold to metastatic cancer. Our experiments in treatment were acceptable by the standards of the community, but were not reproducible by the standards of science. Clinical judgement was our method for designing and evaluating those experiments, but the method was unreproducible because we had been taught to call it 'art'...

(Feinstein, 1967, p14)

Chapter 7

Protocol-based decision support and evidence-based medicine

For those who regard modern medicine as a rational and scientific endeavour, the contention that the efficacy of much medical practice is still not validated may come as a shock. The problem medicine faces is not that it lacks the will or the tools to evaluate treatments. The problem lies in part with the mechanisms that exist for transferring evidence into clinical practice, which are unable to keep up with the ever growing mountain of clinical trial data (Roper et al., 1988; Wyatt, 1991).

For example, the first trial to show that streptokinase was useful in the treatment of myocardial infarction was published in 1958. Convincing evidence mounted in the early seventies, and the first multi-trial meta-analysis proving its value was published in the early eighties. However, formal advice that streptokinase was useful in the routine treatment of myocardial infarction only appeared in the late eighties (Antman et al. 1992). This was a full thirteen years after a close examination of the published literature would have indicated the treatment's value (Heathfield and Wyatt, 1993).

There are many other examples of similar delays in transferring research findings into routine clinical practice. The use of low dose anticoagulants in hip surgery, or inhaled steroids in the treatment of asthma both could have become routine treatments much earlier than they did. If research into the management of such common and important conditions is so affected, it is unlikely that less frequent conditions fare any better. There is thus a bottleneck between the publication of clinical trial data, and its conversion into clinical practice.

Just as there are barriers to research moving into clinical practice, there are barriers that prevent practitioners accessing research findings. With well over a thousand journals publishing each week, practitioners with a particular clinical problem can struggle to find the best advice from the mountains of often contradictory research literature.

Finally, the loop that connects the clinical outcome of a treatment to future applications of the same treatment is weak. The rigours of the clinical trial fit ill with the demands of routine care. Not only is the necessary data for such analysis rarely collected in clinical practice, it is not likely to be in a state that permits statistical analysis.

These pressures have renewed the interest of many in the use of clinical protocols to guide practice. The hope is that if best-practice guidance can be distilled rapidly from the literature, then it should be convertible into a set of protocols that can be made readily and widely available to practising clinicians. The phrase **evidence-based medicine** (EBM) is now used to describe this movement (EBMWG, 1992; Mulrow, 1994).

There are still many growing pains within EBM. Some are cultural, as a proportion of medical practitioners argue against such apparent imposition of controls on practice. Others are technical. Statistical meta-analysis for example, is still an unsure tool. For each notable success, such as with the studies of thrombolytics for myocardial infraction, there are also failures. For example, meta-analysis predicted that intravenous magnesium would reduce the risk of acute myocardial infraction, but a subsequent large scale randomised trial failed to find any such benefit (Sim and Hlatky, 1996).

Prior to the current interest in protocols, they had fallen into relative disrepute for a variety of cultural and technical reasons which we shall return to in later sections. Many of these technical objections can now be circumvented through the application of information technologies. Further, the motivation to establish a more evidence-based practice is believed by many to be sufficiently strong to overcome the cultural objections. With such changes, it seems reasonable to attempt to reintroduce protocol-guided care into routine practice.

Their manner of introduction, and their ultimate role, must be informed by an understanding of the strengths and limitations of protocols as an informatics instrument. In this chapter, the discussion of protocols in medicine will begin with a basic introduction to protocols and their uses. The next chapter will take a look at the issues affecting the design of protocols and the selection of appropriate situations for their use. In the third and last chapter of this discussion on protocols, the role that information and communication technology can play in protocol-based medicine will be explored.

7.1 Protocols

A protocol is a set of instructions. These instructions might describe the procedure to be followed when investigating a particular set of findings in a patient, or the method to be followed in the management of a given disease (Figure 7.1). Clinical protocols are variously called **clinical guidelines, practice parameters** and **care pathways**.

In computer science, a set of instructions to programmatically carry out some task is called an algorithm.

More generally, the notion of protocol permeates most human organisational structures. We talk about following the 'correct' social protocol when meeting a visiting dignitary, or 'having to do things by the book' within an organisation. A protocol is thus usually understood to be advice on the 'best' way to carry out some task. It is the way something should always be done.

Alternatively, protocols may simply represent advice on good practice - what should be done in most circumstances. For example, a recipe is a protocol for cooking a particular dish. Following all of the steps in a recipe should guarantee that a reasonable meal will be produced. An experienced cook will know which steps are essential, and which can be varied.

Clinical uses for protocols

The fundamental value of a protocol is in ensuring tasks are carried out uniformly. It serves as a guide or reminder in situations in which it is likely that procedures will be forgotten, are not well known, are difficult to follow, or where errors can be expensive. Consequently, protocols have a wide variety of uses in healthcare.

Research. Protocols have long been an accepted and integral part of medical research. Whenever the efficacy of a treatment is being assessed, a standardised protocol is drawn up to guide the way that treatment is to be given over the clinical trial period. This maximises the likelihood that the same thing is being done to each patient, and that the data collected are representative of the effects of that particular treatment. It also provides a basis for comparison with other studies that might have adopted variations in the treatment protocol, and obtained different results.

Delegation of responsibility. There is a strong case to be made for comprehensively trained healthcare staff to delegate the care of minor or routine problems. Thus, patients are taught to look after themselves at home for a variety of conditions. Everything from insulin administration to ambulatory peritoneal dialysis can be carried out by patients if they have been given explicit protocols to follow, and instructions on when to follow these and when to seek further advice.

Demarcation of responsibility. A protocol can make clear which tasks are to be carried out by different members of a healthcare team. For example, the roles of a physician, nursing staff, and paramedics can all be defined within a protocol for managing a large scale disaster.

Education. A clinical protocol ensures that, even if there is a variation in ability or training, that a certain minimum standard is adhered to in the delivery of care. Thus, when the general public is trained in the 'ABC' of resuscitation, they are given a simple recipe to follow.

Safety-critical or complex situations. In situations in which errors are likely to have significant consequences, clear guidelines are adhered to, even by highly trained individuals. Thus most clinicians will be able to describe step by step the procedures they would carry out in the management of a cardiac arrest. Equally, airline pilots have pre-takeoff checklists that need to be completed to ensure the aircraft is flight-worthy. Operators of nuclear power plants have defined procedures for every aspect of controlling their plant.

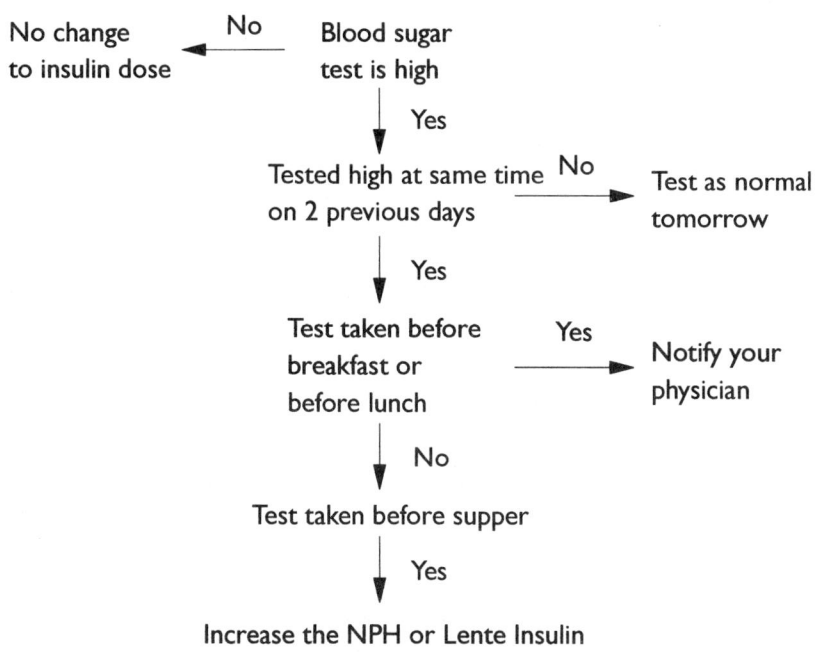

Figure 7.1: In this sample protocol, a guideline is presented for an insulin dependent diabetic's self management of their intermediate-acting insulin regime. Such a flowchart representation of a protocol makes all the choice points and the flow of decision making graphically explicit, but is space consuming, and for trained individuals may be too rigid.

Similarly, when complex machinery is used in clinical situations like the delivery of anaesthesia, then checklists may be valuable.

Uncommon conditions. Protocols are also important when they deal with rare conditions, and it is unlikely that the individuals managing a situation have encountered it before.

Evidence-based clinical practice. Where there is irregularity in the methods applied in the treatment of a condition, then adopting a protocol that represents agreed best practice can help in ensuring uniform standards of care. It can, as a consequence, enhance the likelihood that clinical outcomes will also be uniform. This potential benefit, as discussed earlier, may prove to be one of the major driving forces for the widespread adoption of protocols.

7.2   The protocol life-cycle

In his classic work on clinical judgement, Feinstein suggested that there should be as much rigour applied to the way patients are

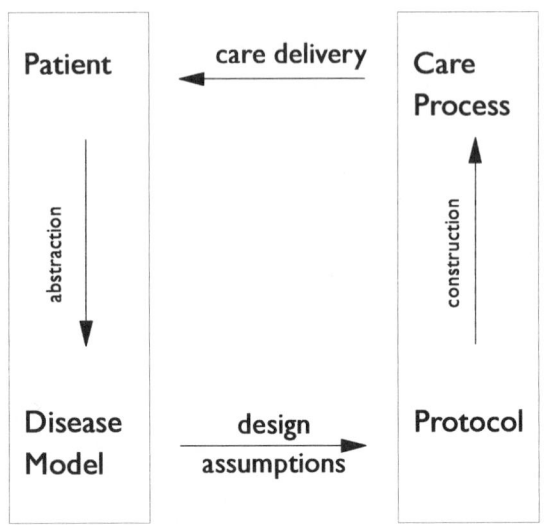

Figure 7.2: *Protocols are designed based upon a set of assumptions both about the nature of the disease that is to be treated, as well as the context within which the protocol will be used. This context of the care process defines who will be delivering care, their available resources, and the local expectations of the goal of care.*

routinely treated as is applied in medical research (1967). The management of every patient could be considered, at an abstract level, as constituting a scientific experiment. Consequently, the results of that experiment could contribute to the advancement of knowledge.

With the advent of evidence-based practice, we are drawing closer to realising that vision. If it is possible to treat most patients using protocols, then it should also possible to close the loop, and use the knowledge gained from each patient's treatment. In effect, every patient treated according to a protocol can be part of a clinical trial.

We are a long way from realising that vision at present, but at its most abstract, the overall form of the system is relatively clear. Recall from Chapter 1 that in modelling the world, the processes of abstraction, definition of design assumptions, and construction all influence the final design of an object. When a protocol is designed, it should be shaped both by an understanding of the best treatments, as well as by the circumstances in which it will be used. Thus the first step in arriving at such a process is to develop a model of the disease process. Then, based upon an understanding of the context in which the protocol will be used, for example about the level of resource or training of staff, a set of assumptions are made. As we will see in the next chapter, these assumptions have a strong

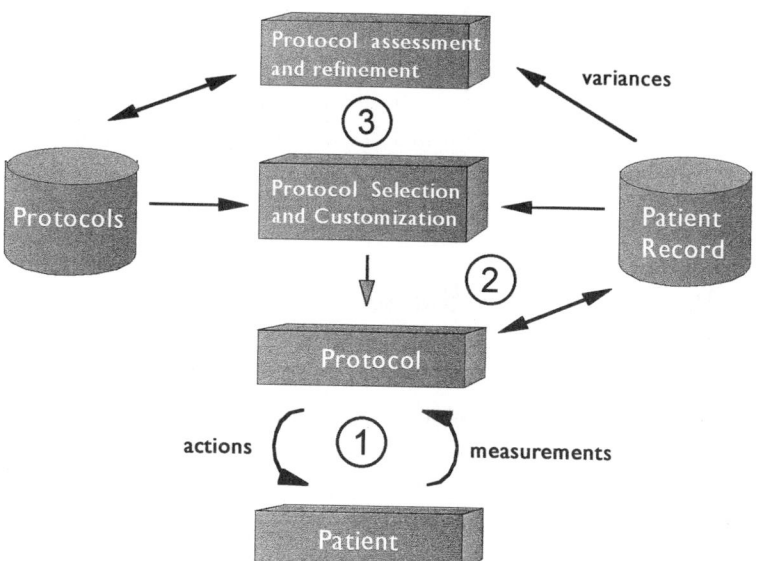

Figure 7.3: The three-loop model describes the way in which protocols can be used to manage individual patients in a uniform way, and use the results of treatment to grow medical knowledge.

influence on the form and content of a protocol's design. The last step is the construction of a care process around the protocol.

Because this is nothing other than the model-measure-manage cycle, the results of protocol application feed into subsequent revisions of the protocol. The overall process of protocol design, creation and application is summarised in Figure 7.2.

The wider use of protocols can be understood through the three-loop model developed in Chapter 4 (Figure 7.3). The information loops are formed around the selection and application of protocols, and the analysis of the protocol's effectiveness.

To commence treatment, a protocol is selected in loop 2, based on a patient satisfying some entry criteria. For example, before being admitted onto a thrombolytic protocol, a patient with chest pain may need to have presented within a number of hours, and have ECG evidence of a recent myocardial infarction (e.g. French et al., 1996).

Once selected, the protocol drives the treatment of that patient. With reasonably sophisticated protocols, there can be variations in treatment captured in the treatment logic. Consequently, based upon measurements of the patient's progress, the management in loop 1 can in principle vary according to the patient's state.

Finally, in loop 3, one assesses the outcome of treatment over a statistically significant population of patients. In formal clinical trials, the methodology will involve comparison of variances in outcome using the protocol group against a control group treated in a different manner. As a consequence, protocols are refined over time, as evidence suggests ways in which they can be improved.

7.3 Departures from the protocol help drive protocol refinement

A common criticism often voiced of protocols is that patient states are too variable to be amenable to such programmatic care. As we will see in the next chapter, attention to design can provide some latitude to accommodate individual variation. Sometimes, however, variations will occur that have not been anticipated in the protocol.

Such **variances** might be due to the patient, to specific treatment choices, or to external factors like resources available in the hospital. A patient, for example, may have an intercurrent illness that makes it difficult to carry out the care designed for a typical patient.

Equally, treatments may be given that are at variance with the planned protocol, for a variety of appropriate or inappropriate reasons. In any case, such treatment changes may change a patient's clinical state. Consequently, the likelihood that the patient is able to fit the expectations implicit in the protocol's design may diminish.

Finally, external factors like the hospital system itself may contribute to variances. For example, it may be that a particular investigation is scheduled to occur on a particular day of the admission. If the laboratory carrying out the investigation is overbooked, then the protocol has to be varied.

Rather than being problematic, identification of variances can become a central part of the way in which protocol-assisted care is given. Firstly, variances are signals to the care team to reassess whether it is appropriate for a patient to be maintained on a protocol, and may indicate that more individualised care is necessary.

Secondly, when variances from a number of patients are pooled, they act as checks on the way in which care is delivered. It may be that recurrent variances suggest that care delivery is sub-optimal, and that changes need to be made in the way staff or resources are allocated.

Finally, and perhaps most critically, variances offer an opportunity to assess the appropriateness of the protocol over time. In this case, variances provide a measurement of the effectiveness of a protocol, and consequently can feed a process of continuing protocol refinement in loop 3.

Chapter summary

1. The mechanisms that exist for transferring research evidence into clinical practice are unable to keep up with the ever growing mountain of clinical trial data, resulting in delays in the transfer of research into practice.
2. Evidence-based medicine is an attempt to distil best-practice guidance from the literature into a set of protocols that can be made readily and widely available to practising clinicians.
3. A protocol is a set of instructions. These instructions might describe the procedure to be followed to investigate a particular set of findings in a patient, or the method to be followed in the management of a given disease.
4. A protocol can ensure that tasks are carried out uniformly. It can serve as a guide or reminder in situations in which it is likely that procedures will be forgotten, are not well known, are difficult to follow, or where errors can be expensive, for example in the face of rare conditions, safety-critical or complex situations, in clinical research, education, and in task delegation.
5. The creation and application of protocols can be characterised as a model-measure-manage cycle, and their overall use in healthcare can be captured within the three loop model.
6. Variations to treatment that have not been anticipated in the protocol are termed **variances**, which can signal the care team to reassess whether it is appropriate for a patient to be maintained on a protocol. When variances from a number of patients are pooled, they can act as checks on the way in which care is delivered.

Chapter 8

Designing and applying protocols

Protocols represent a powerful method for improving the quality of decisions when two main conditions are satisfied. Firstly, it must actually be feasible to prescribe a course of action ahead of time. If the situation in question is novel, constantly changing or in some other way non-deterministic, then it is hard to see how an explicit recipe for action can be predetermined.

Secondly, irrespective of how easy it might be to create a protocol, the conditions at the time of decision making must make it possible to access and apply the protocol. It may simply be that a protocol cannot be easily used in some types of situation. In others, it may be that the effort involved in applying the protocol may be too great.

Failure to meet either of these conditions of **protocol designability**, or **protocol usability** will cause difficulties for the introduction of a protocol. Understanding when they are satisfiable should increase the likelihood that the use of protocols will be successful.

A third broad area of difficulty lies within the culture of medical practice. The introduction of a more regimented approach to care delivery is seen by some, rightly or wrongly, as an intrusion on their clinical freedom to practise medicine in the manner they personally consider most suitable.

In this chapter, each of these three areas of protocol design, application, and cultural clash will be examined in more detail. Firstly, some common forms of protocol representation will be introduced, and the importance of designing a protocol for the context of use explained. Next, the need to ensure usability by incorporating protocol guidance into the heart of the care process will be outlined. With both of these topics, inherent difficulties in the use of protocols will be highlighted. This will act as a prelude to the next chapter in this section, in which the role of information and communication technology in supporting protocol-based care will be examined.

8.1   The structure of protocols

There are a variety of different ways to represent a protocol. Indeed, protocols can vary both in form of their structure and their content, depending upon the context within which they will be used. Variations in the training of those using it, for example, will require protocols to behave in quite different ways. Content will also vary in its level of detail, and number of options available.

Entry criteria define a protocol's context of use

Irrespective of its form, each protocol begins with an **entry criterion** that defines the context within which the protocol is designed to be used. For example, 'patient presents with acute retrosternal chest pain' might be one of the criteria that allow a patient to be entered onto a protocol for the investigation and management of suspected myocardial infarction. If the entry criteria for a protocol are insufficiently precise, then the protocol might be used in inappropriate circumstances.

It is sometimes argued that protocols are of little value in their own right because the decision to use the protocol requires medical expertise. Consequently the argument continues, protocols are of marginal value in permitting non-medical staff to manage significant conditions. It can be argued in those circumstances, that it is more likely that insufficient thought has been put into the design of the protocol's entry criteria. Equally, protocols are valuable precisely in those circumstances in which it is possible to be explicit. If such clarity is not possible, then it is unlikely that the problem is one that is amenable to protocol-directed management.

Protocol form is determined by function

Flowcharts are probably the simplest way to represent a protocol, because they are graphical in nature, and make decision points and the flow of logic explicit (Figure 7.1). Flowcharts can be built up in great detail, especially in areas in which there is a high procedural content to the work, for example in anaesthesia (e.g. Bready and Smith, 1987).

A flowchart begins with an entry criterion, for example 'you are a self-managing insulin dependent diabetic on intermediate acting insulin, and your urine has tested high for blood sugar'. Choice points in the logic are made explicit. Depending upon responses to questions, often with simple 'yes' or 'no' answers, the protocol user is guided through a decision making process. Actions are usually arrived at on the 'leaf' nodes of the decision tree.

Protocols can also be expressed more compactly as a simple set of rules (Table 8.1). If the rule's precondition is satisfied, then the action in the rule should be carried out. Since rules are more compact, they usually require a little more effort to understand than the same information expressed in a flowchart.

If tests are poor 3 Days in a Row	Do this
BEFORE SUPPER	Increase the NPH or Lente Insulin by 2 units on the 4th morning
BEFORE BREAKFAST, but good before supper	Notify your physician. You may need an evening dose of insulin
BEFORE LUNCH, but better before supper	Notify your physician. You many need a mixed dose (NPH or Lente + Regular) in the morning

Table 8.1: The same patient guideline presented in Figure 7.1, this time expressed as a set of rules, (adapted from Krall and Beaser, 1989).

Chunking protocols helps manage complexity

As can be seen from the small examples above, protocols for even relatively simple tasks can begin to be complicated. Consequently, capturing the decision making required to manage a long sequence of

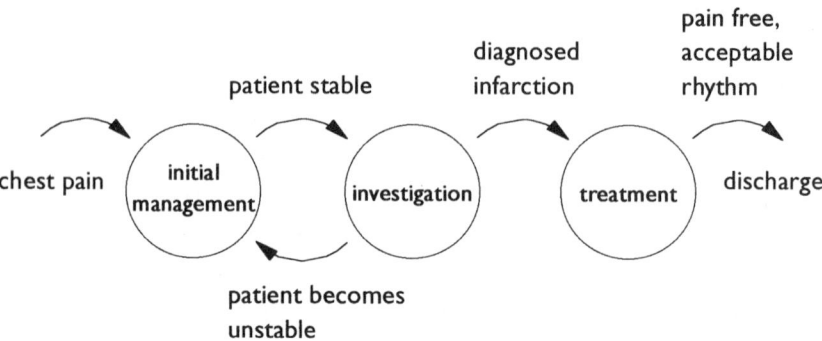

Figure 8.1: Complex protocols can be broken down into chunks corresponding to different states in a process, or in the progression of a patient's condition. Each state within the protocol is entered or exited when a set of conditions is met. Movement back and forth between states can be permitted if necessary.

tasks can result in very complex protocol structures that may be very difficult to use.

One way to manage this complexity is to break the protocol down into a sequence of smaller chunks, each corresponding to a specific task. Each chunk has entry and exit criteria, allowing one to move from one task to the next. In this way, one is not limited to building protocols that are a simple sequence of tasks, but one can create quite complex pathways.

The simplest way to think about such chunks are as **state machines**. Each task grouping corresponds to a particular state of the process of the patient. For example, the states in the management of chest pain might be broken down into initial assessment and management, investigation, and treatment (Figure 8.1). As we saw in Chapter 6, another advantage of breaking a system design down into chunks or functional modules is that it minimises the effects of design change. Thus, in a well-designed protocol, it should thus be relatively easy to change some detail in a particular protocol segment, usually without affecting other segments.

8.2   Care pathways

The process of breaking down treatment into a set of stages or states, each with their own entry and exit criteria is the basis of care pathways. These protocols are at present especially of interest in nursing, where they are often used to support patient care (e.g. Hydo, 1995).

Patient Problem	Day I	Day 2
myocardial ischaemia	Patient at risk of infarct extension I_x: serial ECG cardiac enzymes R_x: thrombolytics	Patient should be pain free
cardiac rhythm	Patient at risk of arrhythmia I_x: continuous ECG monitoring	Patient should have stable cardiac rhythm
cardiac output	I_x: risk of cardiac failure R_x: regular ABP	
fluid balance		Patient at risk of fluid overload I_x: Check volume status

Table 8.2:
Fragment from a sample care pathway for the management of a myocardial infarction. Paths are plotted for each expected problem and plotted out over the expected length of stay. Expected outcomes are plotted across the time course. Special difficulties associated with each problem are recorded in the days they are most likely to occur, along with investigations or treatments that need to be scheduled for that day. (I_x - Investigation, R_x - Treatment).

In a care pathway, a patient's care may be broken down into a sequence of days, corresponding the ideal length of stay in hospital for that condition (Table 8.2). Each day has a set of instructions describing the typical care that should be given to a patient. Each day also has a set of expectations that describe the anticipated clinical state of the patient on that day. For example, 2 days after admission with a myocardial infarction, the pathway might state that a patient should be able to take a short walk. Failure to satisfy these criteria may prevent a patient progressing along the pathway until the conditions are met.

In this way, there is some allowance for individualisation of care depending on a patient's rate of recovery, as well as a check to prevent inappropriate treatment being given. Consequently, the protocol begins to be based on the clinical outcome of intermediate steps in a patient's care. This emphasises the potential for protocols to assist in the process of improving or sustaining quality of care.

Care pathways can have quite complex structures, depending on the nature of the condition being managed. Part of the chunking strategy that can be adopted is to identify individual problems associated with a condition, and chart the management of each problem over the period of the patient's stay. For each problem, one can then identify which tasks occur on which days, and what the outcome of those tasks should be. In the previous example of myocardial infarction, problems might correspond to the patient's cardiac rhythm status, cardiac output, fluid and electrolyte balance, coagulation status and so forth.

8.3 The design of protocols

Perhaps the most common criticism of protocols is that it they are inflexible or rigid, and that individual patients do not always neatly fit the guidance recorded in a protocol. The cause of this apparent rigidity can often be attributed to poor design.

In the last section, several forms of protocol representation were introduced, and the situations in which one could be favoured over another outlined. We can go further now, and state more general principles about design. In particular, the design of a protocol should reflect two things. Firstly, it should prescribe care according to the best evidence available from clinical research and practice. Secondly, it should be crafted to reflect the context within which the protocol will be used. These contextual factors include the following.

The patient. Patients are rarely so accommodating as to present a typical pattern of disease. Medicine would be a simpler and more precise science if that was the case. In reality, patients present at different stages of an illness, with different underlying abilities to recover. They also may have a variety of different concurrent illnesses. These other illnesses may mask the appearance of symptoms and signs.

In such unclear circumstances, it is difficult to launch along a specific course of treatment. Even if it is clear which illnesses are present, the normal protocol for management of an individual illness may have to be changed because it will have adverse consequences for a particular patient. The potential for drug side-effects and interactions are good examples of risks that cause treatment to be varied in individual circumstances. As a consequence, it is often important for a number of treatment options to be included in a protocol. The selection of particular options can then be made to reflect the individual circumstances of a patient.

Treatment goals. The goal of care for the same problem varies with the clinical situation. For example, in disaster situations, triage will be used to ascertain which patients receive immediate treatment, and which are unlikely to survive and therefore should be left untreated. The very same untreated patients may, in the context of a teaching hospital, receive complex and highly intensive therapy. Thus, the immediate circumstances of a situation dictate the goals of treatment. There is thus no absolute 'best' treatment. Notions of best treatment are always constrained by local goals.

Local resources. Local goals are also constrained by the resources available for treatment. Delivery of care in a relatively poor nation will reflect the resources available to it. Thus, there is little point in specifying protocols that cannot be carried out, either because equipment, medications, time, staff, money, or other resources are unavailable. The management of diarrhoea, for example, will vary not just to reflect local disease patterns, but the scale of the problem and the availability of medication. A child returning home to a developed nation with possibly infectious diarrhoea will receive very different treatment to a child caught up in large scale epidemic in an underdeveloped nation. The disease is the same, but the circumstances in which treatment occurs are not.

Staff. The skill level of the individuals required to carry out the protocol also affects the form and content of protocols. This affects everything from the words used in the protocol, which would vary for protocols designed for patients or members of the public, to the level of detail and goals of the protocol. In particular, the ability of an individual to recognise that the entry criteria for a protocol have been fulfilled is essential. There is little point in having a set of finely crafted protocols if it is unclear when they should be applied.

Local processes. Local care processes evolve to reflect not just best practice knowledge, but local resources and goals. A protocol has to be designed with an understanding of how it will be used within such existing processes. Will it simply be looked at as a reference after an initial care plan has been drafted, or will it be used to drive every detail of a care process? In each situation, the requirements for clarity, level of detail, and availability are vastly different. In the former, protocols might be collected together into a small reference manual. In the latter, they might need to be crafted into the basic documentation used to plan and record the delivery of care.

8.4 Protocol design principles

We can now begin to formulate a set of 'good design' principles for protocols, based upon an understanding of the need to acknowledge the context of use.

Principle 1 - Make any assumptions about the context of use explicit.

We saw in the previous chapter that assumptions about the context of use made by a protocol's designer determine its utility in other contexts (Figure 7.2). The clearer one can be about the context within which a protocol is intended to be applied, the clearer it will be to others in slightly different circumstances whether that protocol can be reused. Some of the assumptions about the context of protocol use are summarised in Figure 8.2.

Principle 2 - A protocol should not be more specific than is necessary to achieve a specific goal.

The more closely a protocol matches a specific set of local conditions, the less likely it is to be useful in others. Thus, one needs to determine how many of these local conditions really need to be considered. This will affect how widely the protocol can be applied. As a consequence, protocols intended for widespread general use may need to ignore specific local details.

This is an example of a general principle - the more specifically a method models a given situation, the more useful it will be in that situation, and the less useful it will be to others. The converse principle is that very general methods can be applied across many different situations, but will only have moderate utility in any one of them.

Protocol designers should thus be aware of the reason that a protocol is being introduced. For example, in the clinical trial of a new medication, the specification of the treatment protocol needs to be very detailed to maximise the statistical validity of the study. Such a level of detail may be entirely inappropriate in other circumstances. For example, if the role of protocol is to ensure that a few specific

- What is the goal of the protocol?
- What are the protocol entry and exit criteria, and how will these be determined at the time?
- Who will decide protocol entry, and who will apply the protocol?
- What terminology will be understood by those using the protocol?
- How much time will be available to follow the protocol?
- What treatment resources are available, including medication and biomedical devices?
- Are multiple treatment options to be considered?
- How much detail should be included?
- Which representation is most appropriate (e.g. flow chart, decision tree, rules)?
- Will users wish to, or be able to, access the evidence used in creating the protocol?
- How is the protocol to be used in the care process? For example, how is it to be accessed?
- How is the protocol's performance to be reviewed, and how are variances to be recorded?
- What mechanisms will be available to update the protocol?
- How long should a protocol be in use before it is considered to be out-of-date?

Figure 8.2: A summary list of questions that help identify key assumptions about the context within which a protocol is be used. Once these design assumptions have been clarified, the process of protocol construction can begin.

actions are taken, there is probably no justification for including greater detail. This then is an issue of identifying the appropriate level of detail for the task in hand. Formalisation for its own sake does not necessarily deliver any greater return, and may require unnecessary effort (Martin, 1995). It also may cause the disaffection of the staff who are required to use the protocol.

One method for managing the difficulties of overspecifying detail is to initially specify a protocol only in general terms. The specifics of individual steps are left to be decided based upon the details of individual clinical cases. For example, one might specify a treatment goal rather than a specific action. Thus 'establish normal blood pressure through intravenous fluid replacement' might be an appropriate goal for a protocol, rather than specifying exactly how much fluid is to be given. The actual amount of fluid given would be dependent on the specific needs of a patient. This technique is known as skeletal plan refinement (Tu et al., 1989), and can be used to create quite sophisticated protocols that are highly flexible to individual patient needs.

Principle 3 - Protocol design should reflect the skill level and circumstances of those using them.

The level of description used in a protocol should also match the abilities of those using it. Very simple steps will probably be best for use with relatively inexperienced individuals. For example, protocols for first-aid resuscitation taught to the public are kept very simple. Protocols for trained paramedical or medical staff in exactly the same circumstance may be much richer and more complex, despite the similarities in overall goal.

Further, different protocol representations make different demands on those who use them. Mnemonic representations like the 'ABC' of resuscitation have great value in stressful situations, but may not permit great detail to be recalled. Flowcharts require relatively little reasoning, and can be designed to make the decision logic extremely clear. Thus one might create a flowchart for situations in which the ability to understand the protocol is limited, such as an emergency situation, or when the user has had limited instruction. The flowchart representation can however become too complicated for complex decisions. In such cases, a rule-based representation is more likely to be used as a reminder for individuals who have less time pressure, or are better trained in the management of the situation.

Principle 4 - Protocols should be constantly reviewed.

As we saw in Chapter 6, human knowledge tends to decay with time as circumstances change. Part of the difficulty many people have with protocols is that they represent a snapshot in time of what some people consider the best way to carry out a task. Even assuming that there was universal agreement on that method, as time goes by, new ways will be developed that supersede the original protocol.

It is thus a mistake to consider a protocol as a piece of knowledge in isolation. The three-loop model conveys the manner in which protocols exist as part of an ongoing process of improvement. Protocols are simply the intermediaries in this overall process of treatment refinement based upon outcomes. Thus much of the rigidity that some see in the use of protocols lies not in the protocol itself, but in the failure to update protocols as knowledge evolves over time. Consequently one kind of protocol rigidity arises out of a failure to adapt over time. Introducing protocols, without introducing processes to review the outcome of protocol-based care, is a recipe for guaranteeing that protocols will be perceived to be increasingly inappropriate over time.

8.5 The application of protocols

In the previous section, it was shown how the design of a protocol was heavily influenced by the way it was intended to be used. Indeed, these two aspects of design and use cannot be separated. However, in addition to design, two other issues relating to usability need to be examined. Firstly, some consideration needs to be given to whether it is appropriate to use a protocol in the first place. In some situations, it may actually be counter-productive. The second question relates to the manner in which the protocol is used. How should the protocol be best integrated into process of care?

When should a protocol be used?

The decision tree metaphor captured in flow charts highlights the analytical aspects of decision making. It focuses on what information is needed to make choices between alternatives, based upon some assessment of outcomes. Where people tend to fail, for whatever reason, at this form of analysis, then protocol-based decision support could be helpful. We have already seen that examples of such situations include inexperience of the people making decisions, and complex safety-critical situations.

It is not always the case that protocols are the best way to improve a decision process. For example, Klein and Calderwood (1991) argue that formal decision models (of which protocols are one example), are unlikely to be helpful in the following circumstances.

- When clear goals cannot be isolated, and it is dangerous to make simplifying assumptions in order to isolate goals that would allow a model to be applied.

- When probabilities of outcomes, or the utility of individual decisions, cannot be analysed independently of the particular context in which they are made.
- When end states or outcomes cannot be clearly defined. Doing a 'good job' would be an ill-defined measure upon which to define an outcome.
- When the utilities of different decisions are not independent of one another.

It has thus been strongly argued that there are many situations in which the attempt to formalise decision models like protocols is not helpful and may indeed be harmful. Indeed, when decision making is studied 'in the field' rather than in the laboratory, a very different set of human decision problems is observed. Faced with complex problems, people may not evaluate more than one course of action at a time (Klein and Calderwood, 1991). Instead, once a situation has been recognised, individuals may just follow the first acceptable plan they consider.

This suggests that the main effort that goes into decision making is in recognising and classifying a situation, rather than exploring complex plans to manage the situation. This result is echoed in work on clinical decision making, in which the order in which data that was presented to clinicians had a significant effect upon their reasoning (Elstein et al., 1978). In an analysis of so-called 'fixed-order' problems under experimental conditions, the ability of physicians to generate hypotheses, and to associate data with hypotheses was significantly affected by the order in which data was presented. In other words, their ability to correctly assess the situation was influenced by the way data was encountered.

The implication of this work is that, if the goal is to improve decision making, then the focus should be on improving the ability of individuals to assess situations and not on formalising the decision. In other words, if we are able to help people recognise the nature of the problem they are facing, then they are more likely to be able to handle it.

For situations in which making a good decision is sufficient, then focusing on improving an individual's ability to assess and classify a situation may indeed be most appropriate. The circumstances in healthcare however, are more complex. It may indeed be the case that, given a particular health problem, individuals will usually be able to come up with a 'good' plan, once the problem has been understood. The challenge of evidence-based practice is to come up with the **best** plan, both to maximise the outcomes for populations, and to minimise the cost of those decisions. Improving performance by even a few percentage points over a large number of decisions thus has a large impact on the delivery of health care. The challenge, as should now be clear, is to permit the pool of medical knowledge to be applied in a way that reflects local circumstances.

In summary, the decision to design a protocol to manage a given situation should not be automatic. There are many situations in which protocol application is at the least difficult, and at worst meaningless. Equally, in some situations, if the goal is to improve **individual** decision making, then focusing on improving situational assessment may be more appropriate. When procedures can be identified, and there is a need to improve the analytical aspects of decisions, then protocols are a powerful tool in improving decision outcomes.

How should a protocol be used?

Once a decision has been made that the introduction of a protocol for a given situation is desirable, the next step is to resolve the way in which the protocol is to be used. Indeed, protocols can be used in a variety of ways, depending upon the situation. These approaches to use can be largely divided into **passive** and **active** protocol systems.

In the passive approach, protocols act as a source of information only, and are not intrinsically incorporated into the care process. This is the traditional way in which medical knowledge has been used during care. Thus protocols might only be consulted as a check, at the end of a decision-making process, or as a reference when an unusual situation is encountered. Healthcare workers might carry the protocols around with them as a set of ready-to-hand guidelines, or might have to consult information sources like a library, the Internet, or a telephone help-line to access them.

In contrast, the active use of protocols shapes the delivery of care around a protocol. The steps in a treatment are explicitly guided by protocol, requiring the protocol to be consulted at most steps during the care process. Active use of a protocol might suggest what patient information is to be to captured at different stages, what treatment is to given, or what tests are to be ordered.

In such cases, the patient record system might be crafted around the protocol. In a paper system, specific sheets for the protocol would be created, and data entered according to the sheet's format. A similar approach can be adopted using computer-based systems, albeit with greater potential for flexibility.

The introduction of passive systems is unlikely to cause significant difficulty, since they do not mandate treatment, but just add to the information resources available. One can consider this type of decision support to be **permissive**, in that it permits all courses of action, and only exists as a guide that is accessed as the need arises. In contrast, active systems have the potential to be **prescriptive**, since by definition they are there to actively constrain treatment actions in some way.

Unsurprisingly, the introduction of a new prescriptive process is organisationally difficult. There is an ongoing debate amongst those involved in process engineering over the merits of modifying a new process to reflect existing organisational needs, against the option of redesigning the existing organisational processes around the new one. It has traditionally been considered that it is best to try and modify new processes to suit existing ones - the new system should fit the users and not the reverse.

However, ongoing experience with the re-engineering of corporate information systems seems to suggest that it is ultimately more efficient to start from scratch. In this case, one uses the introduction of a new process as the opportunity to redesign and optimise existing systems. The more radical proponents of this approach suggest that 'users must change their ways in order to maximise profits from automation' (Martin, 1995).

As we shall see in the next section, such a prescription may be too puritanical, and ignore the realities of human nature. Compromises always need to be made to reflect the desires, abilities and concerns of those who have to work with new processes, no matter how desirable the changes may be from an organisational point of view.

8.6   Cultural barriers to the use of protocols

There is a great price placed upon clinical freedom and the 'art' of clinical decisions making in many medical communities. This is not a new tendency (e.g. Cutler, 1979) and it reacts in response to anything that is perceived to infringe upon that freedom. Despite the clear benefits that well-designed protocols can deliver in appropriate circumstances, many healthcare workers resist their introduction.

It seems an obvious statement that this would be reversed if individuals understood why the protocol is in use, and what benefit is expected. In some cases, however, this may be insufficient. It is common with the introduction of any new process that those who are asked to carry out the process may not be the ones who benefit from it. This may be true of treatment protocols, which may seem to bring more work and appear restrictive, despite the benefit of the protocol to others.

Sometimes it is thus necessary to ensure that those using the protocol also benefit directly in some way. For example, in some parts of the United States, if a healthcare worker delivers care according to a recognised guideline, then they will be immune from prosecution in a court of law. This acts as an incentive to the adoption of protocol-based care.

It is also of value to involve those who will ultimately use protocols into the task of protocol and care process design. We have seen from the protocol life-cycle how the use of individual protocols contributes to the wider process of protocol refinement. Allowing protocol users to be participants, for example in the process of variance recording, makes this greater process explicit to them. Thus, rather than simply handing protocols down on 'tablets of stone' and expecting staff to accept them, individuals can be encouraged to own the process of protocol application and renewal.

Chapter summary

1. Protocols are used when a course of action can be prescribed ahead of time and when it is possible to access and apply the protocol. Failure to meet these conditions of **protocol designability** and **protocol usability** will cause difficulties.
2. Each protocol begins with an **entry criterion** that defines the context within which the protocol is designed to be used.
3. Protocols can vary in the form of their structure and their content, depending upon the context of use. Flowcharts make choice points and the flow of decision making graphically explicit, but are space consuming. Rules are more compact, but require more effort and training to interpret. Contextual factors affecting design include the patient, treatment goals, local resources, staff skills, local processes and resources.
4. In a care pathway, a patient's care is broken down into a sequence of days, corresponding to the ideal length of stay in hospital.
5. Some design principle for protocols, based upon an understanding of the need to acknowledge the context of use, include:
    - Make assumptions about the context of use explicit.
    - Protocols should not be more specific than is necessary to achieve a specific goal.
    - Protocol design should reflect the skill level and circumstances of those using them.
    - Protocols should be constantly reviewed.
6. There are many situations in which the attempt to formalise decision models, like protocols, is not helpful and may indeed be harmful. These include situations in which clear goals or outcomes cannot be clearly defined.
7. Protocols systems can be **passive** or **active**. Passive protocols act as a source of information, and are not incorporated into the care process. Active protocols shape the delivery of care.
8. Healthcare workers may resist protocol introduction if they are perceived to restrict freedom, or introduce extra duties. If protocols are seen to benefit workers, they are more likely to be accommodating. Staff involvement in the process of protocol design maximises the likelihood that such benefits are identified.

Chapter 9

Computer-based protocol systems in healthcare

When early computer system designers sought to regularise clinical practice to suit the nature of their systems, this was seen as inappropriate by most healthcare workers. However, with the move to evidence-based medicine, it is now beginning to be acceptable to follow standard assessment and treatment protocols. Consequently, it now seems much more appropriate for clinicians to use information systems to assist them. Indeed, many see the development of protocol-based medicine as the essential cultural change in clinical practice that will permit the design of truly useful clinical information systems (Durinck et al., 1994).

The goal of a computer-based protocol system is to provide a set of tools that allow a clinician to access up-to-date guidelines, and then apply these in the management of patients (Renaud-Salis, 1994). In the previous two chapters, the nature and role of protocols were explored, and we saw how protocols can be used either as passive resources or to contribute actively in the process of care. A consequence of intertwining protocols with active care delivery is that protocols become integral to the design of the electronic patient record.

In this chapter, the role that communication and computer-based systems can play in the delivery of protocol-based care will be examined. The discussion will cover both passive and active clinical systems, and explore the potential for the Internet to contribute to them. Finally, the complex problems of protocol design and maintenance will be touched upon. Without such mechanisms to create protocols, there will ultimately be a bottleneck to the introduction of computer-based protocol systems.

9.1 Passive protocol systems

The Cochrane Collaboration is now perhaps one of the most influential organisations working in the area of evidence-based practice (Goodlee, 1994). It was formed with the intention of creating and distributing evidence-based summaries of best practice, and its first database of systematic reviews covered pregnancy and childbirth research. Yet, despite the relatively high profile of the group, there has been a considerable delay in the uptake of the obstetrics digests (Paterson-Brown et al., 1993; Paterson-Brown et al., 1995). Thus, while evidence-based medicine seeks to formally collate, assess and condense research findings, there still remains the problem of making the results easily available to practising clinicians.

Further, evidence suggests that, even when clinical protocols are available, clinicians forget to follow them, or deviate from them without clear cause (Renaud-Salis, 1994). Forgetting pre-planned management tasks seems to be especially likely in high stress clinical situations (Coiera et al., 1994).

However, it should be possible to make it easy for clinicians to access protocols during routine care, and make it less likely that steps will be inadvertently forgotten or altered. This is the basic goal of passive protocol systems.

With passive protocol systems, the protocols only exist as a source of information. They are not intrinsically incorporated into the process of care, or into any clinical information systems. While they might be accessed as reference material from within a clinical information system, the protocols are not reflected in other functions of the system used during care, such as the entry of patient data (Figure 9.1).

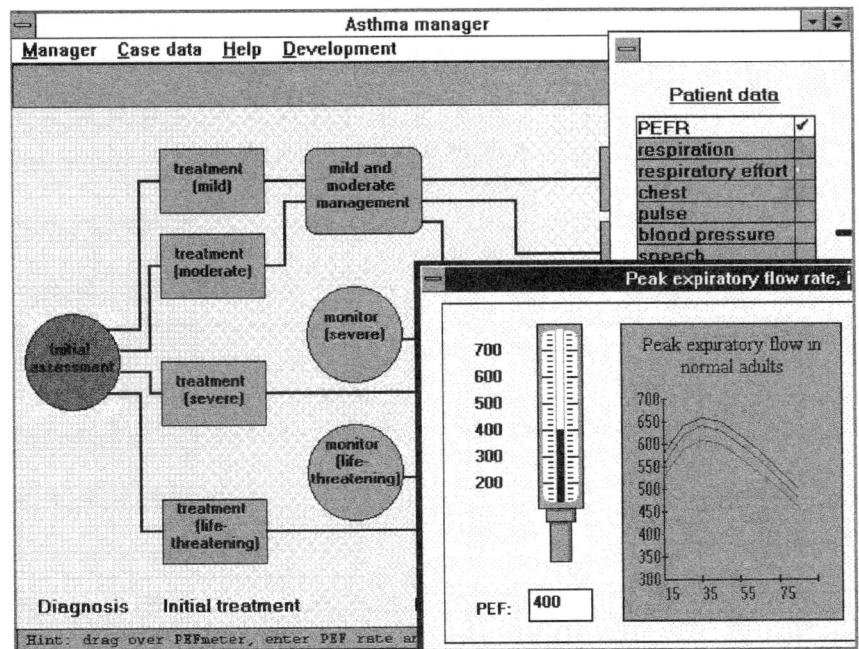

Figure 9.1: A user display from a computerised protocol system for managing adult acute asthma (Fox et al., 1996).

There is growing evidence that providing computer-assistance to improve access to clinical protocols does have a positive impact on adherence to guidelines.

- Lobach and Hammond (1994) reported on a computer system that generated a paper front sheet, outlining customised guidelines for the care of diabetic patients in outpatient setting. The study included 359 patients over 1265 encounters, and 58 providers were randomised to receive the computer-assisted management protocol. The study reported a statistical increase in compliance with guidelines in the computer-assisted group (15.6%) over the non-assisted group (2%).

- Vissers et al. (1996) explored the value of being able to access guidelines from a computer. In their study, resident staff in an emergency room had access to guidance on the management of fractures, which they could access during their initial assessment of a patient and formulation of treatment plan. In a randomised full-crossover trial comparing access to paper and computer versions of the protocols, several results were apparent. Firstly, the residents did not change their treatments significantly more often between the paper and computer-supported protocols.

However, those using the computer had a statistically higher chance that they would change their planned treatment **towards the protocol**. In other words, the computer system was more likely to cause treatment to move towards the protocol recommendations. Overall, there was a 19% better protocol adherence in the computer supported trial. Interestingly, this was despite the residents confidence in the correctness of their own treatment, and their doubts over the value of mandatory protocol consultation.

On the surface these results are encouraging. They seem to suggest that reminding health care workers of the protocol on a case by case basis improves protocol adherence, and that computer tools seem to improve upon paper-based reference materials.

Yet much still remains unclear. If individuals are not reminded to check a protocol for each case, will the advantages of the passive system remain, or will healthcare workers' performance tend towards that without protocols? More importantly, what is it about the way protocols are accessed on a computer that is so beneficial?

The conclusion that a 'computer' protocol is better than a 'paper' one is weak. The complexity of protocol design was underlined in the last chapter, where the multitude of design decisions that could adversely affect a protocol's performance were discussed. There are so many variables involved in making a computer easy to use, that it is conceivable that a well-designed paper system would outperform a poorly designed computer one.

Thus, the question that still remains unanswered is 'what is it about the design of a computer protocol system that results in a positive benefit over a paper system?'. For example, is the computer system faster, easier to access, easier to comprehend, more exciting? It should also be expected that the answers to such questions will vary with the task at hand. For example, in time-critical clinical situations, the speed of a computer system might be a distinct advantage, but in an outpatient setting, other design issues might be more significant.

The role of the Internet

We have so far examined how protocols might be made available in a clinical setting. As important as local access is the question of how those protocols reach the clinical workplace in the first place. How are protocols published and distributed by their authors, who may be geographically far removed from those that wish to use them?

Increasingly, many see the Internet as the vehicle of choice for the distribution of clinical practice guidelines (see Chapter 16). Creating World Wide Web sites on the Internet, as the Cochrane Collaboration has already done, allows anyone connected to the Web immediate access to the guidelines stored there. Placing guidelines on the Web is thus equivalent to immediate global publication on the Internet. The Internet publication model is just as valid if protocols are being created for local distribution across a campus' internal internet (or intranet), as it is if they are being accessed remotely across the global Internet.

As with all things, there are potential drawbacks to using the Internet for protocol distribution. Just as evidence-based medicine might reap enormous rewards from using the Internet, there are forces at play that could, in theory, have the opposite effect to the one intended. In particular, there are at present no formal controls on what can be published on the Internet, and indeed for many that is its great power. This means that while 'centres of excellence' like the Cochrane Collaboration will carefully vet any information they publish, others can publish any material they choose with complete disregard to these standards of care. Worse still, unlike academic journals where there is some sort of peer review process, there are no such checks for a would-be protocol author on the Internet. The Web is in its own way contributing to the confusing growth in medical literature.

Thus, while the Internet offers the technical mechanism for protocol publication and distribution, it does not enforce any particular process. Many now argue that the equivalent of journal peer review mechanisms needs to be established for material that is distributed across the Internet (LaPorte, 1995b).

9.2 Active protocol systems

In contrast to passive systems, which in some respects are simply an evolution of existing methods for providing reference material in the clinical workplace, active protocol systems offer the potential to

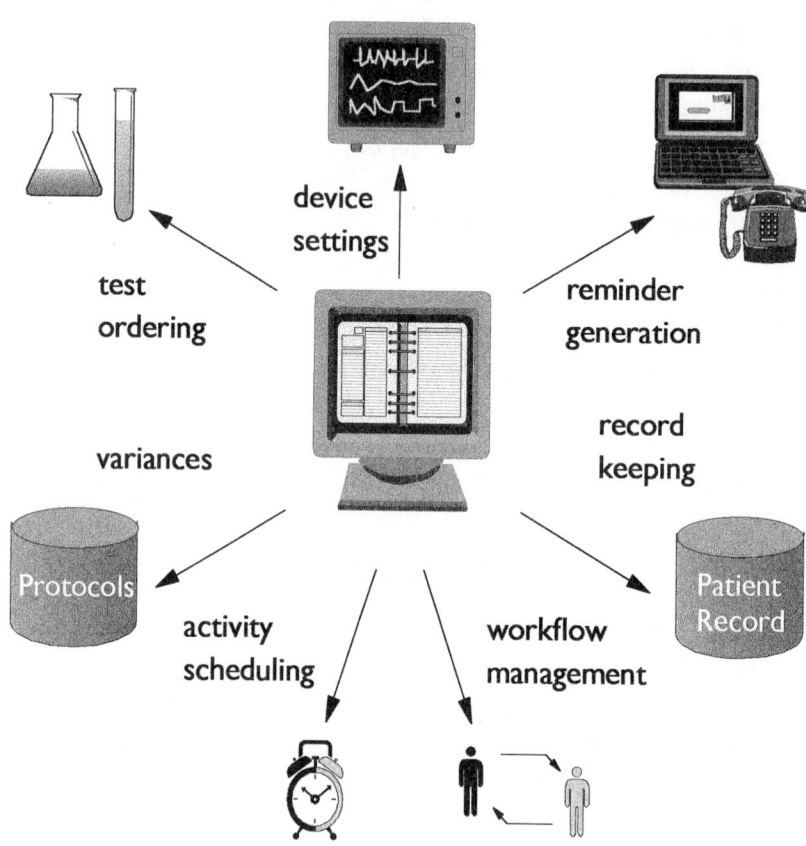

introduce fundamentally different ways of working. Rather than being grafted onto existing processes, in an active system the protocol becomes central to the way care is delivered, and care processes are designed around the protocol. The creation of care pathways, described in Chapter 8, is a good example of the way care processes are re-engineered to both deliver care according to guidelines, as well as capturing variances.

Information systems come into their own in the support of active protocol-based care. Using protocols as a central template, a variety of clinical activities can be supported or automated in some way, with the goal of either improving the quality of care or the efficiency with which care is delivered. These activities range from recording clinical events for the permanent electronic patient record, to driving other clinical events like test scheduling (Figure 9.2). The more important roles of a protocol-guided system will now be examined in more detail.

Record keeping can be semi-automated

Protocol-driven record keeping can guide the entry of routine details into the electronic patient record (e.g. Shiffman, 1994). This has benefits both for those creating the record, as well as those who will access it subsequently. For the individual noting clinical events, indicating that a step in a protocol has been carried out by checking a box on a screen is quicker than having to enter the details from scratch.

For those who wish to access a patient record, protocol-driven record keeping ensures that records reach a minimum standard of completeness and clarity. Firstly, a well-designed system should be quicker and easier to use than a free input system, thereby increasing the likelihood that an event will be recorded. Secondly, by specifying exactly how an event should be recorded, the terms and phrases used in the record can in part be standardised. This becomes especially useful when records are required for clinical audit. Finally, by specifying which data are to be recorded, the completeness of the record is enhanced (e.g. Bouhaddou et al., 1993).

Protocol-driven record keeping is thus a good example of a system that delivers direct benefit both to those who use the system, by reducing their workload, as well as having long term benefits because of improved quality of data capture. This contrasts with systems designed to explicitly code patient events for audit, but that do not improve the lot of those who use them. Systems that are not directly integrated into clinical processes are more likely to cause clinical workers to do extra work, beyond their normal duties.

There are still complexities to be resolved in the design of protocol-driven record keeping systems. For example, it is clear that not all patients will be treated exactly as a protocol specifies. It is thus not possible to exactly specify all the terms that might be used (Heathfield et al., 1995). However, if designed appropriately, such systems should reduce, but cannot eliminate, the amount of free-form data entry that occurs in the patient record.

Reminding can be situational or alert-based

As with passive systems, the first role of active protocol systems is to provide health care workers with reminders of tasks that are routinely associated with patient management. Unlike a passive system, which requires that a worker departs from their routine to check that their actions are appropriate, protocols in an active system should be a natural part of the work flow.

As a result there are two distinct ways in which an active system can remind someone. Firstly, an alert can be triggered by some computer-sensed event, like a laboratory result. For example, warning ranges on laboratory results can be altered to reflect disease specific ranges. Thus, the expected ranges for cardiac enzymes in a patient being managed on an infarction protocol could be different from those of other patients. The alerts generated by abnormal test results can then be flagged when the electronic record is accessed, or be transmitted via a communication system such as electronic mail, or via a paging system. The clinical value of such alerts has already been discussed in Chapter 5.

The second form of reminding is more subtle, but equally as important, and relies on the protocols being a natural part of the work situation. For example, if protocols guide record keeping, then the act of generating a record has the side-effect of acting as a reminder, since the protocol is visible during recording.

The act of structuring the way data are entered into a record has actually been demonstrated to improve clinical performance. In a study comparing the effect of structured data entry forms for patients with abdominal pain against free-form data entry, it was shown that the diagnostic accuracy of staff rose by 7% over baseline (de Dombal et al., 1991). There was also a 13% reduction in use of acute surgical beds at night. These improvements were surprisingly only marginally less than those obtained during the same study, by the use of an expert system for abdominal pain. There are several possible explanations for such results.

Firstly, there is a teaching effect which improves the knowledge levels of individuals participating in such studies. This has been recognised by other researchers too. Discussing the use of protocols for ventilator setting adjustment in Intensive Care, Henderson et al.

(1992) noted that 'although the protocols were complex, the clinical staff learned to anticipate protocol instructions quite accurately, making it possible for them to recognise that a protocol instruction was based on erroneous data'.

Secondly, the ability of individuals to assess a situation may be improved by indicating which data should be collected, the order in which data should be gathered, and presenting them uniformly once gathered. The effects of order of data presentation and hypothesis generation, as discussed in the previous chapter, are certainly a recognised phenomenon.

Variance capture can be semi-automated

Along with a potential to improve record keeping for patient care, protocol systems can also gather broader population data that will contribute to protocol improvement. Whenever a variation in patient management has occurred, it should be possible to include features in the record keeping part of an information system to record the variance and store it for later assessment.

Protocols can drive activity scheduling and workflow management

The facility to enter orders for tests or medications is a basic component of a clinical information system. If such an order-entry function is linked to a protocol, then order generation can in part be protocol driven. For example, as soon as a patient is entered onto a protocol, it should be possible to send requests automatically for the tests or procedures that are specified within the protocol. Thus, one could schedule a stress test several days in advance once a patient has been admitted under a myocardial infarction protocol.

There now exist quite complex and sophisticated computer-based workflow management systems, which find application in a variety of industries beyond healthcare. They attempt to achieve this by using formal descriptions of tasks, the order in which the tasks need to be executed, and perhaps their interdependencies.

The goal of workflow systems is to ensure that work processes are carried about in the most time and cost-efficient method possible.

For example, a process may require a series of steps to be carried out that involve different departments or individuals. The workflow system will try to balance the work requests that arrive at each point in the process so that the most important tasks are completed, or so that each part of the system works to maximum efficiency. The ability to manage scheduling in a more automated fashion may result in a better use of institutional resources, avoiding peaks in which facilities might be overloaded, or troughs of under-utilisation (Majidi et al., 1993).

The degree to which the flow of work in an organisation can be automated depends upon the degree to which tasks can be formalised. At one extreme, we have robot-operated assembly plants which require minimal human intervention, given the high degree of regularity of the assembly process. At the other extreme, every task in an organisation is new, and no workflow automation is possible. Like most organisations, healthcare activities occupy a spectrum in between these two extrema. The degree to which protocols can drive workflow depends upon the sophistication of the protocol care process, and the order-entry and scheduling components of the information system. From the point of view of the care process, it would need to be defined in a quite formal way that lent itself to automation. As we saw in Chapter 4, for some tasks this formalisation will not always be possible or desirable.

The decision to introduce workflow systems will involve revisiting the criteria presented in the last chapter for protocol creation. The prescriptive nature of some workflow systems can make them complex to set-up and they may be overly constraining on staff. However, simple systems that make sure events are scheduled automatically, or that optimise the flow of 'forms' and 'requests' have the potential to yield considerable benefits, if the organisation is willing to formalise its processes sufficiently.

Monitor alarms can be set by protocol

If monitoring equipment is integrated into the protocol system, then it too can be driven in a partially automated manner (Coiera and Lewis, 1994). For example, if anaesthesia is delivered according to computer-resident protocols, then patient monitor alarm settings can be automatically reconfigured, reflecting the changes in alarm bands associated with the different stages of anaesthesia. The computer can detect that a new stage in the protocol has been entered by checking the events noted in the patient record, which can also be protocol driven.

Data display can be modified by protocol

The data required to make decisions vary with tasks, and computer system designers often resort to task specific displays in complex situations (see Chapter 5). If a computer system can be made aware of the current set of clinical tasks, for example, by detecting that a step in a protocol has been executed via a record keeper, then it can prepare itself to generate task-specific data displays.

This is of particular relevance in situations in which large amounts of patient data may need to be filtered, for example in intensive care or anaesthesia. It is also of value in less critical situations, when a large amount of data has accumulated, for example, when patients have long hospital admissions.

Device settings can vary with protocol stage

Protocols can be used either to advise the settings for biomedical equipment (open-loop control), or to control them directly (closed-loop control).

There has been some investigation into open-loop control of ventilators according to standard protocols. For example, protocols have been used to adjust tidal volume and ventilator rate settings for patients with Adult Respiratory Distress Syndrome (ARDS) (Thomsen et al., 1993). One system has been reportedly used for over 50,000 hours on 150 ARDS patients (Morris et al., 1994a). In one sub-trial of 12 patients, 94% of 4,531 protocol-generated recommendations were followed by staff. Of these patients, 52 met extra-corporeal membrane oxygenation criteria (East et al. 1992a). These had a 9% expected survival based upon historical data, but under protocol-directed care achieved 41% survival, 4 times greater than expected (Morris et al., 1994b).

Closed loop-control systems are likely to need sophisticated signal interpretation capabilities, as will be discussed in Chapter 21, in addition to access to protocols.

9.3   Protocol construction and maintenance

In the previous two chapters, two key ideas were introduced. Firstly, protocol creation does not occur at a single event in time, but is part of an ongoing process that assesses a protocol's performance, and refines it accordingly. Secondly, a protocol's creation cannot be an isolated event, but its form and content must be designed to reflect the context within which it will be used. The creation of even a single protocol thus has the potential to become a complex process. If protocols are to be used in only selected cases, then the effort required to create them will probably be significant but manageable.

There are, however, two forces which will cause the process of formalising clinical care to expand greatly. Evidence-based medicine has as its goal the creation of large databases covering most aspects of clinical care, summarising best-practice advice from the enormous and growing body of scientific literature. Secondly, the potential benefits of computer-based protocol systems, outlined above, will see continued pressures to introduce them.

However, computer-based protocols can be complex. For example, the ventilator protocols developed by Henderson et al. (1992) required the efforts of 14 physicians and nurses, covered 25 pages of flow diagrams, and 12000 lines of computer code. Unfortunately the cumulative time required from all the team members to build these protocols was not specified. Thus, whether one is envisioning the creation of large global databases of protocols capturing medicine's best practice or local databases, protocols probably numbering in the thousands will need to be created.

A task on this scale has never been done before. It is also a task that, in all probability, cannot be tackled either without significant human resource, or the use of advanced information and communication technologies. In many respects then, the uniform and rapid transformation of clinical evidence into clinical process represents not just a major challenge for medicine, but it also represents a major challenge for medical informatics (Coiera, 1996b).

Despite the rewards contemplated by those who advocate mass protocolisation, it is by no means yet certain whether it is technically feasible, or even practicable, to do so. For informatics then, the process of protocol creation and application poses a number of significant technical challenges, many of which still have solutions residing in the realms of research. Others thankfully, can be readily solved by the appropriate application of existing technologies.

The degree of technical challenge grows both with the number of protocols contemplated, as well as the inherent complexity of individual protocols. For example, a paper-based protocol to help a diabetic patient adjust their insulin therapy is much simpler than an equivalent protocol that is needed to drive a computer to make the same recommendations.

The major technical steps in the creation of protocols will now be defined, and their associated challenges explored.

Evidence gathering, pooling and dissemination

It still needs to be determined whether it is possible to develop robust methods for sifting through the burgeoning medical literature and creating practice guidelines. Current processes are intensive users of human resources.

The process adopted by the Cochrane Collaboration, for example, is approximately as follows (Wyatt, 1995). To assemble systematic evidence-based reviews for each guideline, a complete literature search has first to be performed. This may involve hand-searching journals from pre-electronic days, as well as doing multiple on-line bibliographic searches. It may even involve contacting authors for access to data supporting their reported results. Reviewers are helped in their search by standards which define what forms of evidence are acceptable. For example, there is a preference for quantitative randomised controlled trials. Where appropriate, the process should also include qualitative research, or case descriptions (Smith et al., 1996).

Progress has already been made by biomedical journals through the adoption of standard formats for article abstracts, ensuring that key aspects of a paper are always present. The data gathering process could be further assisted if all papers were available electronically, and even more so if the data used in a study were also available on line, for example via the Internet (Delamothe, 1996) (see Chapter 16). There are no technical barriers to such proposals, only organisational ones. Key medical journals have begun the process that may eventually see all biomedical publication occurring in electronic form in preference to paper (LaPorte et al., 1995).

However, retrieval of published evidence is not only hampered by limited access to the material. In one study, even if barriers to access had been removed, clear information on specific questions for primary care physicians could only be obtained from the literature in about 50% of cases (Gorman, 1993). Finding such information is both time-consuming and complex. For example, there may be variations in the terminology used, or the papers may not come up to appropriate scientific standards because of variations in the quality of peer review. The solution to such problems is probably as much organisational as it is technological. The adoption, for example, of ICD nomenclature in structured abstracts would reduce the effort involved in bibliographic searches.

Just as there are considerable issues to be faced in the gathering of evidence, there are also difficulties associated with the distribution of protocols and guidelines once they have been created. If they are to be used as passive information resources, then the communication of guidelines can be enhanced through publication on the Internet using the World Wide Web (see Chapter 17).

The model for publication on the Web permits updated guidelines to be almost immediately available, on a world-wide scale. Further, there are no issues associated with multiple editions of a protocol circulating, as is the case with paper-based publication methods. There need only ever be one current version available on the Web, and it can always be regarded as the most current version.

For institutions which have limited communications access, for whatever reason, then regular guideline updates can be delivered on CD-ROM, or other high capacity computer memory devices. This permits very large databases of information to be easily duplicated and disseminated at very little expense. Especially when the rate of change of information is slow, or communication costs are an issue, then this method of publication may prove to be more than adequate.

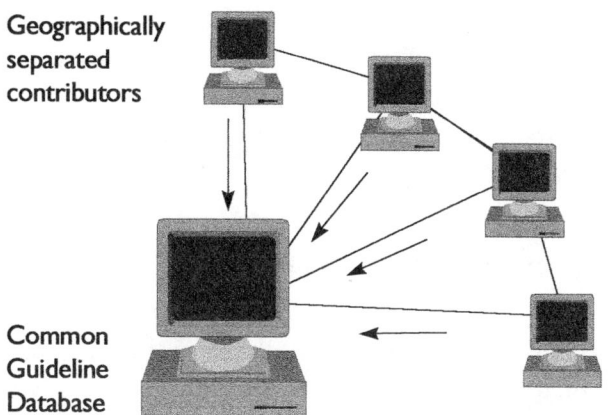

Geographically
separated
contributors

Common
Guideline
Database

Figure 9.3: Long-distance collaboration on protocol creation can be supported by communication technologies like the Internet. Individuals can have shared access to common information sources, permitting computer-supported collaborative working (CSCW).

Consensus review

Statistical meta-analysis is one of the tools used to decide what constitutes 'best practice' based on published clinical studies. There has to be a consensus process in which individual studies are selected to be pooled for such analysis. Equally, where the literature is equivocal about what is the best way to treat a condition, then decisions need to be made based upon other criteria. In both cases, it is important for experts to discuss and reach consensus on the best way forward. In fact, some suggest that such a process is the most important factor in protocol development and use - 'The systematic and careful development of protocol logic and its acceptance by consensus are the most important factors in the success of our medical protocols' (Henderson et al., 1992).

Where discussions occur locally amongst members of an organisation, then the process of organising meetings for consensus review is demanding but perhaps not intrinsically difficult. Where team members live in many different countries, then the process becomes more challenging. As we will see in Chapter 13, communication technologies can help minimise the amount of travel that need occur in such circumstances. They can, for example, provide mechanisms for team members to collaborate remotely, through the electronic sharing of information and documents (Figure 9.3). The Internet, as we will see in Chapter 16, is increasingly being used in this way.

As the number of bodies involved in protocol development grow, and the cost of travel and interaction rise, the use of communication technologies will of necessity increase. This will be driven not just by the need to minimise travel, but to speed up the sometimes lengthy process of creating protocols.

Protocol representations and languages

We have already seen in previous chapters that the representation one uses when writing a protocol has consequences when people come to use the protocol. Decision trees might be useful in some circumstances, for example, but not others. Similar issues arise when a protocol is written for computer interpretation. There is no clear 'best' way of capturing a protocol, and the choice of representational form is dependent on the protocol's intended use.

*Knowledge can be represented either **declaratively** or **procedurally**. In the former, we declare how things relate to one another, but do not specify how we use that knowledge to come up with an answer. In the latter we include in the knowledge how the answer might be derived. See Chapter 20 for a fuller discussion of knowledge representation and reasoning.*

Computer protocols are further complicated because, in contrast to humans who are able to bring much knowledge to bear when they read a protocol, a computer system does not come with such background knowledge. Recall from Figure 2.5 how the more is required of a computer, the more knowledge it must be given about the task it is to accomplish. As a consequence, computer protocols need to be specified in considerable detail. Recall the example of the ventilator management protocol that needed 12000 lines of computer code for its specification (Henderson et al., 1992).

In an attempt to develop a standard method for representing protocols, the American Society for Testing and Materials (ASTM) developed the Arden syntax. This language encodes the actions within a clinical protocol into a set of situation-action rules. The Arden Syntax resembles the Pascal computer programming language, and is procedural in its design. Arden has recognised deficiencies in the type of things that can be described using it (Musen et al., 1995). Further, because it is limited to describing protocols in terms of rules, it has other limitations as far as computers are concerned. Since there is no way to express the knowledge and ideas humans use when they come to read a protocol, there is little tolerance for errors and interdependencies between rules.

Much of the advanced research into protocol languages for computers is aimed at creating ways that ensure that the knowledge is captured in as reliable a way as possible. So, some workers seek to define formal protocol **ontologies** which would then be used to support the writing of specific protocols. An ontology can be thought of as a definition of what is knowable in some context. So, an ontology here would capture all the important knowledge about the things being described in the protocol. An ontology about cardiac surgery would include amongst other things, all the tests and procedures that might be of interest. It might also contain rules about the relationships amongst these, which could then be used to prevent some mistakes when the time comes to write a protocol. For example, it makes no sense to write in a protocol that a patient will be treated with a clinical action that the ontology knows is actually a type of test, and not a therapy. It is this need to create ways of automatically checking protocols for errors that has driven the development of such ontologies (Glowinski, 1994).

PROforma is one such protocol language, whose ontology is structured around the notion of clinical tasks, which are subdivided into plans, decisions, actions and enquiries (Fox et al., 1996). The PROTÉGÉ-II system is similarly structured around an ontology of tasks (Musen et al., 1995). In both examples, the researchers spent much effort in developing ways for people to specify a protocol in a simple way. They also needed to develop mechanisms that translated these descriptions into more formal language for computers. They are thus systems that can be programmed using high-level languages understood by humans, that are then translated into a lower-level language understood by computer.

Protocol terminologies

Implicit in the creation of an ontology that will support protocol writing is the creation of some kind of circumscribed set of words or terminology, that will be recognisable by a computer system. This is not a requirement that is specific to protocol systems, but is in fact, a fundamental informatics need in many areas. Given the importance of the whole subject of terminologies, and their fundamental relationship with active protocol systems, the next three chapters will examine this field.

9.4   Conclusions

In the previous sections, some of the different ways a protocol-system can interact with other components of a clinical information system have been outlined. In many ways, protocol-based systems can provide the glue that can connect these different components together.

Since the goal of protocol-directed care is to improve clinical processes, active protocol-systems are richly entwined with the delivery of care. As with any such marriage, costs and benefits result from the union. Poorly designed systems can have a significant impact upon care delivery. Consequently the emphasis on good design, both of protocols, and the systems that embody them becomes more critical the more deeply they are used to manage the care process.

Striking a balance between prescription and permission, protocol-systems need to be only as formal as is necessary to ensure appropriate outcomes, without restricting the permission needed by clinical workers to vary their work patterns.

Chapter summary

1. Computer-based protocol systems can support passive and active protocol usage.
2. There is growing evidence that providing computer-assistance to improve passive access to clinical protocols does have a positive impact on adherence to guidelines.
3. Using protocols as a central template, a variety of clinical activities can be actively supported or automated. These include recording clinical events for the electronic patient record, reminder generation, adjusting settings on devices like monitors, ordering tests, capturing variances from protocol specifications, scheduling procedures and guiding efficient and effective workflow.
4. The rapid transformation of clinical evidence into clinical process represents a major challenge for medicine and informatics. The degree of technical challenge grows both with the number of protocols contemplated, as well as the inherent complexity of individual protocols. Technical challenges exist in the following areas.
   - Supporting evidence gathering, pooling and dissemination, using systems like the Internet.
   - Facilitating consensus review amongst geographically remote peers through the use of communication technologies.
   - Developing protocol representations and languages that permit large protocol databases to be built with some inherent error checking, and that also support active use of protocols in computer systems.

Part Four

Language, Coding and Classification in Healthcare

By an almost instinctive impulse, similar to that which leads to the use of language, we are induced to collate or group together the things which we observe - which is to say, to classify them. Our intellectual nature and requirements compel us, in fact, not merely to observe the objects and phenomena...and designate them by this or that name, but also to imagine them combined or grouped in a certain order... Accordingly, every science and art has endeavoured to classify as completely as possible the things belonging to it; hence, in our field of enquiry, the objects classified are the phenomena and processes of the living body, diseases, remedies, the hundred influences and agencies of external nature, etc.

F. Oesterlen, *Medical Logic*, (1855).

Chapter 10

Terms, codes and classification

Both conceptually and practically, the study of medical language is inescapably central to informatics. Theoretically, medical languages are the building blocks with which we construct and apply our models of health and disease. As such, they exert their influence at the very foundations of medical thinking.

Practically, administrative bodies increasingly require healthcare workers to codify their records using specialised words to permit auditing of their practices. National and international bodies seem to be constantly creating longer lists of words, often in open competition with one another. The support given to individual collections of words sometimes reaches near religious fervour.

So, the languages of medicine attract great attention within informatics, and their development consumes much resource. In this chapter, the basic ideas behind terminologies, coding and classification will be explained. The next chapter examines some of the more important terminological systems, their uses and limitations. The concluding chapter in this part critically examines the scientific basis of these coding schemes, outlining the difficulties inherent in creating languages, and reviews the likely avenues for future development.

10.1 Language establishes a common ground

Human beings are designed to detect differences in the world. We distinguish different objects, name them, and then categorise them.

This process of discovering a difference between two things, and then giving both names is basic to the way in which we learn about the world, develop language, and proceed to interact with the world (Wisniewski and Medin, 1994). It is canonised in the scientific method, where each new concept is a theory, created to explain away the differences between existing theory and our observations of the world.

Unsurprisingly then, language evolves as we interact with the world, discovering new things about it, and doing different things within it. However, this growth in language is tempered by the need to communicate with others and share our experiences. When members of different cultures wish to meet, they need to establish a linguistic common ground. To do this there must be some shared language, and agreement on the meaning of that shared language. There is little value in each of us developing a complicated set of words if no one else understands what they are intended to represent. Consequently, the sharing of words and the underlying concepts they represent, constitute an important part of human language development. Thus the natural drive to create new words is tempered by the need to communicate.

The story in medicine is similar. Medicine has a long history of discovery and the creation of new ideas. As a consequence, the words used in medicine change both their meaning and form over time (Feinstein, 1988). A physician today has a very different understanding of the meaning of the word asthma to one of even 100 years ago. Further, different cultures have different concepts of illness. Even amongst overtly similar western cultures there can be quite different notions of what constitutes a disease and what is normal. Hypotension or low blood pressure is a routinely treated disease is some European countries, but regarded as within the bands of normality in others.

Even amongst the different medical 'cultures' there are differences. Different groups of heath professionals, from the medical specialities, through to nurses, medical economists and administrators all evolve slightly different words or jargon.

Medicine is a practical endeavour, and so in this respect practitioners want to be able to share the same vocabulary so that they can discuss and learn from one another. In an age where communication and travel have combined to unite the global medical community, the need to share knowledge through a common vocabulary has never been so great.

10.2 Common terms are needed to permit assessment of clinical activities

If the need for a common language was solely to permit discussion amongst different groups, then there would probably be little need for organised intervention. Language can be shared informally simply through common usage at meetings and in scientific publications. However, the enormous resources devoted to healthcare provision have made the need to control the delivery of care inescapable. To do this, there has to be some commonality to the way in which illness and care are described.

Consequently, much of the effort devoted to formal medical language development has been for the purpose of epidemiology, resource management and clinical audit. Audit is the process of assessing the outcomes associated with different diseases and their treatments. We can understand the audit process through the model, measure and manage cycle introduced in Chapter 3, which explains the basic process of system control.

To make all such assessments, it is first necessary to make measurements by pooling patient data. While it is possible to compare patient outcomes based upon measurements obtained from instruments, for example serum biochemistry, these rarely are sufficient to describe a patient's state. In healthcare, language itself is often the basis of measurement. Words are needed to describe observed findings like 'pitting oedema' or 'unconscious' and the diagnoses ascribed to these findings.

Yet the words used by people to describe conditions vary so much that simple analysis of their records is often not possible. Further, the meanings attached to the terms they use may vary. If there was an agreed set of terms to describe the process of care, then data analysis would be much simplified (Ackerman et al., 1994). The goal in developing medical terminologies is to arrive at a consensus on the most appropriate set of terms and the way they should be structured.

Once they have been created, controlled terminologies can also be used in other sometimes unexpected ways. For example, if a set of clinical notes was created using standard words, then a computer system could check the words and issue alerts when it detected anomalies. It could, for example, check a patient's diagnosis against current treatments, and warn of any potentially dangerous side-effects or drug interactions. If a computer system were to try to do the same by interpreting the freely entered text, it would need to be a far more complicated system, able to understand the complexities of natural language. Such systems are still the subject of research, and unlikely to appear in clinical practice for many years, whereas the simpler word-based solution could in principle be applied now.

10.3 Terms, codes, groups and hierarchies

Medical terminologies (or nomenclatures) like all languages start with a basic set of words or **terms**. A term, just like any normal word, has a specific meaning. In this case a term stands for some defined medical **concept** like 'diabetes', 'tibia' or 'penicillin'.

Most languages permit words that have the same or similar meanings, and this is usually the case in medicine too. To permit some flexibility, most medical languages allow the same concept to be named in several different ways. However, since several terms may be used for the same concept, it is usual to define a single alphanumeric **code** for every distinct concept in the language (Figure 10.1).

This gives rise to the process of **coding**, where a set of words describing some medical concept is translated into a code for later analysis. Thus a terminology should contain a separate name for each distinct disease entity, as well as any reasonable synonyms. A coding system may collect many such terms into a single code.

The terms and codes in different terminologies vary, depending upon how they will be used. For example, if the coding system exists for epidemiological analysis, the concepts of interest are at the level of public health, rather than at the level of a particular medical specialisation. The level of detail captured in the codes would be much finer in the latter case, and the concepts would be different.

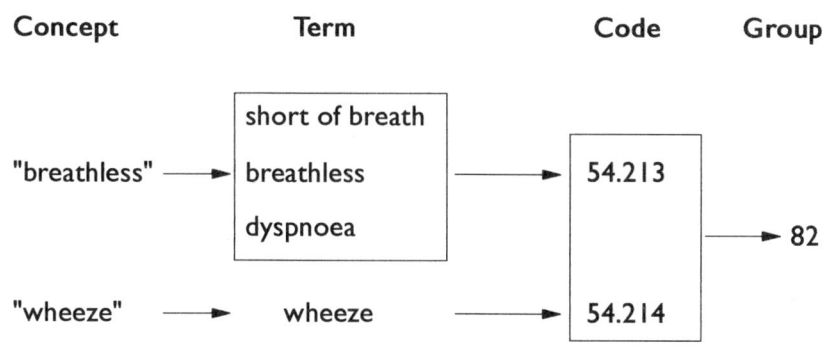

| Concept | Term | Code | Group |

Figure 10.1: Multiple terms may map onto a single numeric code in medical languages. Groups collect together similar codes for more coarse-grained analysis.

While terms and codes are created at a level of detail that is appropriate for statistical analysis or patient management, they may be too fine-grained for other purposes. In particular, the determination of the cost of providing care and the overall determination of patient outcomes usually needs this information to be pooled. A **group** thus collects together into a single category a number of different codes that are considered to be similar for the purpose of reimbursement.

The process of ascribing terms, encoding them, and then grouping them may seem overly complex, potentially inefficient, and to some extent ad hoc. In the next chapter, where specific systems for each are described, this impression will be reinforced. Driven by practical necessity, terminological systems created for one purpose have been adapted, for example through the grouping process, to other quite different ones.

Classification hierarchies

Once a set of terms and codes are collected together, they can quickly become so large that it is difficult to find individual terms. They consequently need to be organised in such a way that the terms can be easily explored.

Most people are familiar enough with alphabetically organised dictionaries as a way of looking up words. It is often the case that the words used by a person might be different to the terms in a system, or the term may not be known at all. Consequently a straightforward alphabetical listing of terms is of limited value. A terminology needs to be organised in a way that permits concept-

Figure 10.2:
Classification hierarchies organise terms in some conceptual structure that gives meaning to terms through their relationship to other terms in the hierarchy.

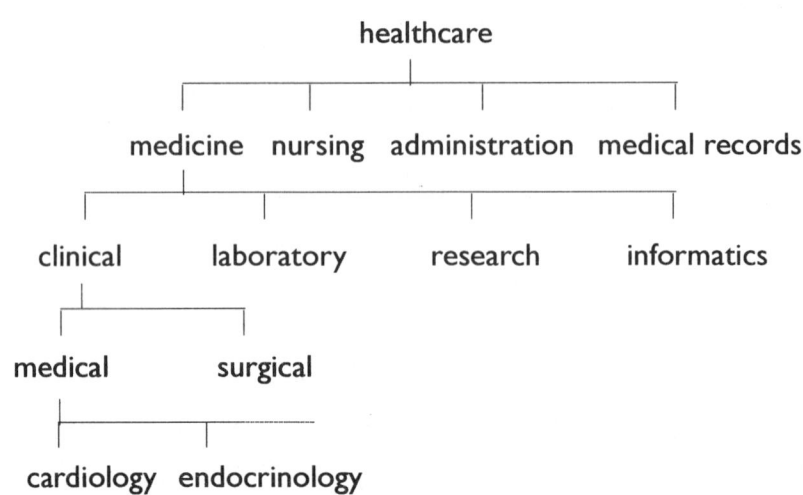

driven exploration. For example, it should be easy to locate the word 'pericarditis' knowing that one is seeking a word describing inflammation of the pericardium. Thus, from a user's point of view, a terminology needs to be more like a thesaurus than a dictionary, organising terms into conceptually similar groupings.

The most common way to organise ideas is to produce a classification hierarchy. Everything from rocks and minerals, through to the elements and the species, are classified in some form of hierarchical structure. The essence of a hierarchy is that it provides a structured grouping of ideas, organised around some set of **attributes** or **axes**. In this way, the hierarchy begins to provide some meaning to terms through the way they are related to others. For example, in Figure 10.2, it is clear without knowing anything more about the term 'endocrinology', that it is a branch of clinical medicine, and not a part of healthcare administration.

Just as a hierarchy may serve as a map to help locate unknown terms, it can help uncover new relationships between concepts. Here the act of constructing the hierarchy is used to help map out possible relationships. A researcher, for example, might try to arrange concepts in such a way that a deeper set of relationships becomes apparent. If this has explanatory power, then the classification system can then be used to direct further research, explain or teach.

Box 10.1 - The basic level

When people are asked to name objects, they instinctively pick words that describe them at a level that is most economic, but still adequately describes their functionality. For example, people will usually use the word 'chair' in preference to the more general word 'furniture' which loses much sense of function, or the more specific description 'dining chair' which adds little.

This cognitively economic level of description has been called the basic level by Elanor Rosch, who developed her classification theory to describe this feature of human cognition (Rosch, 1988).

Rosch proposed that objects in the basic level have the quality that they are prototypic of their class. Such prototypic objects contain most of the attributes that represent objects inside their category, and the least number of attributes of those outside the category. Thus if people were asked to describe 'a chair' they would list a set of attributes that could be used to describe most, but not all, kinds of chair. A stool may be a special kind of chair, even though it does no have a back support which might be considered part of the features of a prototypic chair.

The basic level is thus formed around a natural word hierarchy based upon level of detail of description, coupled with utility of description. The basic level therefore is not absolute, but varies with the context within which a word is used. Sometimes 'dining chair' actually is the most appropriate description to use. Similarly, in some circumstances, it is sufficient to classify a patient as having an 'acidosis'. Clinically however, it is probably more useful to use a description like 'metabolic acidosis', which becomes basic in this context because it is at this level that treatment is determined.

The periodic table of elements, developed by Mendeleev, was used in this way. Atomic weights of the elements, along with some of their chemical properties, were the attributes used to construct the initial classification system. Where no elements were known to exist, gaps were left that were later filled as new elements were discovered. Further, the regularity of the table led to a deeper understanding of the underlying atomic structure of the elements. The table is now a standard way of teaching the basics of atomic structure.

Thus, for most people, classification systems are invaluable in imparting knowledge about the relationships between related concepts, and are commonplace in scientific writing and textbooks.

The meaning of terms in a classification hierarchy is determined by the type of link used

There are many ways in which terms can relate to one another in a hierarchy, depending upon which attributes of the concept are of interest. In each case the meaning of the linkage between terms is different. For example, a hierarchy may describe the way a complex structure is assembled (Figure 10.2). Such **part-whole** description might be used to describe anatomic structures, or the components of a device.

In contrast, in a **kind-of** (or **is-a**) hierarchy, elements are assembled because of some underlying similarity. For example, a drug like penicillin is a kind-of antibiotic. It is also common in medicine to use causal structures to explain how a chain of events might unfold. So for example, in Figure 10.3, a portion of the possible set of events starting with a plaque in a coronary artery and leading to an arrhythmia is described.

Each of these different types of link allows one term to inherit properties from other terms higher up in the hierarchy. What is inherited depends entirely on the type of link. So, for a part-of hierarchy, terms inherit location from parent terms higher in the hierarchical tree. In kind-of hierarchies many different properties of parent terms are inherited by their children terms. Thus there are many chemical and pharmacological properties that amoxycillin inherits from the parent class of penicillins, and that the penicillins inherit from their parent class antibiotics. Equally, in a causal structure one would not expect that the concept 'thrombosis' to be a kind of 'coronary plaque', but only that it takes its temporal ordering in a chain of events from it.

This leads to an obvious but critical point about classification hierarchies. For the meaning of terms in a classification system to be as explicit as possible, the links between terms should be as uniform as possible. In other words, if one is to be clear what properties a term can reasonably inherit from its parents, then the type of link

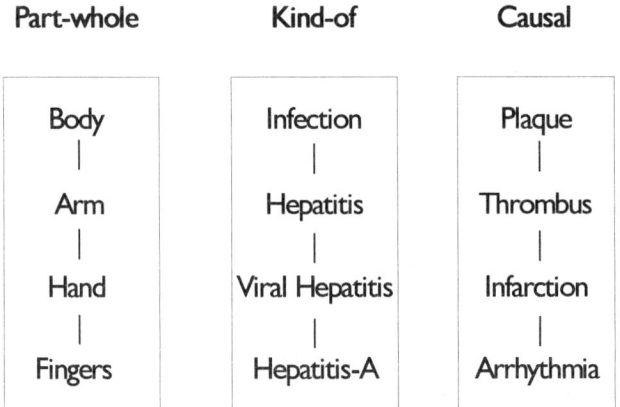

Part-whole	Kind-of	Causal
Body	Infection	Plaque
|	|	|
Arm	Hepatitis	Thrombus
|	|	|
Hand	Viral Hepatitis	Infarction
|	|	|
Fingers	Hepatitis-A	Arrhythmia

Figure 10.3: Depending on the type of attribute used to classify concepts, many different types of hierarchical structure are possible. Each type of link implies a different relationship between the terms in the hierarchy.

being used should be clear. Confusion is easy, and it is common to see classifications mixing part-of and kind-of relations. Ideally, to ensure clarity of meaning, an individual hierarchy should only use one kind of link, and be explicit about the kind of link being used.

Some complex medical terminologies permit multiple axes of classification within them. These multi-axial systems allow a term to exist in several different types of classification hierarchy, which minimises duplication of terms, and also enhances the conceptual power of the system as a whole. So in a multi-axial system a term like hepatitis could exist both as a kind-of infection, as well as a cause of jaundice.

10.4 Compositional terminologies create complicated concepts from simple terms

Most existing coding systems are **enumerative**, listing out all the possible terms that could be used in advance. Terminology builders strive to make such systems as complete as possible, and to contain as few errors or duplications as possible. Understandably, as the numbers of terms in a system move into the thousands, this task becomes increasingly difficult. Especially when there are many people contributing to a terminology, the natural tendency is to create slightly different terms for similar concepts.

This leads to redundancy in terms, or worse, partial overlaps. Equally, it is difficult to make sure that all the necessary terms in a given area have been produced. As we shall see in Chapter 12, these problems are inherent in the process of terminology creation, and to some extent will always exist. There are, however, ways of improving the situation, and minimising these types of error.

One approach is to agree on a basic set of primitive terms, and assemble more complex terms from these as they are needed (Rector et al., 1993). For example, 'acute bacterial septicaemia' represents a distinct medical concept. An enumerative system would have to have a pre-existing code for this concept. With a **compositional** terminology, the system would generate the complex term from a set of more primitive components (Figure 10.4).

Indeed it should be able to generate many such specific conjunctions. In this way, there is no need to explicitly create all the needed terms in an area in advance, but merely to make sure that all the basic building blocks exist. This helps to minimise incompleteness in a terminology, and eliminates duplication or error in the more complex terms.

Since terms are assembled as they are needed, compositional systems need to try to check that the new compound terms are medically sensible (e.g. Glowinski et al., 1991). For example, 'acute inflammation of the penicillin' is a meaningless term, as is 'viral tibia'. To prevent such composite terms being created, compositional systems need to have rules about the way in which terms can be combined. Suggested combinations are then checked against the rules before they are accepted. An example of such a rule might be that 'only a kind-of body part can be a part of another body part'.

In compositional systems there are both terms corresponding to concepts, like diseases and drugs, as well as **modifiers** or **quantifiers**, which describe them. Thus words like 'acute', 'left', or 'proximal' need to be explicitly included in the list of basic terms. It is also necessary to construct rules about the way these modifying terms can be applied. Thus 'a term about duration like acute or chronic cannot modify a drug'. This would exclude a composite term like 'acute penicillin'.

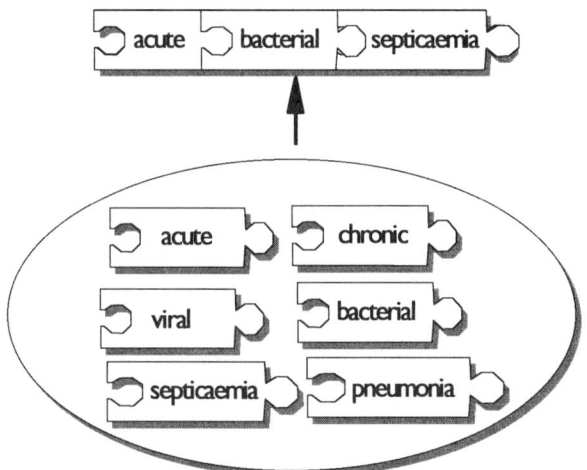

Figure 10.4:
Compositional
terminologies create
complex terms from
libraries of more
primitive ones.

To do this kind of checking, the terminology builder has to say more about each primitive term than if a simple enumerative list was being created. For example, penicillin might be created as a term and the properties that it is a type of therapy, a drug, and a kind of antibiotic would all need to be listed.

Thus each primitive term is classified according to a number of different axes, and this information is used to ensure that any complex terms created from it are sensible. The terminology builder also has to create a library of rules that describes the way terms in the system can combine, which has its own difficulties in terms of completeness and accuracy.

10.5 Using coding systems

The process of using a terminology to generate codes is also complex. In an ideal world, the individual in need of the coded information is actually the person best qualified to assign the code. This is because there is a certain amount of subjectivity in the coding process. Data in a medical record, for example, needs to be interpreted before a diagnostic code is assigned. The act of interpretation will thus affect the codes selected. To ensure that this process results in codes best suited to the task at hand, those who understand that task should be involved in the code selection process.

Such involvement is not always the case. Medical administrators in a hospital, for example, may wish to code medical data in a certain way for an audit. By the time the coded data has reached the administrator, two sets of different people may have each interpreted the data, and potentially introduced distortions into the final codes. Firstly, the clinical staff have interpreted what they believe is important to be recorded when they create a record. Next, the staff responsible for coding then have to re-interpret this and try and find a set of codes that matches what they have understood the record to contain.

The situation is much improved in a primary care setting, where the coding might occur at the time the record is created. Even more ideally, some of the audit will also be carried out by the doctor creating the record and codes.

We can summarise these observations as follows.

- The quality of coding improves the closer it occurs to the point of information capture.
- The quality of coding improves if the individuals involved in the coding understand the task to which the coded data is to be put.
- The quality of coding improves if the staff doing the coding benefit from the coding.

The last point is an important one. If, for example, the burden of coding is shifted to clinical staff at the time of information capture, then they are being asked to carry out an additional task. If this task is for the benefit of others, for example administration, then they are less likely to carry the task out enthusiastically. They would be more enthusiastic if the data was to be used, for example, for a clinical trial in which they were personally involved.

It is one of the maxims of computer system design that if the problem owner is not the same as the user, then there is likely to be reluctance to accept a new computer system. This problem has long been recognised with clinical coding. The chief medical statistician for the World Health Organisation's International Classification of Diseases noted in 1927 that 'administrative statistics have no value in the eyes of practitioners, who as a result are completely uninterested in it; whereas unless these practitioners provide exact

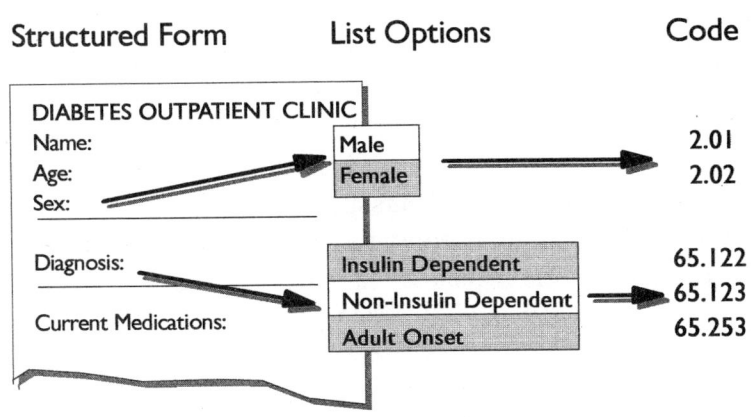

Structured Form   **List Options**   **Code**

DIABETES OUTPATIENT CLINIC

Name: Male   2.01

Age: Female   2.02

Sex:

Diagnosis: Insulin Dependent   65.122

               Non-Insulin Dependent 65.123

Current Medications: Adult Onset   65.253

Figure 10.5:
Structured data-entry forms can offer a predetermined list of acceptable terms for given fields and these can then be converted to codes for later analysis. This minimises, and to some extent hides, the effort involved in coding.

data, then the scientific value of administrative statistics has to be called into question' (Gregory et al., 1995).

It is because of the burden that the coding process imposes that attempts have been made to reduce the effort involved by automating the process. There are actually several different ways that medical information can be converted into a set of coded terms. Each requires progressively less effort from the coder, and more effort from those that design the system supporting the coder.

Free code entry, with no support. This is traditionally how coding has occurred. The coder has access to a list of codes, perhaps in a set of manuals, and access to some information, like a medical record. It is up to the coder to interpret the content of the record, locate codes in the list that seem close to that interpretation, and then assign the codes.

Free code entry with decision support. The situation can be improved with tools to help navigate and explore the terminology system. For example, many medical terminologies are enormous, and finding appropriate codes is time consuming. Success is largely dependent upon an individual's experience and knowledge of the particular coding system. If computer tools permitted rapid exploration of a terminology with word searching and graphic visualisation, then it is more likely that the coder will access the most appropriate codes (e.g. Hohnloser et al., 1995; Tuttle et al. 1995). This can result in a significant increase in the quality of coding (Hohnloser et al., 1996).

Semi-structured information entry. In this approach, the act of coding occurs at the time of information capture. Data is entered onto a structured form, which has fields for the different pieces required. Wherever possible, the list of possible alternatives is specified for each field in the form (Figure 10.5). Thus in a diabetes clinic run by primary care nursing staff, the different types of diabetes would be listed as options against the diagnosis field on the form. Each diagnosis would be a recognised and codable term. Clearly this approach is well suited to computer automation, and different pick-lists of terms can be associated with fields in a form. The benefit of this approach is clear for situations in which there is a clearly defined context, and in which clear procedures are in place.

Automatic coding. In situations in which it is harder to anticipate the type of information that will be captured, or the uses to which it will be put, the structured approach is inadequate. It would be ideal in these circumstances if there were a way to take a piece of text, and automatically encode it, using some type of computer system. To do this the computer coding system would need to be able to work with natural language with all its inherent complexities. It would also need to understand something of the medical context within which the information was recorded, since this too determines meaning. For example, the sentence 'The ventricle was traumatised' changes meaning depending upon whether the patient has had a chest or head injury.

At present, the design of computer systems capable of free natural language interpretation, especially in complex domains like medicine, is a subject for ongoing research. With time, however, systems capable of restricted recognition may be available. It is likely that these will work alongside a human, suggesting appropriate terms, and relying upon the human to select or adjust them as necessary. It may be that the very notion of coding as an explicit task disappears. From the human's perspective, the computer is simply assisting with the completion of the medical record.

Chapter summary

1. Language evolves as we interact with the world, discovering new things about it. This growth is tempered by the need to communicate with others.
2. Medical language develops over time as new concepts emerge. At any one time, medical language varies between different individuals, institutions, specialities, and nations.
3. Most formal medical language development has been for the purpose of epidemiology, resource management and clinical audit. If there is an agreed set of terms to describe the process of care, then data analysis is much simplified. The goal in developing medical terminologies is to arrive at a consensus on the most appropriate set of terms and the way they should be structured.
4. Languages consist of a basic set of words or **terms**. To permit some flexibility, most medical languages allow the same **concept** to be named in several different ways. However, it is usual to define a single numerical **code** for every distinct concept in the language. A **group** collects together a number of similar codes and can be used for coarse-grained analysis.
5. Classification hierarchies are used to organise terms and codes in a way that permits them to be more easily accessed by those who use them. The type of link used in the hierarchy determines what meaning a term inherits from the terms above it.
6. A terminology can be **enumerative**, listing all possible concepts, or **compositional**, allowing complex concepts to be created from a set of more primitive components. In compositional systems, there is no need to create all terms explicitly in advance, but to make sure that all the basic building blocks exist. This helps to minimise incompleteness, and eliminates duplication or error in the more complex terms.
7. Coding of clinical concepts from the medical record can happen in a number of ways. Specialised staff can do the coding, or clinical staff can do it at the time they enter data into a patient record. Computer systems can be used to assist this process, or to automate it partially.

The terms disease and remedy were formerly understood and therefore defined quite differently to what they are now; so, likewise, are the meanings and definitions of inflammation, pneumonia, typhus, gout, lithiasis, &c., different from those which were attached to them thirty years ago...It is evident ... that great mischief will in most cases ensue if, in such attempts at definition and explanation, greater importance is attached to a clear and determinate, than to a complete and comprehensive understanding of the objects and questions before us. In a field like ours, clearness can in general be purchased only at the expense of completeness and therefore truth.

Oesterlen, *Medical Logic*, (1855)

Chapter 11

Medical terminologies and classification systems

Coding and classification systems have a long history in medicine. Current systems can trace their origins back to epidemiological lists of the causes of death from the early part of the eighteenth century. François Bossier de Lacroix (1706-1777) is commonly credited with the first attempt to classify diseases systematically (ICD-10, 1993). Better known as Sauvages, he published the work under the title *Nosologia Methodica*.

Linnaeus (1707-1778) who was a contemporary of Sauvages also published his *Genera Morborum* in that period. By the beginning of the nineteenth century, the *Synopsis Nosologiae Methodicae*, published in 1785 by William Cullen of Edinburgh (1710-1790) was the classification in most common use.

It was John Graunt who, working about a hundred years earlier, is credited with the first practical attempts to classify disease for statistical purposes. Working on his *London Bills of Mortality*, he was able to estimate the proportion of deaths in different age groups. For example, he estimated a 36% mortality for liveborn children before the age of 6. He did this by taking all the deaths classified as convulsions, rickets, teeth and worms, thrush, abortives, chrysomes, infants, and livergrown. To these he added half of the deaths classed as smallpox, swinepox, measles, and worms without convulsions. By all accounts his estimate was a good one (ICD-10, 1993).

It has only been in the last few decades that these terminological systems have started to attract wide-spread attention and resources. The ever growing need to amass and analyse clinical data, no longer just for epidemiological purposes, has provided considerable incentive and resources for their development. Further, with the development of computer technology, there has been a belief that such wide-spread collection and analysis of data are now possible. In parallel, the requirement for clinicians to participate in that data collection has meant that they have had more opportunity to work with terminologies, and begin to understand their benefits and limitations.

In the previous chapter, the basic concepts of term, code, and classification were introduced. In this chapter, several of the major medical coding and classification systems in routine use will be introduced, and their features compared. Some specific limitations of each system will be highlighted. In reality there are a large number of such systems in development and use, and they cannot all be identified here. The systems discussed are however representative of most systems in common use, and can serve as an introduction to them. Throughout, a historical perspective will be retained, since in this case the lessons of the past have deep implications for the present. The more general limitations of all terminological systems will be addressed in the following chapter.

11.1 The International Classification of Diseases

Purpose. The International Classification of Diseases (ICD) is published by the World Health Organisation. Currently in its tenth revision (ICD-10), its goal is to allow morbidity and mortality data from different countries around the world to be systematically collected and statistically analysed. It is not intended, nor is it suitable, for indexing distinct clinical entities (Gersenovic, 1995). The International Nomenclature of Diseases (IND) provides the set of recommended terms and synonyms that correspond to the entries classified in the ICD codes.

History. The ICD can trace its ancestry to the early days of medical terminologies. William Farr (1807-1883) became the first medical statistician for the General Register Office of England and Wales. Upon taking office, he found the Cullen classification in use, but that it had not been updated in accordance with medical advances, nor did it seem suitable for statistical purposes. In his first Annual Report of the Registrar General, he noted:

> 'The advantages of a uniform statistical nomenclature, however imperfect, are so obvious, that it is surprising that no attention has been paid to its enforcement in Bills of Mortality. Each disease has, in many instances, been denoted by three or four terms, and each term has been applied to as many different diseases: vague, inconvenient names have been employed, or complications have been registered instead of primary diseases. The nomenclature is of as much importance in this department of enquiry as weights and measures in the physical sciences, and should be settled without delay. (ICD-10, 1993).'

Farr toiled hard at improving the classification, and by 1855, the International Statistical Congress adopted a classification based on the work of Farr, and Marc d'Espine of Geneva. Subsequently steered by Jaques Bertillon, this developed into the International List of Causes of Death. This was adopted in 1893, and continued to develop through the turn of the century and beyond, and ultimately evolved into the current ICD system.

In particular, the system was expanded to include not just causes of death, but diseases resulting in measurable morbidity. This expansion started with the urging of Farr. It was supported by Florence Nightingale, who in 1860 urged the adoption of Farr's disease classification for the tabulation of hospital morbidity in her paper *Proposals for a uniform plan of hospital statistics*. In 1900 at the First International Conference to revise the Bertillon Classification, a parallel classification of diseases for use in statistics of sickness was finally adopted.

Level of acceptance and use. The ICD today is used internationally by WHO for comparison of statistical returns. It is also adopted by many individual countries in the preparation of their statistical returns. Most other major classification systems endeavour to make their systems compatible with ICD, so that data coded in these systems can be mapped directly to ICD codes. ICD thus acts as a defacto reference point for many medical terminologies.

Classification structure. The ICD-10 is a multiple-axis classification system. At its core, the basic ICD is a single list of three alphanumeric character codes. These are organised by category, from A00 to Z99 (excluding U codes which are reserved for research, and for the provisional assignment of new diseases of uncertain aetiology). This level of detail is the mandatory level for reporting to the WHO mortality database and for general international comparisons.

The classification is structured into 21 chapters, and the first character of the ICD code is a letter associated with a particular chapter (Table 11.1).

Table 11.1: The ICD-10 chapter headings (adapted from ICD-10, 1993).

Chapter I	Infectious and parasitic diseases
Chapter II	Neoplasms
Chapter III	Diseases of the blood and blood forming organs and certain disorders affecting the immune mechanism
Chapter IV	Endocrine, nutritional and metabolic diseases
Chapter V	Mental and behavioural disorders
Chapter VI	Diseases of the nervous system
Chapter VII	Diseases of the eye and adnexa
Chapter VIII	Diseases of the ear and mastoid process
Chapter IX	Diseases of the circulatory system
Chapter X	Diseases of the respiratory system
Chapter XI	Diseases of the digestive system
Chapter XII	Diseases of skin and subcutaneous tissue
Chapter XIII	Diseases of musculoskeletal system and connective tissue
Chapter XIV	Diseases of the genitourinary system
Chapter XV	Pregnancy, childbirth and the puerperium
Chapter XVI	Certain conditions originating in the perinatal period
Chapter XVII	Congenital malformations, deformations and chromosomal abnormalities
Chapter XVIII	Symptoms, signs and abnormal clinical and laboratory findings
Chapter XIX	Injuries, poisoning and certain other consequences of external causes
Chapter XX	External causes of morbidity and mortality
Chapter XXI	Factors affecting health status and contact with health services of a person not currently sick

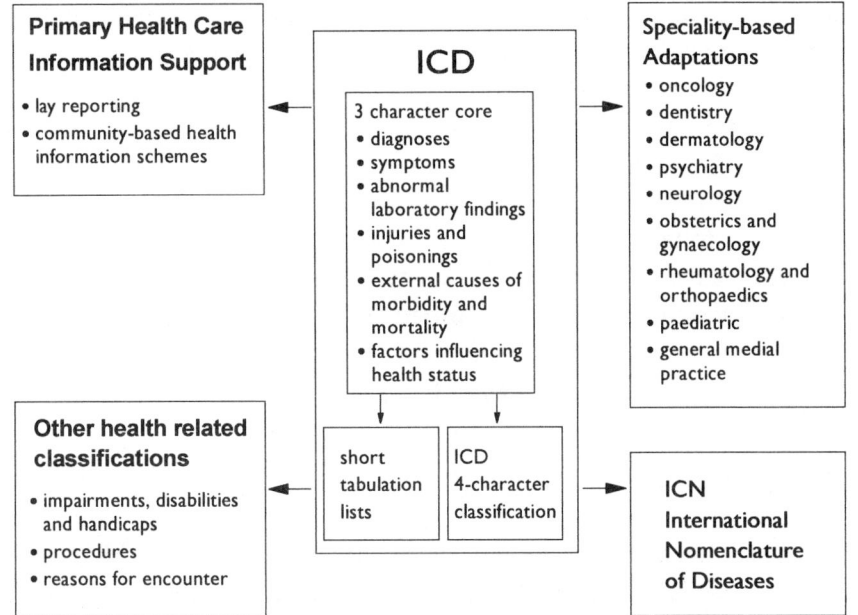

Figure 11.1: *The ICD family of disease and health-related classifications (adapted from ICD-10, 1993).*

Within chapters, the 3 character codes are divided into homogenous blocks reflecting different axes of classification. In Chapter I for example, the blocks signify the axes of mode of transmission and of the broad group of the infecting organism. Within Chapter II on neoplasms, the first axis is the behaviour of the neoplasm, and the next is its site. Within all blocks some codes are reserved for conditions not specified elsewhere in the classification.

When more detail is required, each category in ICD can be further subdivided, using a fourth numeric character after a decimal point, creating up to 10 subcategories. This is used, for example, to classify histological varieties of neoplasms. A few chapters adopt five or more characters to allow further subclassification along different axes.

Since ICD continues to be used for ever wider applications beyond its intent, the WHO decided in the 10th revision to develop the concept of a family of related classifications surrounding this core set. This 'family' contains for example, lists condensed from the full ICD, and lists expanded for speciality-based adaptations (Figure 11.1). It also contains lists that cover topics beyond morbidity and mortality. For example, there are classifications of medical and surgical procedures, disablement and so forth (Gersenovic, 1995).

Limitations. The ICD has developed as a practical, rather than theoretically based, classification. There have been compromises between classification based on axes of aetiology, anatomical site and so on. There have also been adjustments made to it to meet the needs of different statistical applications beyond morbidity and mortality, for example social security. As such, the ICD exists as a practical attempt at compromise between various health care needs. Consequently, for many applications, finer levels of detail may still be needed, or other axes of classification required.

11.2 Diagnosis Related Groups

Purpose. Diagnosis Related Groups (DRGs) relate patient diagnosis to cost of treatment (Murphy-Muth, 1987; Feinstein, 1988). Developed in the United States by the Health Care Finance Administration, DRGs were designed to calculate federal reimbursement for care delivered under the Medicare system. Each DRG takes the principle diagnosis or procedure responsible for a patient's admission, and is given a corresponding cost weighting. This weight is applied according to a formula to determine the amount that should be paid to an institution for a patient with a particular DRG.

DRGs are also used to determine an institution's overall **case-mix**. The case-mix index helps to take account of the types of patient an individual institution sees, and estimates their severity of illness. Thus a hospital seeing the same proportion of patients as another, but dealing with more severe illness, will have a higher case-mix index. An institution's case-mix index can then be used in the formula that determines reimbursement per individual DRG. Unsurprisingly different versions of the reimbursement formula favour different types of institution, and case-mix represents an area for ongoing debate and research.

History. In the mid 1970s the Centre for Health Studies at Yale University began work on a system for monitoring hospital utilisation review (Rothwell, 1987). Following a 1976 trial of a DRG system, it was decided to base the final system on the ICD-9-CM which would provide the basic diagnostic categories. The ICD-9-CM (clinical modifications) classification was developed from the ICD-9 by the American Commission on Professional and Hospital Activities. It contains finer-grained clinical detail than the old ICD-9, and is intended for medical review and reimbursement use.

Level of acceptance and use. DRGs are used routinely in the United States for management review and payment. Given the importance of reimbursement world-wide, DRGs have undergone ongoing development, and have been adopted in one form or another in many countries outside the USA.

Classification structure. Patients are initially assigned an ICD-9 CM code. ICD-9 CM is a multiaxial system closely based on the ICD 9 structure. Diagnoses are then partitioned into one of about 23 Major Diagnostic Categories (MDCs) according to body organ system or disease. The aim of this step is to group codes into similar categories that reflect consumption of resources and treatment (Figure 10.1). Codes are next partitioned based upon the performance of procedures, and then the presence of complications, patient age, and extended length of stay, before a DRG is finally assigned (Rothwell, 1987). There is thus a process of category reduction at each stage, starting from the many thousands of ICD codes to the few hundred DRGs:

$$\text{ICD 9-CM} \Rightarrow \text{MDC} \Rightarrow \text{DRG}$$

Limitations. Given the local variations in clinical practice, disease incidence, patient selection, procedures performed, and resources, DRGs and case-mix indices will always only give approximate estimates of the true resource utilisation. For example, should a hospital that is developing new and expensive procedures be paid the same amount as an institution that treats the same type of patient with a more common and cheaper procedure? Should quality of care be reflected in a DRG? For example, if a hospital delivers good quality of care that results in better patient outcomes, should it be paid the same as a hospital that performs more poorly for the same type of patient?

As importantly, those institutions that are best able to create DRGs accurately are more likely to receive reimbursement in line with their true expenditure on care. There is thus an implication in the DRG model that an institution actually has the ability to accurately assemble information to derive DRGs and a case-mix index. Given local and national variations in information systems and coding practice, it is likely that institutions with poor information systems will be disadvantaged, unless the information infrastructure across a region is a 'level playing field'.

Developments. DRGs are designed for use with inpatients. Accordingly, other systems have been developed for other areas of healthcare. Ambulatory Visit Groups (AVGs) have been developed for outpatient or ambulatory care in the primary sector. These are based upon a patient's diagnosis, visit status and physician time. Given the increasing age of the population in western nations, there is a tremendous ongoing cost that comes from the chronic care needed by the elderly. Consequently Resource Utilisation Groups (RUGs) have been developed to help determine the usage of long-term care resources. RUGs are based upon the time spent by nursing home staff when caring for a patient.

11.3 SNOMED

Purpose. The Systematized nomenclature of medicine is intended to be a general-purpose, comprehensive and computer-processable terminology to represent and, according to its creators, will index "virtually all of the events found in the medical record" (Côté et al., 1993).

History. SNOMED was derived from the 1968 edition of the *Manual of tumour nomenclature and coding* (MONTAC) and the *Systematized nomenclature of pathology* (SNOP). In its current form, SNOMED International is a development of the second edition of SNOMED, published in 1979 by the American College of Pathologists. SNOMED International is reportedly being translated into twelve separate languages (Rothwell, 1995).

Classification structure. SNOMED is a multi-axial classification system. Terms are assigned to one of eleven independent systematised modules, corresponding to different axes of classification (Table 11.2). Each term is placed into a hierarchy within one of these modules, and assigned a five or six digit alphanumeric code.

Module designator	No Records
Topography (T)	12,385
Morphology (M)	4,991
Function (F)	16,352
Living Organisms (L)	24,265
Chemicals, Drugs & Biological Products (C)	14,075
Physical Agents, Forces & Activities (A)	1,355
Occupations (J)	1,886
Social Context (S)	433
Diseases/Diagnoses (D)	28,622
Procedures (P)	25,000 (estimate)
General Linkage-Modifiers (G)	1,176

Table 11.2: The SNOMED International modules (or axes) and the number of terms within each (adapted from Rothwell, 1995).

Terms can also be cross-referenced across these modules. Each code carries with it a packet of information about the terms it designates, giving some notion of the medical context of that code (Table 11.3). SNOMED also allows the composition of complex terms from simpler terms, and is thus partially compositional. SNOMED International incorporates virtually all of the ICD-9-CM terms and codes, allowing reports to generated in this format if necessary.

	Nomenclature				Classification
Axis	T	+ M	+ L	+ F	= D
Term	Lung	+ Granuloma	+ M. tuberculosis	+ Fever	= Tuberculosis
Code	T-28000	+ M-44000	+ L-21801	+ F-03003	= DE-14800

Table 11.3: An example of SNOMED's nomenclature and classification. Some terms (e.g. Tuberculosis) can be cross-referenced to others, to give the term a richer clinical context (adapted from Rothwell, 1995).

Limitations. It is possible, given the richness of the SNOMED structure, to express the same concept in many ways. For example, acute appendicitis has a single code D5-46210. However, there are also terms and codes for 'acute', 'acute inflammation', and 'in'. Thus this concept could be expressed either as Appendicitis, acute; or Acute inflammation, in, Appendix; and Acute, inflammation NOS, in, Appendix (Rothwell, 1995). This makes it difficult for example, to compare similar concepts that have been indexed in different ways, or to search for a term that exists in different forms within a medical record.

Further, while SNOMED permits single terms to be combined to create complex terms, rules for the combination of terms have not been developed. Consequently such compositions may not be medically valid.

11.4 The Read codes

Purpose. The Read codes are produced for clinicians, initially in primary care, who wish to audit the process of care. Version 3 is intended, like SNOMED International, to code events in the electronic patient record (O'Neil et al., 1995).

History. The Read codes were introduced in the UK in 1986 to generate computer summaries of patient care in primary care. In the subsequent revision Version 2, their structure was changed and based upon ICD-9 and OPCS-4, the Classification of Surgical Operations and Procedures. As Version 2 became increasingly inadequate, the UK's Conference of Medical Royal Colleges, and the government's National Health Service (NHS) established a joint Clinical Terms Project, comprising some 40 working groups representing the different specialities. This was subsequently joined by groups representing nurses and allied health professionals. Version 3 of the Read codes was created in response to the output of the Terms project.

Level of acceptance and use. Use of the Read codes is not mandatory in the UK. However, in 1994 it was recommended by the medical and nursing professional bodies as the preferred dictionary for clinical information systems. The Read codes have been purchased by the UK government and made Crown Copyright.

Classification structure. The Read codes have undergone substantive changes through their various revisions, altering not just the classification and terminological content, but also their structure. In Versions 1 and 2, Read was a strictly hierarchical classification system.

Read Version 3 is released in 2 stages. Version 3.0 is a kind of compositional classification system. Like SNOMED, a term can appear in several different 'hierarchical structures', classified against different axes. Unlike ICD or SNOMED, the codes themselves do not reflect a given hierarchy. They simply act as a unique identifier for a medical concept. The 'hierarchy' exists as a set of links between concepts. Terms can inherit properties across these links. For example, 'pulmonary tuberculosis' may naturally inherit from a parent respiratory disorder or a parent infection term.

In Version 3.1, a set of qualifier terms such as anatomical site is added that can be combined with existing terms. When terms are composed, these composites exist outside of any strict hierarchy. To help in the combination of qualifiers with terms, they are grouped into templates. These capture some rules that help describe the range of possible qualifiers that a term in Read can take (Table 11.4).

Object	Applicable Attribute	Applicable values
Bone operation	Site	Bone, Part of Bone
Fixation of fracture	Reduction method	Percutaneous, open, closed
Fixation of fracture using intramedullary nail	Reaming method	Hand, powered rigid, powered flexible, etc.
Fixation of fracture using intramedullary nail	Nail Type	Flexible, Locking, Rigid, etc.

Table 11.4: Example Read Version 3.1 template showing allowable combinations of terms with qualifier attributes, and attribute values (adapted from O'Neil et al., 1995).

Like other major systems, Read offers mapping to ICD-9 codes to permit international reporting, and in some cases also provides ICD-10 mapping.

Although Read Version 3 does not overtly emphasise axes of classification like SNOMED, both systems allow terms to be linked to each other and to inherit properties across those links. Therefore the underlying potential for expressiveness is the same at the structural level. Differences in the number and type of terms, and the richness of interconnections between them are probably greater determinants of difference between these coding systems, than any underlying structural difference. The presence of a fixed hierarchy, as we find with ICD or SNOMED, carries certain benefits of regularity when exploring the system. It also imposes greater constraints when it is necessary to alter the system because of changes to the terminology. In Read, this burden of regularity begins to be shifted to the rules guiding the composition of terms.

Limitations. The Read templates for term composition are limited in their ability to control combination. A much richer language and knowledge base would be needed to regulate term combination (Rector et al., 1995).

11.5 Comparing coding systems is not easy

While it is beguiling to try to compare the utility of different coding systems, such comparisons are often ill-considered. This is because it is not always obvious how to compare the ability of different systems to code concepts found in a medical record. For example, Campbell et al. (1994), reported results of various systems coding terms found in selected patient problem lists from US medical records. They assessed that ICD-9-CM and Read Version 2 'perform much more poorly for problem coding' than either SNOMED or the UMLS systems. As a consequence they concluded that 'both UMLS and SNOMED are more complete than alternative systems' when developing computer-based patient records.

Such generalisations are not meaningful. Firstly, term requirements vary from task to task. Indeed, terms develop out of the language of particular groups on particular tasks. It is thus not meaningful to compare performance on one task and deduce that similar outcomes will result for tests on other tasks.

As critically, term use will vary between user populations. The terms used in a primary care setting will differ to those used in a clinic allied to a hospital, reflecting different practices and patient populations. Differing disease patterns and practices also distinguish different nations. A system like Read Version 2, designed for UK primary care, may not perform as well in US clinics as a US designed system. The reverse may also be true of a US designed system applied in the UK.

In summary, coding systems should be compared on specified tasks and contexts, and the results should only cautiously be generalised to other tasks and contexts. Equally the poor performance of coding systems on tasks outside the scope of their design should not reflect badly on their intended performance.

Chapter summary

1. The International Classification of Diseases (ICD) is published by the World Health Organisation. Currently in its tenth revision (ICD-10), its goal is to allow morbidity and mortality data from different countries around the world to be systematically collected and statistically analysed.

2. Diagnosis Related Groups (DRGs) relate patient diagnosis to cost of treatment. Each DRG takes the principle diagnosis or procedure responsible for a patient's admission, and is given a corresponding cost weighting. This weight is applied according to a formula to determine the amount that should be paid to an institution for a patient with a particular DRG. DRGs are also used to determine an institution's overall **case-mix**.

3. The Systematized Nomenclature of Medicine (SNOMED) is intended to be a general-purpose, comprehensive and computer-processable terminology to represent. Derived from the 1968 edition of the *Manual of Tumour Nomenclature and Coding*, the second edition of SNOMED International is reportedly being translated into twelve separate languages.

4. The Read codes are produced for clinicians, initially in primary care, who wish to audit the process of care. Version 3 is intended, like SNOMED International, to code events in the electronic patient record.

5. Coding systems should be compared on specified tasks, and results should only cautiously be generalised to other tasks, and populations. Equally the poor performance of coding systems on tasks outside their design should not reflect badly on their intended performance.

The problem was that every system of classification I had ever known in biology or in physical science was designed for mutually exclusive categories. A particular chemical element was sodium, potassium or strontium, but not two of those, or all three. An animal might be a fish or fowl, not both. But a patient might have many different clinical properties simultaneously. I wanted to find mutually exclusive categories for classifying patients, but I could not get the different categories separated. They all seemed to overlap, and I could find no consistent way to separate the overlap.

Feinstein, *Clinical Judgement*, p10, (1967)

Chapter 12

The trouble with coding

Terminological systems are usually created with a specific purpose in mind. ICD was created to collect morbidity and mortality statistics. The Read codes were initially developed for primary care physicians, and SNOMED was originally developed to code pathological concepts. As these systems grow in size, and as their use becomes wide-spread within their intended domain, it becomes increasingly tempting to reuse them for other tasks.

As a consequence, some terminological systems have been redeveloped to become general purpose coding systems. It is often a declared intention in the evolution of such general purpose systems that they become complete and universal medical languages. Systems like SNOMED or Read should be able, for example, to describe all the necessary concepts that might be found in a medical record.

Recent advances in terminological research, as well as evidence from related disciplines, does not support such a goal. As we will see in this chapter, current thinking suggests that the goal of constructing a complete and universal thesaurus of medical terms is ill-posed. Terminology evolves in a context of use, and attempting to define a general purpose, or context independent terminology is ultimately implausible. Coupled with this view comes the pragmatic understanding that any terminology we build will always be imperfect.

Each of these important issues deserves to be examined in some detail. This chapter first looks at the theoretical limitations facing all terminology constructors. It then moves on to examine how, given these limitations, terminological systems can be built that perform acceptably and at a reasonable cost.

12.1 Universal terminological systems are impossible to build

The ideal terminological system would be a complete, formal and universal language that allowed all medical concepts to be described, reasoned about and communicated. Some researchers have explicitly asserted that building such a singular and 'correct' medical language is their goal (Cimino, 1994; Evans et al., 1994).

This task emphasises two clear requirements: the ability for the terminological language to cover all the concepts that need to be reasoned about, and the independence of the terminology from any particular reasoning task. A further goal occasionally articulated is that, where alternative terminologies exist, they must be logically related so that one can be translated into the other. For example, if a set of clinical codes is extracted from a patient record, those codes could then be translated into ICD codes or DRGs.

Despite the enormous healthcare investment devoted to achieving these goals, current evidence indicates that they are not possible. There is no pure set of codes or terms that can be universally applied in medicine. There is consequently no universal way in which one medical language can be mapped onto another.

There are two fundamental and related obstacles to devising a universal terminological system. The first is the **model construction** problem. Terminologies are simply a way of modelling the world, and as we saw in Chapter 1, the world is always richer and more complex than any model humans can devise. The second is the **symbol grounding** problem. The words we use to label objects do not necessarily reflect the way we think about the objects, nor do they necessarily reflect defined objects in the real world (Norman, 1993). The cumulative evidence from recent thinking in cognitive science, computer science and artificial intelligence provides a

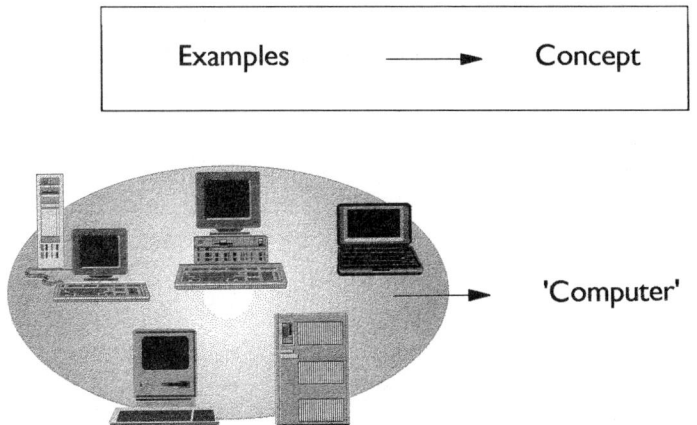

Figure 12.1: Word concepts are created to describe classes of objects that have similar but not identical characteristics. Individual examples of the concept may have unique properties that are not shared by other examples that also fall into their class.

formidable set of supporting arguments. Each of these major issues will now be examined in a little more detail.

Terms are subjective

It is perhaps intuitive to think that the words we use correspond to objective and clearly definable parts of the world. Words should clearly correspond to observable objects. However, cognitive studies of the way people form word categories have shifted us from the view that categories exist objectively. Research suggests that concepts are relative, and are structured around probabilistic prototypes.

These concept prototypes at the **basic level** are the product of pooling many examples observed from the world (Box 10.1). They capture aspects common to all the examples. Equally they exclude aspects that are not universally shared. Thus the qualities of prototypical categories are only generally true of the examples they classify (Figure 12.1). For example, most people would happily say that flight was a property of birds, and cope with the fact that some birds are flightless. The category 'bird' has no pure definition. By implication, the same must be true of the words used by people in medicine. Thus the term 'angina' actually corresponds to a wide variety of different presentations of pain. Students will be taught the classical presentations of angina, but will with clinical experience quickly learn that there are many variations to the general case.

Concept creation is thus a process of generalisation from example. The creation of concept prototypes is an ongoing part of human activity, as language tracks changes in our way of viewing the world (Box 12.1). The way in which people use resemblances amongst a group of examples to create general categories remains an area of ongoing research (e.g. Ahn and Medin, 1992). We also saw in Chapter 10 that different hierarchies can be created, depending on the attributes used to link the terms. Selecting a different set of attributes from the same object will probably result in a different categorisation structure. Categories may also overlap, and objects might fit into several different categories.

From the point of terminological construction, this means that there can be no clean set of terms that clearly demarcate different concepts. Concepts overlap, and so do terms. There thus can be no objective classification model. Many artificial intelligence researchers agree, arguing that there is no objective model of medical knowledge. Much of this is based on their experiences in constructing and maintaining knowledge-based systems (Clancy, 1993a and 1993b).

Terms are context-dependent

A consequence of this process of category formation is that there is no stable notion of the 'correct' category for objects or events. The best category to describe an object depends entirely on the context within which it is applied. Thus a patient might be categorised as 'elderly' if they are over the age of 70. If however, a woman is having a first child, the term 'elderly' primpara might be given to them if they are over 35. The notion of elderly varies with the context within which one operates. We thus choose attributes of an object or event that are of interest to us in a given context, and use these to place it in a category.

Context-dependence has several implications. Firstly, automatically extracting coded terms from a medical record will be difficult. This requires the ability to understand the wider context surrounding a term. Is a 'ventricle' in the heart or the brain? In the sentence 'I spoke to him' the meaning of the word 'him' depends on information that exists outside the sentence.

Box 12.1 - The dominant design

What defines our notions of prototypic concepts like a typewriter, a computer or a car? We know from the way basic level descriptions are used that words are preferred when they become prototypic of the functions of a wider class (Box 10.1).

It is an interesting feature of the marketplace that the introduction of a new class of product at first usually sees a great variety of competing designs enter the market. Each competing design has new features, or different combinations of existing ones. After a period however, such variety almost completely disappears, and most producers end up creating products which have remarkably similar features.

Thus, the first typewriter was produced by Scholes in 1868, and was followed by a host of competing designs. However, 1899 saw the introduction of the Underwood Model 5 typewriter which today we all would recognise as a modern typewriter. Soon after its introduction, because of its immense popularity, all other manufacturers found themselves forced to approximate the Underwood design. Indeed, the design persisted throughout the first half of the twentieth century. It was not until the introduction of electronic typewriters, computers and word processors that radically different sets of designs and functions were introduced.

The evolution of the modern personal computer followed along the same path, with an initial flurry of different designs. Eventually the marketplace settled upon a set of prototypic features that most people would expect when they bought a personal computer (Figure 12.1).

This stable design point in the history of a product class is known as a **dominant design** (Utterback, 1994), and has many interesting parallels with Rosch's basic level. The dominant design 'embodies the requirements of many classes of users of a particular product, even though it may not meet the needs of a particular class to quite the same extent as would a customized design.'

Further, even though a dominant design may after a time become obsolete, its wide-spread adoption and individuals' investment in learning to work with it make them reluctant to shift to a better design. So, even though there are probably numerous better designs than the QWERTY keyboard, most people who have learnt to use one are reluctant to shift to using a better design. Thus, once in place, the dominant design remains fixed, not because newer designs do not offer benefits, but because changing to them incurs unacceptable costs. Only when the cost-benefit trade-off shifts heavily the other way will a new product class become acceptable.

As a result, a computer system would need to have a considerable amount of knowledge about medicine and language before it could successfully interpret much of the medical record. Secondly, if a set of terms is used in a variety of different contexts, then the same term may have a different meaning across these contexts. Pooling data coded by terms thus might risk grouping together quite different things.

Terms are purposive

We have already seen that categories can be quite indistinct things, and that category assignment varies depending on context. Both these issues are reflections of the underlying principle that words are created with the intention that they will be used in a particular way. Language is created for a purpose.

This perspective was illuminated by the philosopher Wittgenstein, who started his career searching for pure philosophical propositions, but soon rejected this search. He was unable to conceive of concepts or language independently of the purpose for which they were created. He thus came to understand that even fields like philosophy or mathematics were actually sets of techniques. They were not collections of objective truth, but knowledge about ways of doing things. It followed that their words were no less subjective.

He invented what are known as **language games** in which a language was created for some tightly defined purpose. The essential point of these games was that one could not describe the language without mentioning the use to which it was put. Wittgenstein used these games to help free us from considering language in isolation from the purpose for which it was created (Wittgenstein, 1953; Monk, 1990).

Medicine, unlike mathematics or philosophy, has always been an applied field. Here, more than in most areas of endeavour, it should be clear that our technical terms and words are created to be applied. Even the apparently most precise medical concepts usually have edges that are demarcated through use. The concept of a bone fracture for example, may seem to be a quite distinct concept, but the dividing line between a normal and a fractured bone is quite unclear. As we move from plane X-rays to CT and MRI scans, the ability to categorise a bone as being fractured increases. The limit to definition is thus actually dependent on the limit to detection.

Further, the lengths one goes to in the detection of a fracture depends entirely on the purpose at hand, which is usually to treat. Thus, if cellular studies of bone activity could detect fine fractures that were not visible by other means, would patients investigated in this way be classed as having a fracture? If their management was quite different, then perhaps they would be categorised in a quite different way.

In medicine, one way to deal with this lack of clarity is to create artificial definitions of disease concepts with a purpose in mind. The purpose is to identify patients so that they can be treated. These definitions are usually based on observations or measurements. They are constructed in such a way that most patients with the condition, based on statistical studies, will be included within the definition. In this way, medicine is seen to replicate in a formal way the innate human process of category formation, which is also founded on some quasi-probabilistic basis.

The implication here is that terminologies are most likely to be of value if they are created with a specific purpose in mind. Consequently, a general purpose terminology will always fail to meet many of the specific needs of different situations, because these cannot be anticipated without specific examination of individual uses.

This is true both of the kinds of concepts represented in a terminology, as well as the level of detail of terms. In general, people choose categories to describe events or objects at a level of description that is most appropriate for thinking about them in a given situation (Rosch, 1988). A general purpose terminology will thus always have difficulty matching its level of detail to that needed in specific situations.

This also means that general categories are of little use. It is understood from the field of knowledge representation that the more general a concept is, the less it says about the world, and the weaker its descriptive power. The corollary is that more specific concepts have a much greater power of description. Consider the difference between describing a patient as being 'sick' and as 'hypertensive'. Both might be correct, but the one that is most specific to the patient is the most useful. The general category of 'sick' would describe most patients, and so carries very little descriptive power with it.

Consequently it does not make sense to think of terminological systems developing independently of a context of use. Even those who seek to build a canonical medical terminology are forced to select a clinical application to set a context before they can meaningfully proceed (e.g. Friedman et al., 1995).

Terms evolve over time

Medicine's terms have evolved over many years and are subject to the same process of cognitive evolution that affects all human language. Disease entities exist for as long as they are useful mental constructs, and are replaced as better concepts emerge. There is no static body of medical knowledge.

Not only are new concepts added, often the very structure of medical knowledge changes as concepts are internally re-organised (Feinstein, 1988; Clancy, 1993b). Many diseases that were commonly discussed a century ago would not be recognised by health care workers today. Indeed, since the first ICD was created at the turn of the century with several hundred concepts, the growth in medical knowledge has expanded the current ICD to contain over 6000 concepts. More recently the process seems to have accelerated. ICD-9 and 10 are substantially different systems, partly because of the changes in medicine over the 15 year period in which ICD-10 was built (CCC, 1995).

A consequence of the changing state of medical knowledge is that any attempt at modelling medical knowledge by the imposition of a structure on its terms will decay in accuracy over time (see Chapter 6). As soon as a terminology is created, medical knowledge begins to evolve away from that structure (Hogarth, 1986; Tuttle and Nelson 1994).

Different systems may not correspond directly

Equally, there is no reason to expect that there is any uniform mapping between terminological systems developed in different contexts of use (Glowinski, 1994; Tuttle, 1994). Should one expect for example, that it is natural that every concept in ICD should find a corresponding concept in Read or SNOMED? While there are often clear correspondences, the mapping is never complete. The greater the difference in purpose for which these systems are created, the greater is the mismatch.

The reason that the ICD seems to serve as a common reference system is that it is created at relatively general level of description. Other systems like Read or SNOMED tend to be more fine-grained in their terms. Consequently it is more likely that one can find a general ICD category that matches a more specific category within these other systems. Such a translation from specific to general will lose some of the detail and meaning from the original term. As long as this suits the purpose of the translation, then this is tolerable. For example, if one wanted to convert a detailed coding of a patient created for clinical purposes into more general ICD categories to create a morbidity report, then the loss of detail is appropriate.

However, even when the systems are of similar construction, problems are encountered when one tries to translate knowledge expressed in one form into another. The authors of one study concluded that the sharing knowledge between terminological systems 'does not seem to be easily achievable' (Heinsohn, 1994).

12.2 Building and maintaining terminologies is similar to software engineering

While coding systems can never be truly canonical, they still provide a practical basis for managing the language of medicine. However, it has to be understood that they define a limited and consensual language that will have to be modified continually. This modification is a predictable consequence of the subjectivity of knowledge. Whenever a knowledge base is applied to a task outside its intended use, it will require change (Clancy, 1993).

SNOMED, for example was initially developed to classify pathological items. It has now been expanded to produce a general purpose system for all of medicine. However a study of SNOMED's utility in coding nursing reports found it coded only about 69% of terms, with the implication that the missing terms would need to be added (Henry et al., 1993). Such additions are required every time a terminology is applied to a new area, making the task of updating problematic (Cimino and Clayton, 1994).

Eventually, as a terminology is continually expanded into new areas, its fundamental organisational structure will be altered to reflect the different structure of these new areas (Clancy, 1993b). The process of terminology growth and alteration introduces huge problems of maintenance, and the very real possibility that the system will start to incorporate errors, duplications and contradictions.

If we simply think of terminologies as computer programs then we already know that continued modification is a poor development strategy. Software engineering tells us that the best time to modify a program is early in the development cycle. In Figure 12.2 the cost of error removal is shown to grow exponentially during the development of a computer program. Further, the times at which errors are introduced and detected are different. Thus an error introduced during the initial functional specification of a program is likely to be detected only when the system is completed and in regular use. At this time, the users will suggest ways in which the system's actual functionality, and the functionality they expected, differs.

Introducing changes into a mature system thus becomes increasingly expensive over time (Littlewood, 1987). As a corollary, maintaining a terminological system will become increasingly expensive over time. Consequently, we have probably reached the stage where uncontrolled addition of terms to existing large thesauri will soon no longer be acceptable. Those who pay for their maintenance will be faced with ever increasing costs. To manage these costs, one would need to measure the performance of a thesaurus on a particular task, and then determine whether proposed additions or alterations will improve that performance, and at what cost.

12.3 Compositional terminologies may be easier to maintain over time despite higher initial building costs

In the longer term, new approaches are needed. Most existing coding systems are enumerative, listing out all the possible terms that could be used in advance. In the compositional approach introduced in Chapter 10, terms are created from a more basic set of components

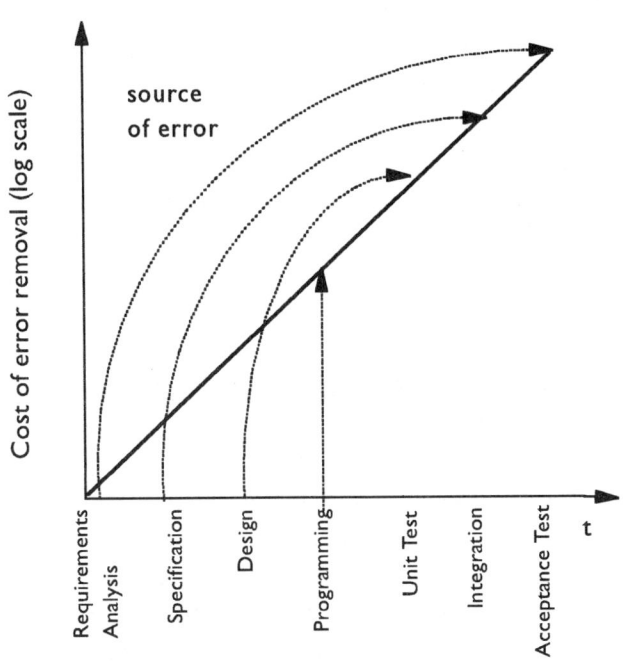

Figure 12.2: *The cost of removing an error in the different stages of software development increases logarithmically. Errors introduced at the beginning of the specification phase are likely to only be detected during the use of the product (after Cohen, 1986).*

that may be more practical to build, maintain and use (Rector et al., 1993; Glowinski, 1994).

There are two broad hypotheses behind the compositional proposal. The first is an engineering hypothesis - that compositional systems are easier and cheaper to maintain and update than enumerative ones. The second one is that compositional systems somehow represent a deeper form of knowledge. While the first hypothesis has merit, the second is somewhat more contentious. Each of these claims will now be examined in some more detail.

The costs of maintaining compositional terminologies may be lower than for enumerative systems

As we have seen, terminological systems continually require extensions and alterations that will over time introduce inconsistencies to the system. As an enumerative terminology gets bigger, the cost of finding and repairing these inconsistencies increases.

Any change in a concept must also be reflected throughout the enumerative system. For example, if a disease entity is redefined into two related diseases, then every term that exists for the original disease will need to be changed. In contrast, most terms in a compositional system are generated from simpler ones. Thus, one may only need to change the core terms associated with the disease. These alterations can be immediately reflected in any new term generated. As a consequence, fewer changes will be required in a compositional system (Figure 12.3).

The initial investment in a compositional system may be higher than for an enumerative system

Thus the costs of maintaining a compositional system, as measured by the number of changes needed, should theoretically be lower over time. In contrast, the initial stages of building a compositional terminology are actually much more complex than building an enumerative one. The compositional approach starts by defining a core set of terms, and the rules about the way those terms can be combined. It thus requires more information about individual terms and the ways they could combine.

There are no such burdens imposed upon the builder of an enumerative system. Here the cost will be paid later on as the number of terms grows. In theory then, the investment in the compositional system is initially higher, but begins to pay off over time, as it requires less effort to maintain and enlarge (Goble et al., 1993a; Glowinski, 1994). Eventually a point is reached where the total investment in the compositional system becomes less than for a comparable enumerative one (Figure 12.4).

However, the cost of maintaining a system does not just come from the need to update the system as knowledge changes. For any large system it is usually the case that it will contain errors that are introduced when terms are created. The cost of detection and correction of such errors, as we have already seen, is high and grows as a system matures. Current research suggests that this cost of error checking may be reduced in compositional systems (Gobel et al., 1993b). Since each term needs to be defined in some detail to permit checking when terms are assembled, this information can also be

Enumerative

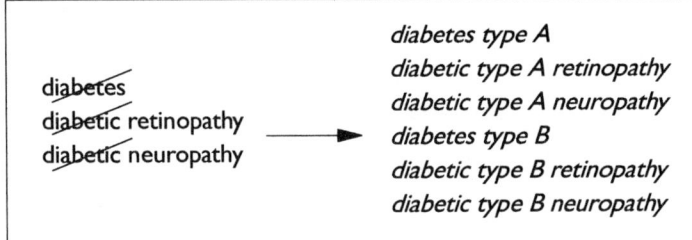

Compositional

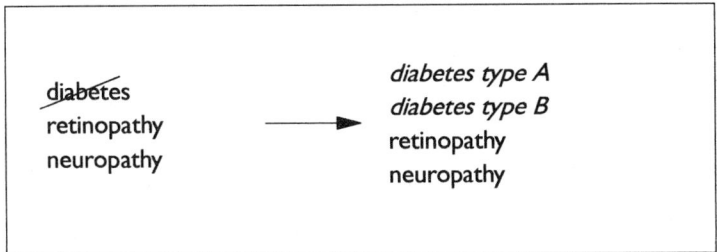

Figure 12.3: The number of changes required when altering a concept is greater for an enumerative terminological system than for a compositional system.

used to check for errors. Checking rules can be constructed to look over the database of terms whenever new terms are introduced, to make sure than the addition does not introduce new inconsistencies.

There are computational and search costs when using terminologies

Another cost with any terminological system is associated with the time and computer resource needed to retrieve a term from the system. These can be broken down into two broad costs. The first is the cost of searching the terminology for a term. Clearly as the terminology grows it will take longer to search it. The more expressive and complete an enumerative system is then, the slower it is to use (Heinsohn, 1994). In this respect, since a compositional system should have a smaller set of terms it will be quicker to search through than an enumerative one.

However, there is a second cost that is related to the computation needed after searching. There is no such cost associated with an enumerative system. Once a term has been found no further work needs to be done. In contrast, the cost of using a compositional

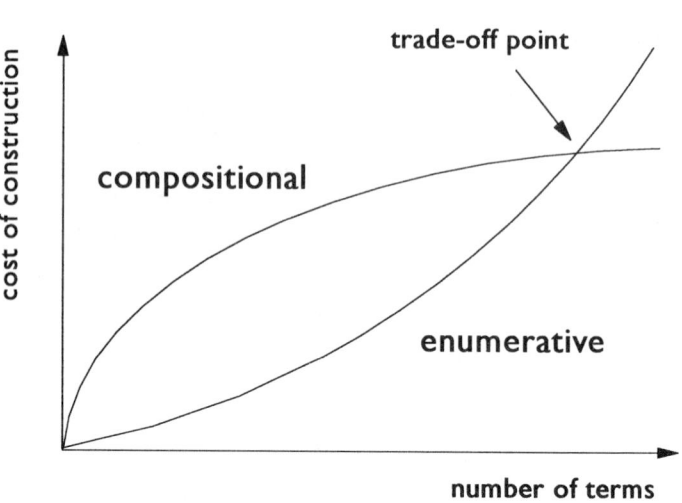

Figure 12.4: *The cost of constructing and maintaining a compositional system may initially be higher, but as the number of terms grows, the enumerative approach may become more expensive. This graph is illustrative only, as the actual shape of these cost functions still remains to be determined.*

system it is that each answer has to be derived from 'first principles'. Simple terms have to be assembled into complex ones, and then checked against rules to see if these constructions are reasonable.

Both searching and composing require computer time, and their effect on usability of a terminology depends upon the performance of the computer system used. One of the engineering trade-offs to be explored in the future will be to decide whether a compositional system is quicker to use than a larger enumerative one. The current hypothesis is that, as enumerative systems grow to be too large, the enumerative search costs should outweigh the compositional computation costs.

Evidence from other disciplines supports the contention that the compositional approach will eventually be fastest. For example in computer engineering, so called reduced instruction set computer chips (RISC) have a small set of basic operations that can be combined to do more complex operations. These chips are much faster than traditional ones that have a large enumeration of operations to cover many eventualities.

Mapping across terminologies may be easier if they are compositional

The fundamental difficulties with mapping between terminologies and coding systems have already been described. While there seems

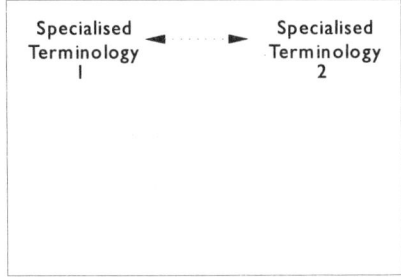 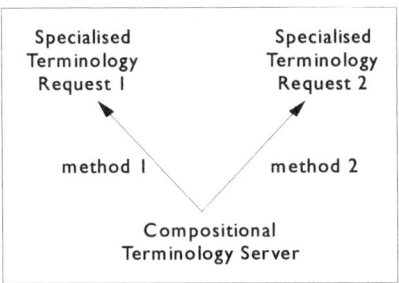

Enumerative Terminologies

Compositional Terminologies

Figure 12.5: Enumerative terminological systems are developed independently of each other. Compositional systems try to use basic terminology building blocks along with specialised methods to generate terms for specialised needs. Mapping between specialised terms is not uniformly possible with enumerative systems, but inherent in the design of compositional systems.

to be no fundamental solution to this general problem, there may be ways of minimising it through term composition. By definition, since compositional terms are generated from the same core terms and the method of generation is known, they should map onto one another logically.

This means that if terms are created for quite different purposes, but come from the same compositional system, then it should be possible to create a mapping between them (Figure 12.5). However, the degree of success possible from such an approach is still unmeasured. It should theoretically be better than customised mappings that are individually developed between independently created terminologies.

Depth of knowledge

The second major compositional hypothesis is a scientific one and is more controversial. It states that there exists a 'deep' set of medical knowledge upon which the core terms can be based, and from which new terms can be composed (Friedman, 1995).

The quest for 'deep' knowledge has been a focus for considerable effort within the artificial intelligence research community, especially in relation to the construction of expert systems (see Chapter 19). In the end, the term 'deep' has fallen into disuse, as it has become clear that it provides little value in distinguishing knowledge (Coiera, 1992a). Like all models of the world, it is more useful to characterise the differences in knowledge bases based upon their level of detail, generality, or point of view.

Thus compositional systems, like their enumerative counterparts, are only models of the world. They suffer the same issues of model fidelity and subjectivity. While they intrinsically capture a richer set of relations between terms than in an enumerative system, there is no greater 'depth' to the knowledge they encode. It is either just more detailed, more general, or different in point of view.

12.4 The way forward

It should be clear by now that the task of creating, using and maintaining medical terminologies is a highly complex endeavour. It should also be clear that, while it is deceptively easy to start to create a terminology, one soon encounters some of the most subtle and difficult problems at the heart of philosophy, language and knowledge representation.

Nevertheless, in the short term administration agencies are keen to obtain aggregate clinical data are so are driven to adopt existing systems, even if they are imperfect. This has lead to much debate amongst those supporting particular systems of their merits over competing ones (e.g. Tuttle and Nelson, 1994).

What is really needed to help rational choice in the longer term is impartial empirical research, comparing the cost and efficacy of different systems in support of well-defined **tasks and contexts**. For example, in a recent study comparing the utility of different coding schemes in classifying problem lists from medical records, none of the major systems were found to be comprehensive (Campbell and Payne, 1994).

The Board of Directors of the American Medical Informatics Association have suggested that it is not necessary or desirable to have all codes coming from a single master system. They suggest that one should embrace several existing and tested approaches, despite their imperfections, to progress quickly. A first phase system could be created by borrowing from the different existing code systems, each created for and therefore better suited to, different subject domains (Ackerman et al., 1994).

The longer term need will be to introduce more maintainable and extensible systems, as the cost of supporting existing systems becomes insupportable. We have seen that the introduction of compositional terminologies may be the next step in achieving such a goal.

Further on, a solution based in part on multiple compositional systems might be feasible. Since any general medical terminology will only cover a small part of the specific vocabulary of any medical speciality, separate systems may need to developed for use **between** specialities and **within** specialities. 'Vocabularies need to be constructed in a manner that preserves the context of each discipline and ensures translation between disciplines (Brennan, 1994)'. Vocabularies developed in this way will be openly based upon the specific needs of specialities. They can more naturally reflect the context and purpose behind specialist terms.

Indeed over a century ago when Farr constructed the classification system ultimately resulting in ICD, he noted that 'Classification is a method of generalisation. Several classifications may, therefore, be used with advantage; and the physician, the pathologist, or the jurist, each from his own point of view, may legitimately classify the diseases and the causes of death in the way that he thinks best adapted to facilitate his enquiries' (ICD-9, 1977).

Compositional systems could thus be constructed to agree on a restricted subset of terms necessary for the passage of information between specialities - an Esperanto between different cultures. Work on such communication standards is at present still in its infancy (e.g. Ma, 1995) and more substantive work should be expected in the future. At present, terms for some of the larger terminologies are being created without explicit tasks in mind in the hope that all unseen eventualities will be served. As we have seen this is a risky strategy, and inter-speciality systems would probably need to be tightly task based to ensure maximum utility.

It is at this point that the importance of evidence-based medicine also becomes very clear (Chapter 7). Treatment protocols are constructed with an explicit task and context in mind. They are written by experts within a speciality, who arrive at a consensus on the management of a specific condition. In the process of doing so they have to define their terms. The communication of information to another speciality can also be defined in the same manner - in the context of a patient on a protocol, what information is needed by an allied specialist? It is clearly the case that good terminologies will be needed to construct computer-based protocol systems (Glowinski, 1994). Equally, the discipline of writing protocols will constrain the terminology problem sufficiently so that a well defined and relevant set of terms can be agreed upon.

Such a strategy will permit languages to be developed in a way that is optimised for those that will use them. It is still unclear what strategies will best handle the evolution of language once a terminology has been constructed. Not only will terminology developers want to extend and refine a system as it proves inadequate, they will also want it to reflect changes in knowledge. Even if systems are built for narrow specialities with tasks in mind, this imperfection of classification will always remain.

One knowledge acquisition strategy is to accept that terms are created in a given context, and should thus only be used within that context. In the 'ripple-down rules' methodology, experts add knowledge to an expert system every time it fails to perform its task (Compton and Jansen, 1990). The new knowledge that 'repairs' the system's performance is attached to the portion of the classification tree that failed. Thus, this new knowledge is placed within the context of the failure of the old knowledge. Over time the classification system grows, always driven by use rather than abstract principles of form. As one would expect, eventually some parts of the system are used less and less, as new classification 'paths' replace more obsolete ones. Despite a process that seems to produce quite large and messy classification systems, ripple-down systems are much easier to build and maintain than normal expert systems, and perform just as well (Compton et al., 1992).

Such an approach might well be suited to medical terminology construction, where terms are added when the existing system fails to provide an appropriate term. Whenever this happens, the reasons for the failure are noted and kept with the new term, which is then placed in the portion of the classification hierarchy that failed. When the system is used next, this contextual knowledge allows the utility of the new term to be judged against the given need. If it suits the need, then it can be used. If it does not, then another new term can be created and added to the system.

One of the other benefits of the ripple-down method is that it does not require great panels of experts to debate the knowledge that will go into a system. Since it is created in an ongoing fashion as a result of the way it is used, individuals can themselves own this process. Absolute notions of knowledge being right or wrong are replaced by appropriateness to the circumstances at hand.

Such an idea may seem modern in its embrace of controlled anarchy, but as with all such ideas, has been anticipated long before.

'And since, for all the reasons above adduced, our language and forms of expression scarcely admit of any further fixation, explanation, or definition, without risk of greater danger than utility, it appears more advisable to give a clear, searching **history** of each of these expressions - e.g., of fever, inflammation - of the names of several disorders, and the like. In this way, our ideas of these matters might be most thoroughly fixed and elucidated, by showing how these expressions were first arrived at, and why the must now be received in a sense different from that which was originally attached to them, and why in this sense and no other (Oesterlen, 1855, p330).'

Chapter summary

1. There is no pure set of codes or terms that can be universally applied in medicine. There is consequently no universal way in which one medical language can be mapped onto another.
2. There are two fundamental and related obstacles to devising a universal terminological system. The first is the **model construction** problem - terminologies are simply a way of modelling the world, and the world is always richer and more complex than any model humans can devise. The second is the **symbol grounding** problem. The words we use to label objects do not necessarily reflect the way we think about the objects, nor do they necessarily reflect defined objects in the real world.
3. Terms are subjective, context-dependent, purposive, and evolve over time.
4. The process of terminology growth and alteration introduces huge problems of maintenance, and the very real possibility that the system will start to incorporate errors, duplications and contradictions. Introducing changes into a mature terminological system becomes increasingly expensive over time and as a consequence maintaining a terminological system will become increasingly expensive over time.
5. Compositional terminological systems are intended to be easier and cheaper to maintain and update than enumerative ones. Early on in their construction, the cost of building a compositional system will be higher than for an enumerative one, but over time will be lower as maintenance costs are comparatively smaller.

Part Five

Communication Systems in Healthcare

It is through the telephone calls, meetings, planning sessions ... and corridor conversations that people inform, amuse, update, gossip, review, reassess, reason, instruct, revise, argue, debate, contest, and actually constitute the moments, myths and, through time, the very structuring of the organisation.

Boden, (1994)

Chapter 13

Communication system basics

It has long been recognised that good interpersonal communication is an essential skill for any healthcare worker. Indeed, this need for effective communication is central to the smooth running of the healthcare system as a whole.

It is now the case that the care of patients involves many different individuals, in part due to increasing specialisation within the professions. It is also due to an increase in patient mobility, which means that they no longer live in the same area for the whole of their life. Supporting clinical encounters now also often involves the efforts of many others who work away from patients, from laboratory and radiology staff through to administrators. These trends, amongst others, have significantly increased the need for healthcare workers to share information about patients and to discuss their management.

The sheer scale and complexity of these interactions within the healthcare system put a heavy burden on the process of communication. Unsurprisingly, miscommunication can have terrible consequences. At the level of patient care, simple communication errors may result in dangerous errors in treatment. At the administrative level, the poor communication of information can have substantial economic consequences.

Over recent years, there has been an increasing understanding of the importance of providing good communication systems in healthcare. It is now clear, for example, that the healthcare system suffers enormous inefficiencies because of the poor quality of communication systems that are often in place. One recent estimate suggested that the US health system could save $30 billion per annum if it improved its telecommunication systems (Little, 1992).

A recurring theme throughout this book is that the specific needs of a given task drive the choice of technology used to assist with that task. This is equally appropriate when considering the application of communication technologies to healthcare. It is clearly inappropriate in an emergency, for example, to send a letter in the post when a telephone call would be a better choice. Up until recently, the scope for such choices has been relatively limited. Consequently most people still tend to devote limited attention during their working day to the consequences of choosing one communication option over another for a given task. However, the available range of communication options is now becoming quite rich. Computer networks, satellite links and mobile telephony, for example, are now commonplace. In contrast, our understanding of the specific roles they can play in healthcare is lagging behind.

As a consequence, there is an apparent delay in the widespread adoption of the newer communication options within healthcare. Whilst there is some significant advanced research in highly specific areas like telemedicine, the adoption of even simpler services like voicemail or electronic mail is not yet commonplace in the health services of many developed nations.

Two things are needed to allow the informed use of any set of technologies. The first is an understanding of the basic problems that need to be solved. Secondly, one needs a solid understanding of the available solutions. In this chapter, the basics of communication and the technology of communication will be explained. The fundamental concepts of a communication channel and a service will be presented first. Several different communication services like voicemail and e-mail will then be examined, along with more traditional forms of communication like the telephone. The next chapter in this section will turn to examine some specific communication technologies, explaining their technical operation and identifying their benefits and limitations. The final chapter in this section examines the specific types of communication problems that arise in healthcare, and

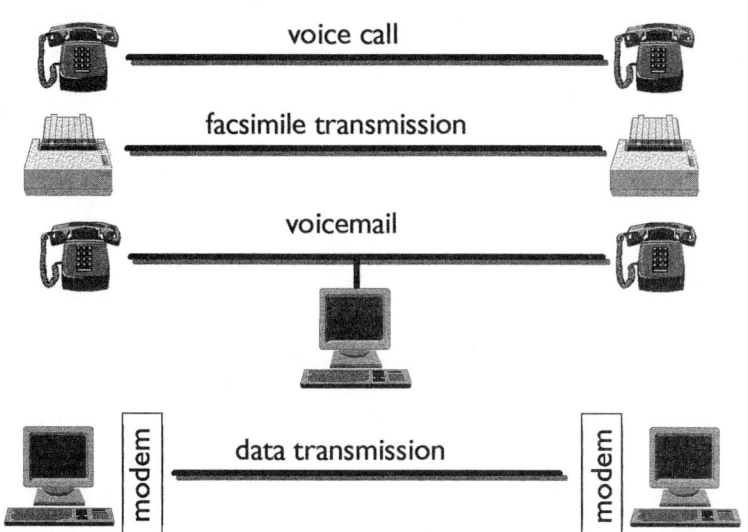

Figure 13.1: A communication channel can support many kinds of communication service. Public switched voice circuits support voice transmissions, but through the use of additional components, can support many other services like fax, voicemail and e-mail.

suggests ways in which communication technology in the guise of telemedicine might be able to improve matters.

13.1 A communication channel can support multiple services

At its simplest, communication occurs when two or more parties exchange information. Unaided by any form of technological intervention, communication occurs when individuals are engaged in a face-to-face conversation. This is often not possible, however, and alternate methods are needed to mediate the act of communication. In these situations, information exchange occurs across a communication **channel**. Thus, a telephone line is as much a communication channel as is a letter. Both are bearers of information between individuals, although they have very different characteristics, and are used in different ways.

One should next separate the notion of a communication channel from the **communication service** that is provided over it. Essentially, a service defines the type of interaction that will occur over a channel. Thus voice communication is only one of the many services available across a telephone line (Figure 13.1). Fax

Table 13.1:
Communication needs can be characterised by the separation of participants over time or distance (after Johansen et al., 1991).

	same time	*different time*
same place	face-to-face meeting	local message
different place	remote conversation	remote message

transmission of documents is an entirely different kind of service that uses the same underlying channel. As we shall see later, electronic mail, voicemail, and video conferencing are amongst the new types of service that can, if desired, be provided over telephone networks.

Shared time and space define the basic contexts of communication

Each of these services mediates the act of communication in different ways, with different costs and benefits. The benefits of a given combination of channel and service depend on the needs of the individuals at the time they need to communicate. In other words, the value of a service depends upon the context within which it is used, and the task to which it is put.

The simplest way to model the different contexts in which communication acts can occur is to note that individuals can be separated either by time or by distance. The nature of the separation changes the characteristics of the exchange, and in part defines the type of channel and service that are needed (Table 13.1).

Same time, same place. A face-to-face conversation is the most obvious example of communication benefiting from shared location and time. The participants in the dialogue are able to both hear and see each other, and share whatever materials they have to hand. Because they can see and hear so much of each other, the opportunity for exchanging complex and subtle cues is high. In whatever other situations communication occurs, one often seeks to replicate the effectiveness of face-to-face communication. Consequently, the strengths and weaknesses of alternative channels can be weighed up against this gold standard.

Despite the richness of face-to-face conversation, devices are often still used to augment the interaction. Everything from slide projectors in an auditorium, to shared computer workspaces in classrooms all provide additional channels to enhance immediate communication.

Same time, different place. Separated by distance, conversations can nevertheless occur in the same time. Channels that support communication in real time are known as **synchronous channels**. Telephone lines provide perhaps the commonest example of a two-way synchronous channel. Broadcast television provides a unidirectional synchronous channel, which thus prevents it being used interactively in support of a conversation.

When conversations occur across large distances, there is less likelihood that the parties are also involved in frequent face-to-face conversations. This means that in these circumstances the channels and services bear the full brunt of the communication burden.

In such cases, channels may be chosen that support richer communication interaction. While voice telephony is usually sufficient for most conversational needs, it might be necessary in some circumstances to see the faces of the participants. In this case, video images can be transmitted along with voice to permit a **video-conference**. The interaction can be enhanced further with data services. For example, one can work remotely on a common document, or use shared electronic white boards. One can thus use a combination of media from sound, image and data, depending on the specific needs of the communication task. The use of such multimedia is still an area of ongoing investigation, as the specific advantages of individual mediums for given tasks is identified.

Different time, same place. In contrast to synchronous communication, when individuals are separated by time they require **asynchronous** channels to support their interaction. Since there can be no simultaneous discussion, conversations occur through a series of message exchanges. This can range from Post-it™ notes left on a colleague's desk, to sophisticated electronic messaging systems.

It is a common characteristic of these local message exchanges that they are often brief, since they represent ongoing conversations between working colleagues who also have other opportunities for face-to-face conversation.

Different time, different place. In many ways, this is the most challenging of the four quadrants, since neither location nor time are shared by the communicating parties. Asynchronous messaging is clearly needed in this circumstance.

The object of such communication might, for example, revolve around the co-ordination of a group of individuals all working at the same location but working different shifts. For example, a team of physicians working in a hospital might meet only once during the day as a group, and communicate non-urgent information for the remainder of the day through written messages, voicemail or e-mail.

Message services are often provided across computer networks, and are sometimes also known as **store and forward** systems. For example, a radiology image stored in a radiology department computer system, can be forwarded along with a report, to the requesting physician, who reads it at a convenient time.

If the correspondents do not often meet in the same location, there is a potential need for richer services than simple message exchange. For example, messages may need to contain complex documents with text, voice or video records.

Services vary in the media they employ

The time and place classification presented earlier separates synchronous and asynchronous services. Services can also be understood in terms of the different media they employ. Some for example, are designed only for voice, whilst others may carry images or data (Table 13.2).

Unsurprisingly, the value of one medium over another is also context dependent (Caldwell et al., 1995). The nature of a particular task, the setting in which it occurs, and the amount of information that a medium can bear all seem to have effects on human performance on a communication task (Rice, 1992). For example, relatively information-lean media like electronic mail (Rice, 1992) and voicemail (Caldwell et al., 1995) can be used for routine, simple communications. In contrast, it seems that for non-routine and difficult communications, a richer medium like video, and preferably face-to-face conversation, should be used.

	sound	*image*	*data*
synchronous	telephony	video-conferencing	shared electronic white boards, shared documents
asynchronous	voicemail	letters and notes, computer image store and forward	paging, fax, e-mail

Table 13.2: Communication services can be classified according to the media they support, and whether they are asynchronous message based systems, or operate synchronously in real time.

This may be because in routine situations, individuals share a common model of the task and so need to communicate less during an exchange. In contrast, in novel situations a significant portion of the communication may need to be devoted to establishing common ground (Clarke and Brennan, 1991).

In simple terms, since the participants do not share a common model of the task at hand, they are unable to interpret all the data passing over the channel. This means that during the conversation, there are additional demands upon the channel to also support the transmission of task models. Since this is a complex communication task, individuals may need to check with each other repeatedly throughout the conversation that they are indeed understanding each other.

13.2 Communication services

We have now seen that the context of communication affects the choice of channel and service. In this section, several basic combinations of service and medium will be examined in more detail, with an emphasis on the type of communication they are best able to support.

Voice telephony

Undoubtedly the backbone of any organisation's communication system, the apparent simplicity of voice telephony belies the richness of the communication it can support. In contrast to asynchronous

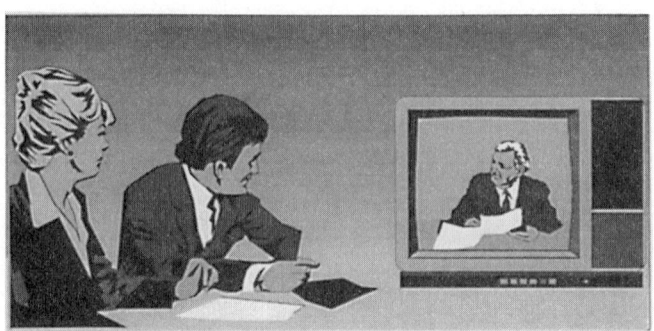

Figure 13.2: Video-conferencing permits face-to-face interaction when participants are geographically separated.

Voice telephony

Undoubtedly the backbone of any organisation's communication system, the apparent simplicity of voice telephony belies the richness of the communication it can support. In contrast to asynchronous systems, real-time interaction allows problem solving and negotiation to take place. Voice is also a rich enough medium for many of the subtle cues needed to develop a shared understanding to be exchanged (Clarke and Brennan, 1991).

Perhaps because it is so commonplace, voice telephony is often taken for granted, and people do not look for new or innovative ways with which it can be used. However, innovative use of the telephone can make significant improvements to the delivery of care. For example, patient follow up can often be done on the telephone, in preference to bringing patients into the clinic (Rao, 1994).

Undoubtedly the biggest change in voice telephony in recent years has been the expansion of mobile telephony. Mobile communication reduces the effort required to locate and speak to people. The combination of mobile telephony and paging systems can reduce the 5-10 minutes out of every hour many clinicians spend answering pagers (Fitzpatrick, 1993).

Video-conferencing

The addition of video to voice telephony is seen by many as one of the next major advances in mass telecommunication. It is perhaps surprising then, that despite being available in one form or another networks. Consequently, video-based systems can only appear after a significant investment in higher capacity networks. However, the costs involved in this process mean that video seems relatively expensive for the extra benefit it gives the average consumer. As cable television services to the home become commonplace, this should change, since fibre-optic cables are capable of supporting the much higher data capacity needed for video.

Video-conferences permit face-to-face interactions when participants are geographically separate (Figure 13.2). This permits richer interaction than is possible by voice alone. However, interactions are not necessarily 'natural'. There may be time lags between events being shown or discussed, depending upon the capacity of the channel being used, and the amount of image data that is sent.

It remains unclear in which situations the increased cost of using video delivers a proportionate increase in benefit (Whittaker, 1995). For most conversations for example, it may be that voice is a sufficiently rich channel that little extra benefit is conferred through the addition of video. Indeed, video-conferencing seems to be more similar in its characteristics to audio-only channels than face-to-face conversation (Williams, 1977).

One study suggests that the ability to see lips in addition to hearing voice makes only a modest improvement to understanding of meaningful communication. However, it significantly improved an individual's ability to disambiguate meaningful sentences from garbled or anomalous ones. The addition of gestures to face and voice seemed to not help further with meaningful conversation, but slightly improved the handling of anomalous data (Thompson and Ogden, 1995).

More recently, the 'video-as-data' hypothesis suggests that one of the main benefits that video brings is the depiction of complex information about shared work objects, creating a shared physical context for conversations (Whittaker, 1995; Ramsay et al., 1996).

E-mail

Electronic mail, or e-mail, is typically used to send short textual messages between computer users across a computer network. It is one of a number of electronic data exchange services available to those with access to a computer network.

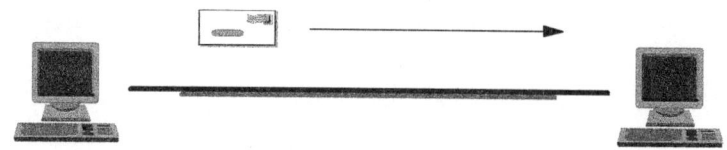

Figure 13.3: E-mail is used to send messages to specified addresses of individual users on a computer network.

E-mail systems can be confined to local computer networks, for example covering a university or hospital campus. However, when separate local networks are connected, messages can be exchanged across much wider areas. As we shall see in Section 6, the Internet permits local networks to join onto an international network, giving electronic mail services a global range. Already in some populations, access to e-mail via the Internet is high. Fridsma et al. (1994) in California found that 46% of their patients at a clinic already used e-mail, 89% of which was through their place of work.

E-mail can be used in a variety of ways. It can, like voice telephony, be used for personal communication. It can also be used for the distribution of information. For example, a central resource like a laboratory can use e-mail to distribute test results, and associated alerts or warnings. The benefits of such exchange need not be confined to within large institutions like hospitals, but can be used to communicate information within smaller groups, like primary care groups. It is also a simple but effective means for communicating between different sectors in healthcare. For example, patient data can be sent from hospitals to primary care physicians after discharge. Drug alerts can be communicated by regulatory bodies to the medical community at large.

E-mail continues to evolve in sophistication, and it is now common to find e-mail programmes that allow complex messages. For example, it is possible to use many different media like voice, still images or video when composing a message. Thus an e-mail could contain a brief explanatory text note, along with a file containing documents from a medical record, dictated voice message, and some images.

Voicemail

Similar in conception to electronic mail, voicemail allows the asynchronous exchange of recorded voice messages. The commonest

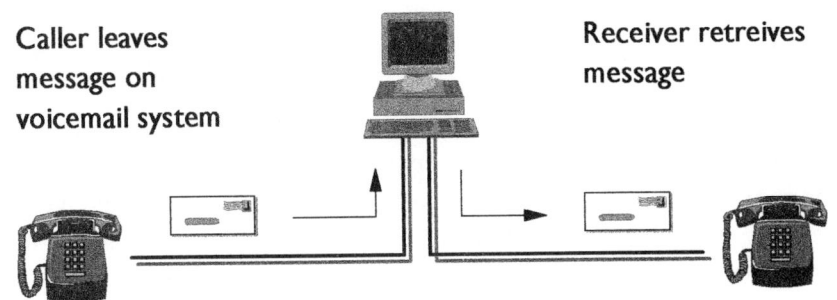

Caller leaves
message on
voicemail system

Receiver retreives
message

Figure 13.4: Basic
voicemail allows a
caller to leave a
recorded voice
message. The receiver
calls up the voicemail
system, accesses their
own private mailbox,
and retrieves any
messages put there.

use of voicemail is to collect messages when a phone is unanswered. In contrast to simple answering machines attached to individual telephones, voicemail systems permit relatively complex message handling. Firstly, it acts like a collection point for many different individuals, each of who might have a private 'mailbox' on the system. This is possible because voicemail systems are created and operated on computers connected to the telephone system, for example through an organisation's switchboard. Secondly, messages can be tagged with different levels of urgency, forwarded to others with additional information, or stored for later review.

Inexpensive voice messaging can deliver simple but powerful services over existing telephone networks. Voicemail for example, has significant potential for improving the process of care (Constable, 1994). Voicemail can be integrated into many existing processes. For example, it is common for many radiology or pathology reports to be prepared by dictation, then transcribed and committed to text. Eventually much of the transcription will be automated through computer voice-recognition systems. In the absence of that, the dictated reports could be distributed to the ordering physician by voicemail, well in advance of the report being transcribed and arriving through a paper-based mail system.

Quite sophisticated functionality can be incorporated into telephone services based upon voicemail. For example, an answer message can incorporate call logic that offers a pre-programmed range of options to the caller. The caller can interact with the system, and indicate their preferences. This interaction can happen by collecting information from the caller using the dial tone created when different digits are pressed on a telephone (so-called dial tone multi-frequency or DTMF tones). Computer-based voice recognition systems can look for specific words in the caller's response to determine their preferences.

From such seemingly simple elements, many different services can be constructed. For example, a patient could call in to a health information line that begins by playing a pre-recorded voice message. Depending upon the information needs of the caller, the system then plays different messages on a variety of health topics. If the recorded information is insufficient, the system could either allow the caller to record a message registering a more specific request, or put them through directly to someone who is able answer their questions.

Voicemail systems are thus in some ways a misnomer, since they can be programmed to do much more than send and capture messages, and can be programmed to provide a variety of information services. They also can be designed to capture and exchange more than voice recordings. For example, DTMF is a simple way of exchanging data across the voice channel.

13.3 Conclusions

We have briefly covered some of the basic elements of communication and the way in which technologies can be used to support it. In the next chapter, we shall delve more deeply into the specifics of current and emerging communication technologies. It may often appear that simply introducing technology will quickly improve poor communication processes, but this is not necessarily the case. Since the introduction of such technology changes existing processes, the success of the introduction is as dependent on the technology as it is on the appropriateness and complexity of re-engineering these processes. This is a theme we shall return to in Chapter 15 where we examine specific ways that technology can and cannot help the process of communication in healthcare.

Chapter summary

1. Information exchange occurs across a communication **channel**.
2. Many different **communication services** can be provided over a channel. For example, voice and fax transmission are both available over a telephone line.
3. Communication systems can support communication between individuals separated either by time or by distance.
4. Channels that support communication in real time are known as **synchronous channels**. Channels that support communication over different times are known as **asynchronous channels**.
5. Voice telephony forms the backbone of an organisation's synchronous communication system. This is now enhanced through routine use of mobile telephone systems, and the addition of video capabilities that can permit video-conferencing.
6. Electronic mail, or e-mail, is an asynchronous data service available over computer network channels, typically used to send short textual messages between computer users across a computer network. It can be used for the exchange of messages and distribution of information. For example, a central resource like a laboratory can use e-mail to distribute test results, and associated alerts or warnings.
7. Voicemail allows the asynchronous exchange of recorded voice messages. It can be integrated into many existing healthcare processes. For example, dictation radiology or pathology reports can be distributed by voicemail in advance of being transcribed.
8. Video-conferencing adds video to voice telephony. It remains unclear what benefits this additional video brings, since video-conferencing is more like using a telephone than having a face-to-face conversation.

The simple contrivance of tin tubes for speaking through, communicating between different apartments, by which the directions of the superintendant are instantly conveyed to the remotest parts of an establishment, produces a considerable economy of time. It is employed in the shops and manufactories in London, and might with advantage be used in domestic establishments, particularly in large houses, in conveying orders from the nursery to the kitchen, or from the house to the stable...The distance to which such a mode of communication can be extended, does not appear to have been ascertained, and would be an interesting subject for inquiry. Admitting it to be possible between London and Liverpool, about seventeen minutes would elapse before the words spoken at one end would reach the other extremity of the pipe.

(Charles Babbage, 1833, p10)

Chapter 14

Communication technology

In the previous chapter, a broad view of the different communication channels and services was presented. In this chapter, these different technological options for communication will be discussed in more detail. While the complex technical details of channel construction and operation are not of interest here, it is helpful to understand the basic channel types, and some of the terms associated with their operation.

In this respect, this material will be a departure from the content of other chapters, which have sought to de-emphasise technology, and focus on its principled application. However it is at present difficult to get a concise description of communication technology basics. Tanenbaum (1996) provides a comprehensive introduction to the area of computer networks, which will only be touched upon here.

This chapter should thus serve as a technological introduction for those who need a deeper understanding of this area. Those without such an interest can move directly to the final chapter in this section, where we shall turn to examine communication problems in healthcare, and assess the roles that particular technologies can play in solving them.

14.1 Communication channels can be dedicated or shared

A channel provides a connection between the sender and the receiver of a communication. The simplest way to create such a channel is to

Figure 14.1:
Dedicated lines connect communicating parties in a circuit-switched system. In contrast lines can be shared by exchanging data packets from different conversations across a common channel.

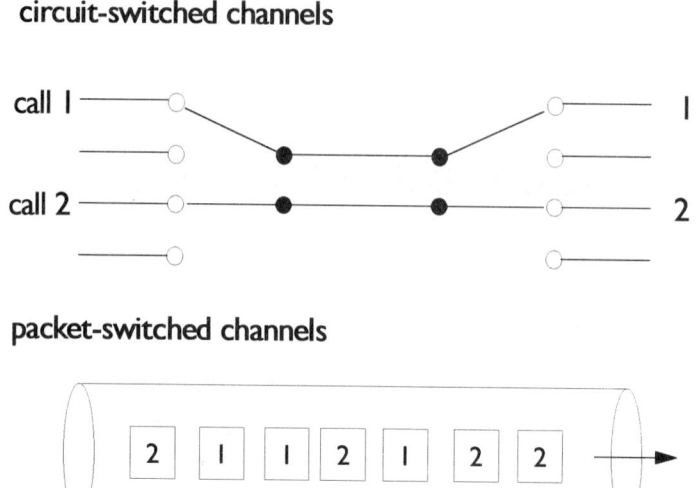

completely dedicate a wire to the transmission. Local telephone systems work in this way, with each telephone number having a dedicated telephone cable running from the telephone unit to the local exchange. Systems like these are called **circuit-switched**, since they make connections by establishing a completed circuit between the communicating parties.

Circuit-switched systems are not very efficient ways of transmitting data. If the dedicated circuit is used only infrequently, it results in inefficiency during the idle periods. If there are many people who want to use the same circuit, a bottleneck is created, since once a circuit is in use it is unavailable to others.

Common channels can carry data packets

One solution to this problem is to try to share the resources on a circuit. This can be achieved by allowing a channel to carry packets of data which may come from a number of different sources. Such systems are called **packet-switched** systems.

Here a message is broken down into a number of discrete packets, and these are sent one after the other down the channel's circuit. On the circuit, the packets mingle with packets from other messages. Each such packet is small, and contains the address of the place it is

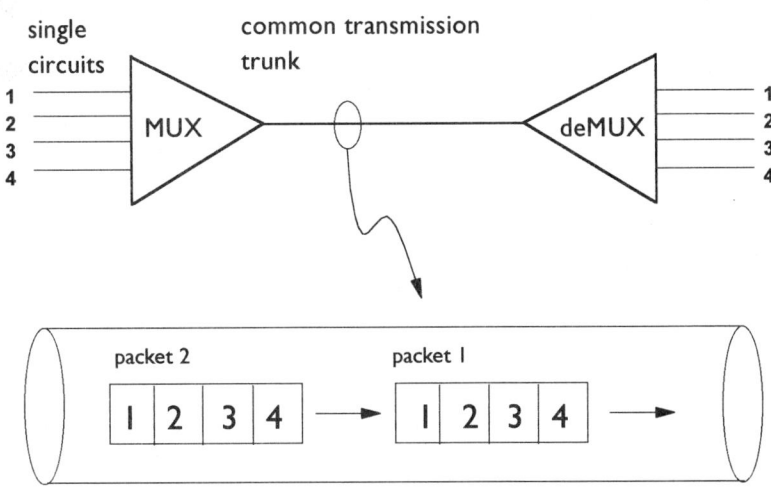

Figure 14.2: To increase the efficiency of transmission, the signals on single telephone circuits are concentrated onto common trunk lines. The concentration is achieved by assigning each circuit a time slot on data packets or frames, which are sent down the line. This concentration of signals is performed by a multiplexer (MUX).

being sent. In this way many packets, each destined for different locations, can pass down the same wire over the same period (Figure 14.1). When the packets reach a switching point in the communication network, the address is read, and the packet is then sent down the right part of the network towards its final destination. By and large, all computer networks are packet-based.

In telephone networks common channels are multiplexed according to time or frequency

A similar general principle is used in voice telephony. Since a segment of voice from a conversation is reducible to digital data, it too can be broken down into a number of packets. As long as the packets are sent and reassembled in a short enough time, then the speaker and listener will not realise that they do not have a dedicated circuit to themselves.

Once voice data has travelled down a dedicated circuit from a customer's premises to a local area exchange, the data is shipped along a high capacity common trunk. Each packet is passed along the trunk using a technique called multiplexing (Figure 14.2) which is another method for combining a number of calls in order that they may all be transmitted along the same single cable (Lawton, 1993).

Figure 14.3:
Channels can combine multiple calls by allocating each call a different slot from the frequencies available on the common channel.

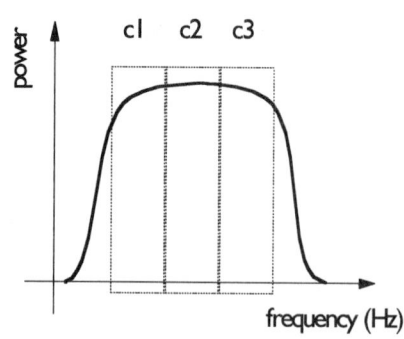

One way of multiplexing a number of different conversations is to time the arrival of data, and to divide time into a series of repeating 'slots'. Each call is pre-assigned a different time slot on the same circuit. The receiver of the multiplexed signal knows which conversation occupies which specific time slot, and reconstructs individual conversations as their specific packets are taken from their time slot (Figure 14.2).

The second way in which a number of calls can be multiplexed together is to allocate each a frequency slot rather than a time slot. This is possible because, for analogue channels, there is a spread of possible signal frequencies that can be used to transmit data. The band of possible frequencies is broken up into a number of smaller bands which then becomes a call slot. Each individual call is then allocated one of the frequency slots on the channel (Figure 14.3). Thus, in contrast to a time multiplexed system, each frequency slot carries its information at the same time down the common channel. The call is limited to occupying a few of all the possible available frequencies on the common channel frequency band.

This explains why one measure of a channel's capacity to carry data is called its **bandwidth**. The wider the range of frequencies available on a channel, the greater the opportunity to break it up into separate bands, each of which are able to carry data independently. Channel bandwidth is calculated in Hertz, which is a frequency measure, and the wider the bandwidth, the greater the channel's capacity to carry signals. In contrast to an analogue channel, the capacity of a digital channel to carry data is measured by the number of data bits per second that can be transmitted by the channel. Unsurprisingly, it is possible to relate a channel's bandwidth to its data rate. For example, a normal telephone line can carry up to 64 kbytes per second, based upon a 3.4 kHz voice requirement for the transmission of intelligible speech (Lawton, 1993). In contrast, a common trunk on a telephone network may handle between 1.5 and 2 Mbits per second.

14.2 Channel types

The current explosion in services in the communication industry is as much a product of the increase in capacity and variety of channels, as it is due to the emergence of innovative ways of using their capacity. These channels can be created either by establishing connections through wired physical circuits, or by establishing wireless links.

The great number of different systems competing in the telecommunications sphere can make the area a difficult one to understand. Each system usually offers slightly different technical and economic advantages over its competitors, and the basis for choosing one system over another is rarely straightforward. One may need to compare attributes like bandwidth, cost, reliability, flexibility, call set up time and so forth. As a consequence, only some of the major and emerging communication systems can be reviewed here. The discussion should give a clear indication of the types of technologies now available, and of their varying ability to support communication.

Wireline channels

The majority of the world's communication infrastructure is based on physical networks, whether they be made of copper wire of fibre-optic cable. Just as important as the difference in the transmission characteristics of these physical media is the method used to transfer information across them. We saw earlier that using a circuit-switched network meant that only one 'call' could use a wire at any one time. Packet-switched and multiplexed systems in contrast, because they handle information exchange in a different way, result in a more efficient sharing of network resources.

Figure 14.4:Wired channels - Plain Old Telephony Services (POTS) across public telecommunication networks are the basis for most communication. Integrated Services Digital Network (ISDN) provides a digital connection with twice the bandwidth of POTS. Asynchronous Transfer Mode (ATM) systems are designed for high bandwidth computer networks. When higher bandwidths are needed private trunks like E1, provide guaranteed connections. (V-voice, D-data, c-control.)

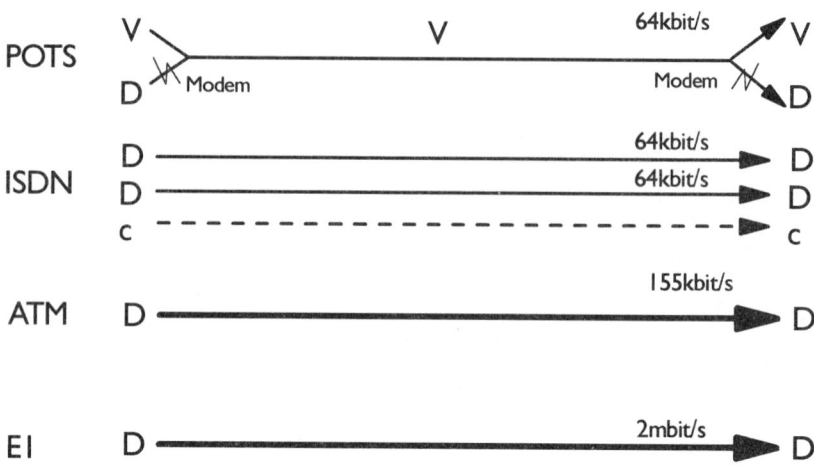

Consequently, when discussing the capacity for information carriage over any particular system, both the physical attributes of the system, as well as the type of protocol used to carry data over it contribute to the eventual data rate achieved. The technical details of these specific protocols are well beyond the scope of this discussion. However, two in particular - ISDN and ATM will be introduced given their increasing importance in telecommunications.

Integrated Service Digital Network (ISDN)

We have already seen that the public switched telephone network was initially developed to carry only voice but is now used to carry fax and data over it. As the desire to provide ever more intricate services across the telephone network grows, it has become increasingly clear that the existing system, developed over the last 100 years, is now reaching its limits.

ISDN, in contrast to normal telephone circuits, provides direct digital connection between a subscriber and the telephone network. Thus, while on a normal analogue telephone line one needs a modem to carry data across the voice channel, no such device is needed when using ISDN. (A modem converts data into a series of tones that are carried across the voice channel, and then are converted by another modem back into digital format.)

Secondly, ISDN provides two independent data channels to a subscriber (Figure 14.4). One channel could be used to carry a voice conversation, while data were transmitted across the second. Thus, for example, one could be discussing a patient on the telephone, and simultaneously transmitting and sharing data about that patient. A third signalling channel allows the user's equipment to communicate with the network, allowing for rapid call set-up, and exchange of other information (Lawton, 1993). For example, caller identification information can be transmitted and read before deciding to accept a voice call.

ISDN services are now available in many countries. They have been slow to be adopted partly because of the costs to users, and partly because the need for the higher speed data services of ISDN to the home has only recently arisen, especially with increased home connection to the Internet (see Section 6).

Asynchronous Transfer Mode (ATM)

Whilst ISDN represents a significant improvement on existing telephony, it has a relatively limited bandwidth, being roughly twice that of a normal 64 kbit/s telephone line. For some tasks, like the transmission of high resolution moving images, this is insufficient. In anticipation of a need to provide such high bandwidth channels, the so called B-ISDN or broadband ISDN system has been developed. The upper transmission rate that will be made available to broadband users will be from 1.5 Mbits to 100 Mbits/s (Handel and Huber, 1991).

Along with the anticipation that there would be a consumer need for such transmission rates, B-ISDN has also been driven by the development of fibre-optic channels. These are able to sustain high bandwidth transmission, up to several hundred Mbits/s.

One of the main criteria in shaping the design of the B-ISDN was the realisation that the demand for data capacity would be highly variable from different customers. Recall that in normal telephony, a channel can be created by assigning a specified time-slot in a sequence of packets that are transmitted down a common channel. This is an example of a **synchronous transfer mode**. For largely

Figure 14.5:
Asynchronous transfer mode (ATM) transmission uses a packet transmission system by variably assigning different channels to a given packet, based upon the requirements of individual channels at any given time. Each ATM packet (or cell) carries information in a header segment that describes its particular contents, which are located in the main body of the cell.

synchronous transfer mode

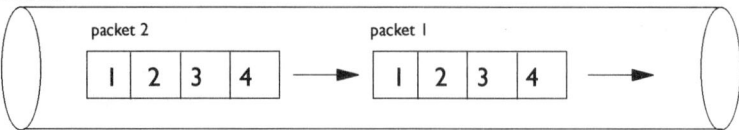

asynchronous transfer mode

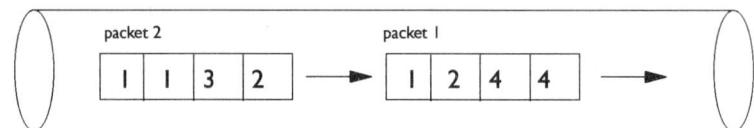

ATM packet structure

header with routing data	field carrying information from multiple user channels

voice based systems, because there is a fixed demand on capacity for each given channel, this synchronous system suffices.

If the network is used for other forms of data such as video, then another approach is required. The irregularity with which a user might need to transmit large volumes of video data means that a synchronous method becomes inefficient for broadband services. This is because the large dedicated packets needed to accommodate video might often remain relatively under-utilised if they were used for voice. As a consequence, rather than assigning fixed capacity communication slots, an asynchronous system based on the transmission of data packets, (or cells) is needed. The method for transmitting these packets is call the **asynchronous transfer mode** (or ATM).

In ATM, each packet is filled with information from different channels in an irregular fashion, depending upon the demand at any given time. Since each packet contains information about the specific channels it is carrying data for, they can be reassembled upon arrival. In other words, ATM allows a communication system to be divided into a number of arbitrarily sized channels, depending upon demand and the needs of individual channels.

ATM systems are currently being testing in many nations, but are not at present routinely available for public use. As the demand for broadband services like high quality video image transmission, or video-telephony grows, the economic case for the widespread deployment of ATM will become stronger. The deployment of ATM is also dependent on the rate with which high-capacity fibre-optic cabling is laid in the community, since it cannot run across the existing smaller capacity circuitry.

For many in the telecommunications field, healthcare is an example of an area that could adopt ATM, because it is perceived that telemedical video services will be of high benefit (e.g. Cabral et al., 1996). Whether this is an example of a technology seeking problems to solve, or an appropriate solution for healthcare's communication needs is an issue that shall be returned to in the next chapter.

Wireless channels

While wireline networks have now been developing over an extended period, and now provide affordable voice and data communication channels, developments in wireless communications systems have been somewhat more recent. The goal of any wireless system is to provide individuals access to voice and data channels, irrespective of their location or mobility. The technical requirements that these channels must meet vary according to the data rates expected of them, the mobility patterns of those using the system, and the reliability expected of the system. For example, a cordless telephone system that will only be used within a home can be built to far less demanding specifications than a mobile telephone system designed to be used across a continent, in a moving car, or to support simultaneous calls.

Radio provided the first wide-area wireless communication technology, followed later by the provision of television services over broadcast radio channels. Over the years the exploitation of the radio frequency spectrum has continued relentlessly. Microwave and satellite communication links are now commonplace replacements in situations in which the laying of cable connections is inappropriate or expensive. Radio technology, in the form of mobile analogue and digital cellular telephony, is now freely available to the public at relatively low cost in most western nations.

In contrast to this wide-area use of wireless channels, one can also exploit wireless communication at very short distances. In these circumstances, the wireless system might be providing channels for local telephony and paging. It can also be used to provide wireless links for computer terminals. For example, a hand-held computer terminal can connect to a hospital local area network over a wireless link. This allows the user to move over the local area freely, but still be able to interact with information on the network.

For very close distance communication within a room, or between individuals in close proximity, one can exploit the infra-red light spectrum. Infra-red links can be used for example, to allow devices like a computer and printer to communicate with each other.

Of all of these areas, the rapid growth in mobile telephony has been the most spectacular and significant, in terms of adoption rates. Some cellular telephone systems have in recent years experienced staggering growth rates of between 35 and 60% per annum (Cox, 1995). There are several competing standards for the provision of mobile telephony arising from Europe, Japan and the United States, and arguments over the benefits of these systems are as much driven by political and economic imperatives as by technical issues. All these systems deliver more or less the same basic set of services, including voice communications, data communications, and messaging or paging functions (Padgett et al., 1995). Over the last couple of years it has become clear that one of these, the GSM system, is likely to be most widely adopted on a global scale. For this reason, it will be reviewed here in some detail.

The Global System for Mobile Communications (GSM)

GSM was initially developed in Europe, but has in recent years been adopted across much of Asia-Pacific, and is beginning to be adopted in some sections of the United States. The digital nature of GSM allows it to service many more users in a local area than is possible with older analogue mobile systems. The GSM system was initially intended to be deployed around the 900 MHz radio band. It is now

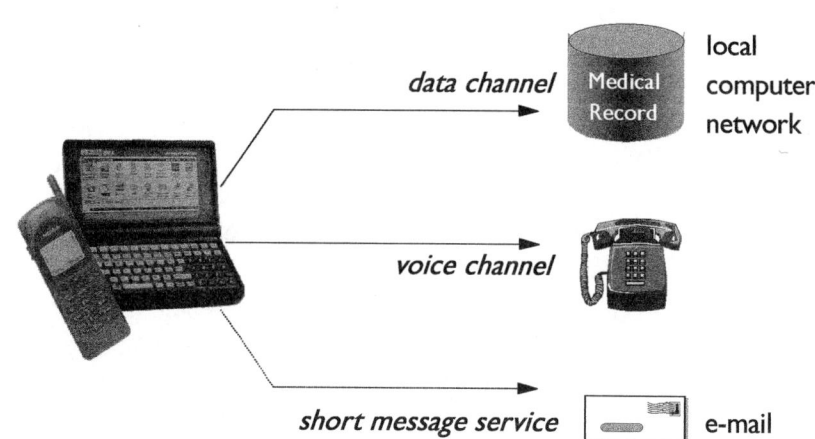

data channel

Medical Record

local computer network

voice channel

short message service

e-mail

Figure 14.6: The GSM mobile digital cellular system provides channels for voice and data connections. The data link allows a mobile computer to connect remotely, via the mobile telephone, to local computer networks. An asynchronous short-message system provides a mobile text-based e-mail service.

also deployed at 1.8 GHz where it is called DCS 1800 (Digital Cellular system 1800) or Personal Communication Networks (PCN). One of the obvious advantages of the widespread adoption of the GSM system is that it offers the ability to roam widely while still using the same handset. Thus a mobile telephone registered to a GSM network in the United Kingdom can be turned on and used on a GSM network in Australia. This contrasts with the situation in some nations where roaming with a network is only possible within the boundaries of a city, because adjoining networks are based on different technologies.

The GSM system provides users with several digital channels (Figure 14.6). One synchronous channel is available for voice communication, and one for data communications offering a 9.6 kb/s data rate. In addition, an asynchronous packet data channel, known as the short-message service (SMS), provides a form of e-mail for GSM users. In addition, services like fax and voicemail are supported over the synchronous channels.

This combination of channels and services makes a digital system like GSM quite powerful. The SMS system for example, can act as an e-mail or paging system. Combined with a voice mailbox on the network, this gives individuals a significant set of channels through which they can be contacted. The mobile data channel allows a GSM telephone to be connected to a mobile computer. Whilst mobile, one can send and receive fax messages over the GSM system. Equally one could use it to connect to a computer network while being remote from the site. This would, for example, permit a doctor to retrieve patient data or gain access to Internet services.

Since the GSM system encrypts the data over its channels, it is also a relatively secure system. Unlike analogue systems, it is not possible to listen in to GSM conversations.

There are still several problems that may affect routine use. For many, battery life between recharges remains an issue, but there is steady progress in improving this aspect of handset design. Perhaps more importantly, use of GSM is limited indoors. The geometry of walls and ceilings means that radio signal reception may not be good. In such circumstances, alternative local systems may be more appropriate. In particular, modern cordless telephony systems like CT2 (Cordless Telephony 2) and DECT (Digital European Cordless Telecommunications) can offer superior in-building performance, but at the cost of installing the whole network privately on a campus (Padgett et al., 1995).

Like any other cellular system, a GSM network is created by dividing up a geographic area into a number of 'cells'. Each cell has its own radio transmitter to receive signals from handsets, and to transmit these to the network's control centre. As a user moves from one cell, the call is handed over to the nearest cell with the strongest reception of the handset. Thus, the territory over which GSM can be used is limited by the size of the local networks. If radio base stations have not been installed to create cells in a given region, then no network coverage is possible in that area.

Especially for sparsely populated areas, GSM coverage may thus be problematic. Indeed, as GSM systems are deployed, it is routine to first establish cells in major cities and along transportation routes like highways. Then, over time, coverage is rolled out to less densely populated regions. Consequently, when coverage is an issue, as it is in territories without dense GSM networks, then satellite-based mobile telephone systems may provide a useful alternative.

14.3 Computer and communication systems are merging

Despite technical difference, one abiding impression from the preceding discussion should be that computer and communication systems are in many ways similar. In fact, the separation of communication and computer systems is breaking down.

While there are significant differences in the ways both types of system are optimised, they are being put to similar uses. Computer networks are increasingly being used for communication, and communication networks are becoming ever more reliant on computers to deliver complex communication services. Thus, while the telephone network is designed for voice, it is also used to ship data between computers, acting as an extension to local computer networks. Using the Internet, multitudes of local networks have been connected together to create a global computer network that rivals, and sometimes overlays, the existing telecommunications network.

Equally, computer networks like the Internet, once designed to exchange data, are now being used to carry image and sound. Indeed, it is now possible to use packet-switched systems to deliver voice telephony. Recall that most voice traffic on a telecommunications network is already broken up into small packets and reassembled without the speakers being aware. Whilst the methods used are highly optimised to deliver voice, as computer packet networks grow in bandwidth and reliability, they are being used to carry voice calls, independently of the telephone network. To say that this is a challenge to the existing shape of the telecommunications industry is an understatement.

All these signs point to a growing convergence between computer and communication networks. Both have had traditional strengths and weaknesses. Through the convergence of these two quite different systems, new architectures are emerging that try to capture the best aspects of both (Figure 14.7). Computer networks, for their part, are highly flexible. One can buy software and deploy it onto a personal computer, without any constraints from the network to which the computer is connected. The network itself is relatively simple in the way it provides connections between computers, since it traditionally has been designed around packet-based asynchronous data transfer. The net effect has been that it has been very easy to deploy new programs (or 'services' in telecommunication parlance), whilst connectivity has been expensive, with local organisations having to build their own networks.

Figure 14.7: The architecture of telecommunication networks favours centralised control of services, whilst computer networks favour a distributed local ownership. As these architectures converge, emerging systems will begin to inherit characteristics from both.

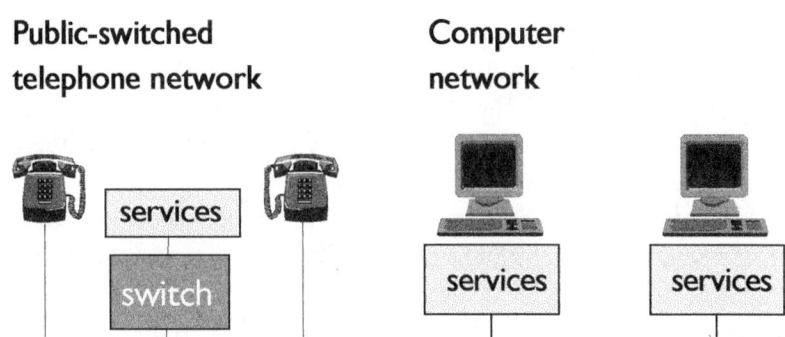

Public-switched telephone network

Computer network

services

switch

services

services

In contrast, telecommunication networks traditionally provided an immediate and rich network of connections to subscribers. This was achieved through relatively complicated and sophisticated public switching systems. All the communications services such as 0800 numbers resided in these centralised switching systems. The user's personal terminal (in this case the telephone) depends entirely upon the network to provide any new services. Thus one cannot go out and buy a new program to load into a private telephone. The consequence of this has been that telephone services are controlled by telecommunications companies, are expensive to develop, and evolve very slowly in comparison to computer network services.

One can summarise the differences by noting that the service 'intelligence' in a computer network is distributed across the computers attached to the network, whilst in a telecommunications system the intelligence is centralised within the network.

One can immediately see the need for a system that offers high speed reliable connections to a global network, with the flexibility of a service deployment of a computer network. Indeed, the telecommunications industry has struggled with these issues for several years, working on so called **intelligent network** architectures that might one day supersede the existing one.

In the meantime, the computer industry has quietly side-stepped these issues by fashioning the Internet into a system that will soon have most of the desired characteristics of this hybrid network. This has caught many in the telecommunications industry by surprise. As we shall see in Section 6, the implications of the Internet are thus as fundamental to the existing telecommunications and computing industries, as it is to those who use their services.

Chapter summary

1. A communications channel can be operated either as a dedicated circuit, or as a shared resource. **Circuit-switched** networks provide a complete circuit between the communicating parties. **Packet-switched** systems transport separate packets of data that can come from a number of different sources on a common channel.

2. A channel's capacity to carry data is called its **bandwidth**, usually measured in bits per second.

3. The type of data transfer protocol used over a communications network contributes to the eventual bandwidth. The Integrated Service Digital Network (ISDN) and Asynchronous Transfer Mode (ATM) systems are currently the most important standard protocols for communicating with multimedia.

4. There are several competing standards for the provision of mobile telephony arising from Europe, Japan and the United States. All these systems deliver more or less the same basic set of services, including voice communications, data communications, and messaging or paging functions. Of these, for the present the GSM system is the most widely adopted on a global scale.

5. There is a growing convergence between computer and communication networks, with merged networks like the Internet now providing both communication and information services.

Chapter 15

Clinical communication and telemedicine

With such a long history of application of information technologies in healthcare, it is surprising that communication technologies have only recently become a focus for attention. It is difficult to explain this difference, but it may well reflect the perception that communication processes for the most part are considered human processes. Technology, when it has been used, has been relatively simple and disappeared into the background. The telephone, for example, is an unremarkable and commonplace item in most people's working day. The enthusiasm and novelty associated with its introduction in the last century have disappeared. In contrast the development of information technologies has dominated most of the second half of this century.

It is only in the last decade of this century that developments in communication technologies have again accelerated. As the limitations of information technology have become apparent, and the potential for communication technologies has emerged, it is no surprise that many have now returned to examine how communication technologies can be applied to healthcare.

In this closing chapter of the Communication section, various human and organisational problems with communication will be explored. With the understanding of communication technologies developed in the previous chapters attempt will be made to assess critically when these technologies are of benefit.

15.1 Telemedicine supports clinical care with communication technologies

Most of the effort in deploying communication technologies in healthcare is associated with the field of **telemedicine**. Definitions of telemedicine abound. For many, it has a particularly narrow technological definition. Specifically, it is seen by some to be the use of video-conferencing techniques to deliver consultation and care at a distance. Unfortunately, technology-driven definitions usually end up focusing more on the technologies than the problems that need to be solved. In particular, they miss the many opportunities for solving problems that do not encompass a given technology. So it is with telemedicine. Healthcare has many and varied communication needs, and video-based technologies are only one of many solutions that should be explored. Indeed, many solutions to communication problems are never technological, but require changes in human and organisational processes.

The essence of telemedicine is the exchange of information at a distance, whether that information is voice, an image, elements of a medical record, or commands to a surgical robot. It seems reasonable to think of telemedicine as the **remote communication of information to facilitate clinical care**. And it is not a new enterprise - Einthoven experimented with telephone transmissions using his new invention, the electrocardiograph at the beginning of the century (Nymo, 1993).

At its inception, telemedicine was essentially about providing communication links between medical experts and remote locations. It is now clear that the healthcare system suffers enormous inefficiencies because of its poor communication infrastructure and telemedicine is seen by many as a critical way of reducing that cost. Consequently, telemedicine has now become a significant area for research and development.

As one might expect, the renewed interest in telemedicine also has much to do with the excitement of new technologies. At present the press is flooded with articles about the information superhighway, the Internet, and the rapid growth of mobile telephony. Telemedicine is often presented in the guise of sophisticated new communications technology for specialist activities like teleradiology and telepathology. These are championed by telecommunication companies because they have the potential to become highly profitable businesses for them (Bowles and Teale, 1994). Perhaps influenced by these forces, much of the research in telemedicine is driven by the possibilities of technology rather than the needs of clinicians and patients.

Yet the communications infrastructure used by healthcare will not necessarily need to be special. The telecommunications market is competitive and the evolving options are numerous. Healthcare providers will be able to utilise the services of cable television, mobile cellular carriers, and telecommunication companies. Further, communications technology does not need to be sophisticated to deliver benefit. For example, simple but appropriate use of today's telephone can make significant improvements to the delivery of care. Consequently, we will examine telemedicine from a problem-driven point of view, and only then examine the role that technologies have to play in their solution.

15.2 Communication needs in healthcare vary widely

Communication tasks vary widely across the healthcare system. The needs of a doctor working as part of a close-knit team in a major hospital are very different from those of a nurse working in the community visiting patients in their homes. Consequently, the stresses placed upon communication are as varied.

It is helpful to separate communication needs into two groups. Firstly, specific **intra-organisational** needs exist within particular groups, such as hospitals or primary care centres. Secondly, there are significant **inter-organisational** needs that occur at the interfaces between significantly different organisations (Figure 15.1). The communication boundary between primary care givers in the community and hospital based health services, for example, are characterised by the widely differing task styles and organisational structures of individuals within the two groups.

Figure 15.1: Major communication interfaces exist between primary care delivered in the community and tertiary institutions like hospitals, as well as between these and patients receiving care in the home.

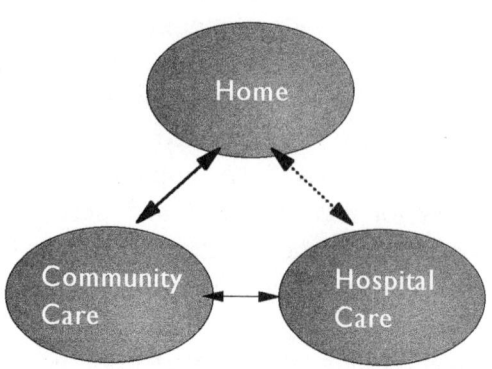

In the following sections, current work devoted to supporting communication within each of the areas of home, community, and hospitals will be reviewed. Wherever possible, work that addresses communication at the interface between these sections of the healthcare system will also be presented.

15.3 Communication and home healthcare

The delivery of health care in the home continues to grow as a proportion of the total healthcare sector. With ever increasing bed-costs, patients are being discharged from hospitals earlier, or having care once associated with in-patient stays delivered entirely as an outpatient. Equally, the benefits of being in a familiar environment, and away from risks such as hospital-acquired infection means that home care carries many added therapeutic benefits.

Typically, long-term home care patients might be managing a chronic illness like insulin-dependent diabetes, or undergoing home dialysis for renal failure. The delivery of chemotherapeutic agents in the home is also an option for some cancer patients. Short-term care at home might be appropriate following early discharge from hospital after an operation.

Consequently, for some patients, care in the home can span many years for a single condition, whilst for others it represents a brief episode. In either case, communication can support both patient and carer. Patients have a need for information about their care, which is to a greater or lesser extent self-managed in the home. As well as requiring access to factual information about their therapy, patients may simply need to interact with healthcare workers to assure themselves that they are managing their own care well.

For their part, carers will need access to data about the patient's physical as well as mental state to ensure that they remain well managed. The ability of patients to communicate this information themselves depends on their condition, their understanding of the process of care, and its complexity. One thus might expect a young adult insulin-dependent diabetic to be able to be deeply involved in the communication of information, whilst an elderly patient may need much more assistance and simpler interactions.

Remote monitoring of patients at home

The most obvious way for health care workers to monitor the progress of individuals at home is to visit them in person. Approximately 1.5 million such home visits take place in the USA each year. However, it is said that in many of these visits, hands-on care is not needed.

For this reason, some have advocated that such interactions can occur over communication links, rather than through physical visits. The proposed benefits are economic, as well as an improvement in the efficiency of staff who would spend less time travelling, and presumably more time communicating with patients.

The simplest way one can carry out such remote monitoring is to schedule a regular telephone call. Leirer et al. (1991) used a voicemail system to automatically telephone medication reminders to elderly people at home, and showed that it did reduce both tardiness and complete forgetting.

Using more sophisticated technology, nursing staff in another study used interactive video to do things like verify compliance with medication regimes, assess mental and emotional status, or check measurements like blood sugar levels. Despite a high acceptance with nursing staff, 40% of patients in this study felt a face-to-face visit would have been preferable because it might have altered the care that was delivered (Allen et al., 1996).

Despite the uncertainties in even this simple form of remote care, others are advocating much more complicated monitoring systems.

For example, it is technically possible to install monitoring equipment in the home. Measurements like blood pressure and cardiogram data can then be transmitted to a remote monitoring station (Rodriquez et al., 1995, Doughty et al., 1996).

This type of monitoring service is seen as way of allowing patients in hospital to be discharged early, for example post-infarction or post-operatively, or for the management of elderly or chronically ill patients at home.

The arguments for and against such communication services to the home are still unresolved, and await further study. Much of the impetus behind many home communication proposals seems to be either economic or technological.

Where resources and staff are limited, or patients are in remote locations, they may indeed prove to be useful alternatives to routine care. It is equally clear that these arguments omit the clear need of some patients in the community to occasionally interact face-to-face with healthcare workers.

Patient access to healthcare workers

In normal circumstances, a combination of routine home visits and access via channels like the telephone may be sufficient for most patients. In difficult circumstances this arrangement may break down. For example, elderly patients may have a need to communicate with carers in an emergency, but might be unable to reach a telephone once the emergency has occurred. Fractures of the hip, strokes, and heart attacks are all common problems that can leave elderly patients in a vulnerable position in their own home.

To combat this risk, many elderly people have a personal alarm system, connected to the public telephone system. There are many variations of this type of system. Usually they involve an individual wearing a pendant-style personal transmitter that can be activated with a simple button push. This activates an alarm at a control centre, which is then relayed to healthcare workers who will respond. Personal alarm systems serve over 1 million people in the United Kingdom, and 2-3 million people elsewhere (Fisk, 1995).

Patient access to information

Until recently, apart from the near ubiquitous use of the telephone, communication technology has only played a small role in information provision for patients. This is rapidly changing. For example, in the previous chapter we saw how one could use an interactive telephone system to deliver specialised information services. For example, patients could ring up an automated information system, and request it to fax them back specific pages of information.

Whilst this type of information service may seem to suit the provision of only very general information, similar services have already successfully used for more chronic illness. In France, for example, many diabetic patients have had access to specialised information for quite some time. The service is based upon Minitel, which is a small video-text terminal supplied free in France to all telephone subscribers. Using Minitel, some diabetic patients have had access to email and an expert system customised to give individualised dietary advice based upon information supplied by the patient regarding diet and exercise. Patients also had access to libraries of information, for example recipes. In a randomised trial, patients with access to information through the system demonstrated improved diabetic knowledge, improved dietary habits, and improved metabolic markers of disease control (fructosamine and HbA_1) (Turnin et al., 1992). Similar services can be easily provided across the Internet, which has a much richer functionality than the older Minitel system (see Chapter 16).

Clearly, for patients to master such relatively complicated communication and information resources, they have to be well trained, motivated and physically able to use these resources. Thus, independently of whichever technology is being employed to deliver information to patients, the most critical factors affecting compliance and correct usage will probably be human rather than technical.

15.4 Communication and primary care

There are significant organisational and communication challenges facing those delivering healthcare in the community. The model of shared care often adopted means that many different healthcare professionals may be involved in the management of an individual patient. During the course of routine management, a diabetic patient may for example, interact with a primary care physician, a diabetic specialist nurse, a podiatrist and a dietician. There is thus a clear need for communication between these team members.

Working against this is the decentralised manner in which community services are organised. Unlike a large hospital, team members are unlikely to work in the same building, and may not even work in the same local area. Further, many workers will on occasion be on the move outside their office, for example carrying out home visits.

Consequently, the primary care sector has requirements for solid communication processes be in place. These processes should support both routine updates between workers, allowing team members to keep track of patient progress, as well as communication in unpredictable circumstances.

At present there has only been a minimal attempt at applying communication technology to improve these processes. This is probably due to a lack of clear understanding of the intra-organisational communication needs in primary care. For example, when healthcare workers are working outside their office, do they have difficulties accessing their colleagues or is access to patient record data more important? Without such an understanding, one would not be able to recommend that a primary care group invested in mobile computing to access patient data in preference to mobile telephones.

The interface between primary care and specialist services

There has been a great emphasis in telemedicine on the interface between primary care and specialist services. There is a clear need for patient information to be exchanged between hospitals and primary care physicians upon admission to and discharge from hospital. The use of existing processes like the postal system to deliver such information is often criticised for tardiness and unreliability. In contrast, rapid communication of hospital discharge information using electronic data transfer mechanisms has been shown to be beneficial for general practitioners (Branger et al., 1992).

There has been significant recent effort in promoting methods that permit primary care practitioners to manage patients whom they would normally have referred to specialist centres, by supporting them with access to remote specialist advice.

In one study, direct telephone access to a hospital-based cardiac monitoring centre was provided to primary care practitioners. They were able to consult with a cardiologist as needed, as well as transmit a 12-lead ECG (Shanit et al., 1996). The centre in this study provided a 24 hour continuous service.

Possible outcomes of the discussion were that the practitioner continued to manage the patient, that the patient was referred to a cardiology clinic, or in the case of suspected myocardial infarction, rapid hospital admission was arranged with pre-warning of hospital medical teams. A trial of 2563 patients over 18 months indicated that the service was perceived to be valuable, but no comparative cost-benefit analysis was performed.

In a pilot of video-based consultation for dermatological problems, the primary care practitioner was able to discuss patient cases interactively with a dermatologist, with the patient present. Over half of the patients were then able to be dealt with by the general practitioner immediately after consultation (Jones et al., 1996). Common wisdom sees this type of service as a useful means of screening patients prior to being seen by specialists, especially if travel is involved. However, in this study the patients suggested that they preferred an initial face-to-face consultation with the specialist dermatologist, and that the teleconsultation would have been better used for subsequent review of their progress.

Similar studies in Norway have identified other benefits to this type of remote telemedical consultation. The skill level of isolated practitioners was raised through repeated interactions with remote specialists and through having to manage cases that were previously referred (Akelsen and Lillehaug, 1993). This may arise through the dynamics of the relationship between remote practitioner and specialist. Unlike most educational settings, both are motivated to form a coach and apprentice relationship for the immediate management of a patient.

In the last chapter we saw that it is still unclear in what precise circumstances video-based consultations are most appropriate. While there are some benefits in accessing remote expertise, there are limitations to the current technologies. It is well known for example, that during a clinical encounter, a significant component of the information conveyed between practitioner and patient is non-verbal (Pendleton et al., 1984). Tone of voice, facial expression and posture all convey subtle information cues which are interpreted by the patient. Technology can act either to distort these cues, or to filter them out. In some cases this might be beneficial. A patient may be less distressed if they are unable to pick up cues that the practitioner is worried about a situation. Equally, a patient's distress might increase if cues are misinterpreted because they are unfamiliar with the dynamics of the video consultation. These effects will vary with the type of communication channel used, and the practitioner's skills at using the channel. Having a good 'video manner' may well soon be as important as having a good telephone manner.

15.5 Communication and hospitals

Telemedical systems, as we have seen, have been actively explored at the interface between hospital-based specialist services and primary care. Similar problems exist between small hospitals, which may not have access to the highly specialised personnel that can be found in larger institutions like teaching hospitals. Indeed, with the growing number of sub-specialities in clinical medicine, it is now unlikely that any one institution has a representative from every feasible medical sub-speciality within their institution. For this reason, there is a need to share highly specialised expertise across different hospitals, sometimes involving large distances.

Inter-hospital communication

There is now some evidence that remote consultation, using telemedical facilities like video-conferencing, is able to assist with this problem of distribution of expertise (e.g. Doolittle and Allen, 1996). It has been shown for example, that when a general radiologist is able to consult with a remote specialist, sharing views of X-ray images using low resolution video, then the general radiologist's diagnostic accuracy improved (Franken and Berbaum, 1996). It now seems accepted that with appropriate technology, digitally transmitted images can in principle match existing imaging methods (e.g. Martel et al., 1995, Franken et al., 1995). The cost of achieving such results varies with the type of imaging task being attempted.

Triage models, similar to those explored in primary care, can limit the number of patients who need to be seen by limited sub-speciality resources. For example, in one study, general pathologists reviewed and reported on cases, and referred difficult cases to remote specialists by sending them high-resolution images (Bhattacharyya et al., 1995).

In another study, patients were offered access to specialist medical practitioners in a different country. Patients were able to travel there or to have a consultation by video-link. Choosing the video-conferencing option changed patients' desires to travel overseas. Of those seeking consultation, 20% initially wished to travel for treatment, but after the tele-consultation only 6% chose this option (Richardson et al., 1996).

Most of these studies throw up evidence that advanced communication systems and services are valuable. What remains unclear is whether there is any real cost-benefit from this approach. Indeed, it is becoming clear that the application of such technologies is only beneficial in particular sets of circumstances.

For example, comparing the costs of providing a rural population with radiology services from a small community-based unit, against a teleradiology system, the communication option fared poorly in one study (Halvorsen and Kristiansen, 1996). The study showed that the existing community-based system was the most cost-efficient, and the telemedical option the most expensive. The inconvenience caused when patients had to travel for specialist investigations was not factored into the study, nor was the possibility that some communities might not have access to local expertise.

Overall, the cost savings from installing any communication system must vary for different communities. The amount of resource saved, however measured, depends upon many variables. These include:

- the size of population served,

- the utilisation rates of the services that are being augmented by the communication option,
- the distances workers or patients might otherwise need to travel,
- the effectiveness of local services in comparison to the telemedical options.

There is also evidence that some types of task are not entirely suited to the remote consultation model. Microbiologists, for example, probably need 3 dimensional image information, as well as non-visual data like smell, before remote interpretation of microbiology specimens becomes feasible (Akelsen et al., 1995).

As always, it is important to not overlook simpler solutions to communication problems, if they exist. It is not always appropriate or necessary, for example, to use video-based consultation. In many cases, the communication needs of a specialist consultation may be met by use of the telephone alone (McLaren, 1995). Rather than purchasing systems permitting real-time video conferencing, images can be sent across computer networks. Standard email systems are capable of transmitting text and image, and are more than able to manage the task of sending still images, such as pathological slides or X-ray images (Della Mea et al., 1996). Once images have been received remotely, they can be viewed simultaneously and discussed over the telephone. Simple methods now exist to enhance this further, so that viewers can mark or point to sections of an image, and have these markings appear at the remote site.

Intra-hospital communication

Almost all current telemedical research is focused on the interfaces between hospitals and community services or the home. Very little work has been done to understand the internal communication dynamics and requirements of hospitals. Yet it should be apparent that any hospital is a complex organisation, and that good communication processes must be fundamental to its operation.

Thus, while much effort has been devoted to developing the electronic patient record, there has been minimal exploration of what communication systems can be developed to support hospital operation. However, a critical examination of the characteristics of the hospital as a workplace can identify clear areas in which there is significant potential for improvement. Two areas in particular deserve discussion - the need to support mobility, and the need for asynchronous messaging.

Mobility. In contrast to other populations such as office workers or clinic-based healthcare workers, hospital workers are highly mobile during their working day. Nursing staff are perhaps least mobile, spending most of their day moving around their home ward. Medical staff may have to move widely across a hospital campus. Senior medical staff may also have to move off campus, to attend other hospitals or clinics. Nevertheless, it is important that staff remain within reach during the working day.

At present the commonest solution to this problem of contacting mobile staff is provided by radio-paging. Pagers are almost ubiquitous in modern hospitals, and staff may carry several of these. For example, a pager might be issued to each individual. Other pagers are issued to members of teams, for example a 'crash' team that needs to respond to critical emergencies like cardiac arrests within the hospital. Pagers thus serve to permit communication both with named individuals, and individuals occupying labelled roles like 'surgeon on call' (Coiera, 1996b; H.T. Smith et al, 1991).

Pagers have several drawbacks. Invariably in a busy work environment, people move about and telephones are a pooled resource that quickly become engaged. As someone is paged, they answer the call to find either that the number given is now engaged, or that the caller has moved on to another ward location. The end result is often a game of 'telephone tag'.

The provision of mobile telephones bypasses many of these problems. The call set-up delays inherent in paging are eliminated, and the number of communication access points is multiplied through personal handsets. The value of mobile communications in a clinical environment is starting to be appreciated, but at present remains an under-utilised option (e.g. Fitzpatrick and Vineski, 1993). As with any technology there are some drawbacks. At a practical level, some healthcare workers can choose to hide behind a paging system, effectively choosing which calls to answer based upon their current state. This form of call-screening may no longer be possible if individuals have personal mobile telephones. The reduced costs of contacting colleagues and increased benefits of being contactable may be at the cost of decreased control of communication and increased interruption. At present it appears that the benefits significantly outweigh the costs, but formal studies are needed to confirm this.

Asynchronous communications. Hospitals are highly interrupt-driven environments (Coiera, 1996b). Interruptions to the normal flow of work are caused by the paging and telephone systems, as well as the result of impromptu face-to-face meeting by colleagues (e.g. being stopped in the corridor). The team-based nature of work also demands that subjects communicate frequently with team members throughout the working day.

The consequence of such frequent interruptions is that hospital workers have to repeatedly suspend active tasks to deal with the interruption, and then return to the previous task. Suspending tasks and then returning to them imposes a cognitive load, and may result in tasks being forgotten, or left incomplete. There thus is a cost in time and efficiency arising out of the interrupt-driven nature of the hospital work environment.

In part, the interruptive nature of hospitals is a result of the communication practices and systems in place in these organisations. For example, many hospitals do not at present routinely offer asynchronous channels like voicemail or email. It is likely, however, that many of the interruptions delivered through synchronous systems like the combined telephone and pager system could be handled by asynchronous channels. For example, updates on patient results or non-urgent requests to complete tasks could be sent by voicemail or email. As long as it is felt by those sending such messages that they definitely will be attended to, then some of the cause of interruption can be shifted onto these asynchronous systems. There thus seems to be a need for a concomitant change in communication process as well as the technology for such changes to be effective. The evidence that such asynchronous systems are of genuine benefit is slowly accumulating (e.g. Withers, 1988).

One of the limitations to the introduction of email systems is the lack of access points around a campus, for many of the same reasons that access to telephony is limited. The mobility of workers is perhaps one of the main issues. It is for this reason that mobile computers are being introduced into the hospital environment (Forman and

Zahorjan, 1994). Connected by wireless links, these small devices provide access to the hospital computer network.

The main driver for introducing such systems is to provide an easy way to capture clinical data and enter it into the hospital record system, or to retrieve data from it (e.g. Labkoff et al., 1995; MacNeill and Huang, 1996). One additional benefit of mobile computing will be mobile access to email. However, more advanced systems will be able to provide even richer services. Integrating mobile telephony, paging, and access to the hospital network through lightweight portable devices, newer systems can combine the functionality of the telephone with that of the computer (e.g. Coiera, 1996b).

15.6 Researching clinical communication

While the potential for the clinical application of communication technologies is indeed great, there is much still to learn. In particular, the relationship between telemedicine and informatics needs to be explored in greater detail. Informatics focuses on the use of information and telemedicine on its communication. Although seemingly disparate endeavours, they are intimately linked, since the goals of communicating information and deciding on its content cannot be separated (McCarthy and Monk, 1994).

Several key research questions are apparent. Firstly, clinical practice already revolves around communication, often by telephone, and important information exchanged in this way is often lost because it is not documented (Stoupa, 1990). As we saw in Chapter 4, much of this information is in an informal form. Capturing the informal information currently lost in healthcare's communication channels may soon become an important issue for those developing the formal electronic patient record. How one decides what information is important and how that information is made available are non-trivial questions involving issues of confidentiality, security, as well as the technology of storage and retrieval of voice recordings. The implications of this change in emphasis for the form and role of the electronic medical record are significant. Equally, the role of communications systems in supporting information retrieval should be reassessed. The telephone is an information system, albeit an informal one.

Secondly, our understanding of the effects of technology on communication is still in its infancy. Researchers in the field of human-computer interaction feel that before these technologies can be successfully introduced, the way in which individuals communicate needs to be understood (McCarthy and Monk, 1994). In one recent study, the presence of a computer during doctor-patient consultations had detectable negative effects on the way doctors communicated (Greatbatch et al., 1993). While they were at the computer, doctors confined themselves to short responses to patient questions, delayed responding, glanced at the screen in preference to the patient, or structured the interview around the computer rather than the patient.

Probably the most important issue for immediate research will be to understand the effect of introducing technologies that allow asynchronous communication. At present, devices like telephones and pagers interrupt individuals when communication is desired. The messages sent across asynchronous services like electronic mail and voicemail do not need to be answered immediately and so have the potential to significantly reduce the number of interruptions experienced by clinicians. Such messages may nevertheless carry important information. It will be critical to understand how such services can be designed to ensure that healthcare workers do not miss critical information, and equally are not inundated with a flood of irrelevant messages.

Finally, along with new communication possibilities, there come new medico-legal implications. The medico-legal position for tele-consultations is similar to that of telephone, fax, email or letter. These all amount to the provision of advice from a distance, and the normal standards of care and skill will apply (Brahams, 1995). There thus may be circumstances when it is considered inappropriate **not** to use tele-consultation. For example, if moving a patient puts them at risk and tele-consultation is available, then the communication option may be most appropriate. Equally, in some circumstances it may be inappropriate to use it, perhaps because there is a likelihood that management will be sub-optimal compared to face-to-face care. Until the evidence accumulates to identify which situations are most suitable for tele-consultation, its appropriateness in any given circumstances will have to be argued on a case-by-case basis, quite probably in the courts.

In the United States the courts have already decided that radiologists are negligent if they fail to inform clinicians personally of a diagnosis. 'Communication of an unusual finding in an X-ray, so that it may be beneficially utilised, is as important as the finding itself'. Further, leaving a message with an intermediary is not enough - 'certain medical emergencies may require the most direct and immediate response involving personal consultation and exchange' (Kline and Kline, 1992). The fact that such communication requirements are beginning to be mandated reflects the community's changing perceptions of best medical practice.

The rapid arrival of telemedicine suggests that the benefits of good clinical communications practice are beginning to be identified, and the costs of poor communication realised. The next few years should see the research in telemedicine mature. The main focus will become the application of communication technologies rather than their development. This represents the same shift in focus that was required of medical informatics, which also initially spent much effort in developing technologies specifically for medicine.

Chapter summary

1. Telemedicine is the exchange of information at a distance, whether that information is voice, an image, elements of a medical record, or commands to a surgical robot. It seems reasonable to think of telemedicine as the **remote communication of information to facilitate clinical care.**

2. Communication needs fall into two groups. Firstly, specific **intra-organisational** needs exist within particular groups, such as hospitals or primary care. Secondly, there are significant **inter-organisational** needs that occur at the interfaces between significantly different organisations.

3. Communications systems have a role in home healthcare, providing patients with access to information about their care and the ability to interact regularly with healthcare workers to assure themselves that they are managing their own care well.

4. In primary care there are communication needs at the interface between primary care and specialist services, and between primary care and patients. Video-based telemedical consultations are a possible solution to some of these needs, but their value still remains uncertain.

5. Very little work has been done to understand the internal communication dynamics and requirements of organisations like hospitals. There are clear needs, however, to have support for mobile and asynchronous communication.

Part
Six

The Internet

Telegraphs are machines for conveying information over extensive lines with great rapidity. They have generally been established for the purpose of transmitting information during war, but the increasing wants of man will probably soon render them subservient to more peaceful objects.

Babbage, p36, (1832).

Chapter 16

The Internet

The rise of the Internet presents us with a defining moment at the end of the millennium. Some see it as a technological revolution rivalling Gutenberg's invention of the printing press. Others see it as just another tool that, like the telephone or television, will soon pass into common usage, leaving our lives relatively unchanged (R Smith, 1996a).

However, the Internet defies such simple analysis. It is not a single entity, but represents the conjunction of several quite different technological and social forces. Consequently, its implications for the way information is created, distributed and accessed are wide ranging. For medicine in particular, the implications for the way healthcare is delivered, and the way it will evolve are significant.

In previous sections of this book, the two fundamental informatics strands of information and communication were developed. In this section on the Internet, we will see how information and communication systems can combine, and the power that results from that combination. The following chapters offer a snapshot of the Internet as a complex system in transition. This chapter will begin by introducing the Internet, and explore the technical and social forces shaping it. The next chapter will look at the World Wide Web, its technological basis, and its implications for informatics. The section will conclude with a chapter specifically looking at the way the Internet, and Internet technologies, may be used in healthcare. It ends with some particular challenges and opportunities that the Internet poses for healthcare.

16.1 The Internet has evolved through four stages

From a relatively humble beginning, the Internet has transformed completely in size, form and function. Historically, one can think of the Internet evolving through four relatively distinct stages, each one shaped in turn by its predecessors.

It began in the United States in the late 1960s as a cold-war military research project, designed to ensure that communication lines remained open after nuclear strikes. This system slowly evolved in size and complexity until, in the mid-eighties, the Internet had become a global computer network.

At that time it was used by many academic institutions, and a few commercial companies. During this second phase, its main use was for electronic messaging and the transfer of computer files. What

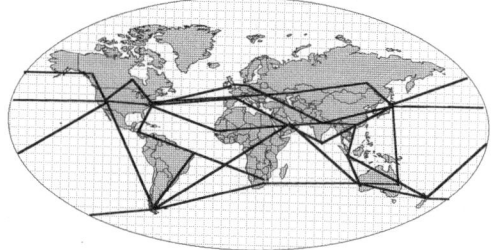

Figure 16.1: The Internet is a global computer network that evolved out of a US military project in the 1960s, and is now in a steady state of growth as new links are added, and new subscribers join.

followed next was a period of steady growth, as the population of users slowly expanded beyond industry and academia.

It was not really until the third phase, with the introduction of the World Wide Web onto the Internet, that the massive growth today associated with the Internet occurred. The Web (WWW or W3) provides a simple and standard way to find and view documents on the Internet. Its ease of use, along with an ever growing store-house of publicly accessible information, combined to transform the Internet into a tool that the public at large was able to appreciate and wanted to use.

The fourth phase has followed on relatively rapidly. It is characterised by the commercial and institutional exploitation of the Internet and its technologies. A constant stream of innovation in the way in which the Internet is being used, as well as in its underlying technologies, guarantees that change will be a feature for quite some time.

Box 16.1 - The end of the ice age

In the Victorian era, there was a global market in ice. The ice was harvested in cold countries like North America, and shipped around the world as far as the Indian sub-continent. Transported in specially constructed ice-ships, the ice was then stored in huge warehouses upon arrival. Every good home had an ice chest in which they kept this precious commodity, and used it to keep food cool.

In the 1860s competition in the form of artificial ice-making plants began to appear. Today that ice trade has disappeared. We no longer need to ship ice because technology has caused the nature of the market to change. Rather then shipping ice, we ship the stuff needed to make ice - energy. Energy is transported across great power grids that originates in huge power stations. The fundamental market need has not changed - we still want the ability to cool our food. What has changed is the way in which that need is met. The power industry and refrigerator manufacturers are the economic inheritors of the ice industries.

We can draw interesting economic parallels between the demise of the ice industry and the fate of printing. Books today are created in printing houses, and from there shipped around the globe, eventually to be stored in the huge warehouses we call libraries.

If the world of publishing is equivalent to the ice industry, then the Internet is equivalent to the power industry. The Internet does not ship documents printed on paper. It ships information down its data grid, which can be reconstituted into documents upon arrival. Just as a refrigerator sits at the edge of the power grid and takes in energy to produce cold, computers sit at the edge of the information grid, and take in information, converting it as needed into other forms. The parallel is striking.

While, the needs met by the 'information market' are the same before and after the arrival of Internet, the nature of that market has changed. The Internet thus heralds fundamental economic change. Old industries will disappear and new ones will emerge.

While some changes will be rapid, others will undoubtedly be very slow. Libraries for example, will still be needed - at least until all their contents have been converted into electronic form. That process may be slow and expensive, and for some works the demand may be so small that it is easier to continue to warehouse them in libraries.

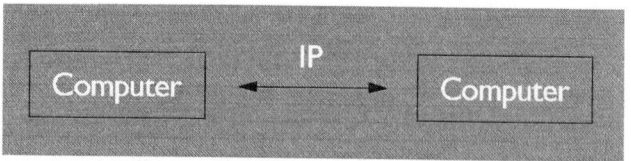

Figure 16.2: The Internetworking Protocol (IP) was developed to ensure that computers connected together in a network were able to communicate with each other in a reliable fashion, even if some elements of the network failed.

With such a background of rapid change, it can be difficult to understand just what the Internet is, and in what ways it is being used. For many healthcare professionals, unused to information and communication technology, it can be particularly difficult to assess the validity or importance of all the claims being made about it. It is thus helpful to examine the technological, social and economic forces shaping the Internet in turn. More importantly, understanding each of these issues will help develop an understanding of the particular ways in which the Internet affects healthcare.

16.2 The Internet as a technological phenomenon

Essentially a network of networks, the Internet permits computers across the globe to communicate with each other. It evolved out of the Advanced Research Projects Network (ARPAnet) developed by the United States Department of Defence in the late 1960s (Lowe et al., 1996).

ARPAnet was built with the intention of developing computer networks which would be capable of surviving nuclear war. The challenge at that time was to develop methods for sharing information across diverse sites, and to keep these connections operational even if a disruption occurred at individual sites.

The result of this work was a standard Internetworking Protocol or IP, which regulated the way in which computers communicated with each other across the network. Throughout the 1970s and early 1980s the Internet grew, as more and more small, mainly academic networks were joined onto it using the new IP.

Initially the information transmitted across the Internet consisted of text-based electronic mail, or computer files that were shipped from one site to another. However, it became clear in the late eighties that it would be desirable to send many different kinds of media, not just text, across the Internet. This **multimedia** added still and moving images and voice to basic text.

Work that began at the European Particle Physics Laboratory (CERN) in 1989 resulted in a set of communication standards and software that provided Internet users with a simple way of creating and accessing such information. These standards allowed users to create and exchange text, image and video documents. The model for the way one could interact with these multimedia files also began to evolve. In particular the notion of **hypertext** became important. Here a computer file included links within it to other files, possibly located on a distant computer somewhere else on the Internet. Activating a hypertext link on a document permits a reader to view the document attached to the link.

This work at CERN was successful in a way that was probably not foreseen by those who commenced the original research project. As we will see in the next chapter, these standards were responsible for the appearance of a large number of interlinked multimedia files that were distributed across the Internet. This expanding global collection of interconnected information sources became known as the World Wide Web.

Today, these standards for interacting with information, and communicating across the Internet are in a state of constant evolution. It is unlikely that the Internet's creators could have foreseen, for example, that the Internet would be used for voice telephony, or that one could one day interact with virtual reality worlds across it. Equally, they could not have foreseen the size of the present Internet or its present rate of sustained growth. Perhaps of greater surprise is that the basic internetworking protocols developed out of the ARPAnet sustain a collection of networks far in excess of the number that was ever intended.

16.3 The Internet as a social phenomenon

While it has been around for most of the 1980s, mostly as a global academic network, the Internet has only recently come into public consciousness. It was probably the advent of the World Wide Web that triggered the recent public growth of the Internet. The Web permits users to navigate easily across the global Internet. Here they

Figure 16.3: The rapid growth in Internet use is shown through the rise in total monthly accesses to the Oncolink World Wide Web Site, which commenced service to the public in March of 1994. (http://cancer.med.u penn.edu/)

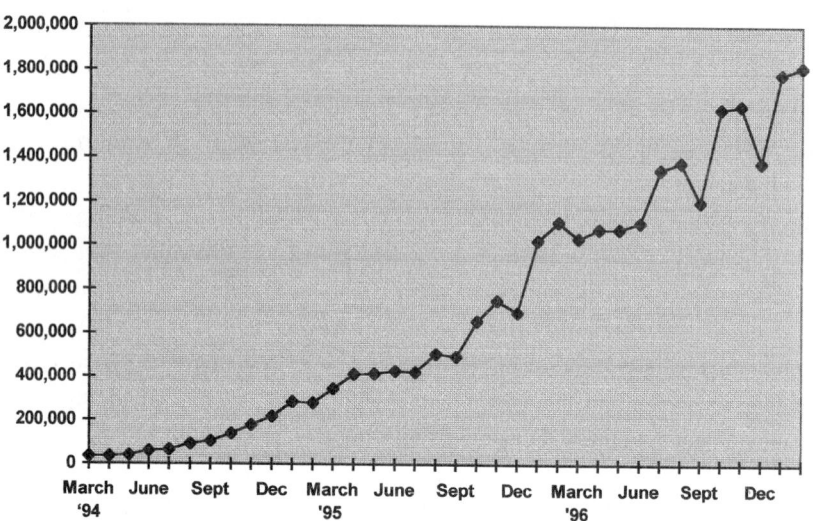

can view a bewildering variety of information, from the bizarre and inaccurate, to the most up-to-date information available from scientific bodies, newspapers and academic journals. It was probably a combination of improved ease of use, along with the amount of information available on the Web reaching a critical mass, that brought the Internet to the public's attention.

At present, the Internet is in a phase of massive expansion, with monthly growth rates of well above 15%. This is largely because, where before its value for most people was marginal, it now offers communication and information services that surpass those possible with plain telephony or television. The OncoLink information resource, for example, provides oncologists with up to date clinical trial and treatment information, as well as acting as an educational resource for cancer patients and their families. At its inception in March 1994, OncoLink was reportedly accessed 36,000 times (Buhle et al., 1994). The figure for February 1997 was 1,813,310 accesses (Figure 16.3).

As more of these information services become available, even more people are being persuaded to join. It is the same phenomenon of technology adoption reaching a critical mass that we have seen in the past with other technologies like the telephone, the CD and the personal computer. When only a few people possessed them, there was insufficient market to develop the services and economies of scale that would make them mass market items. Once a certain threshold of ownership is exceeded, however, the market develops rapidly.

Associated with the growing public interest in the Internet is a brand of more extreme social futurism. Words like cyberspace and virtual reality combine with aspirations for social change to create predictions about the shape of a future society based on a commerce of information (e.g. Negroponte, 1995). As unsurprising is the intellectual backlash of many who reject visions of a world in which people preferentially interact with others across computer networks rather than in more 'human' ways. Because of the heat such discussion generates, it is attention-grabbing and often is the way in which the public is first exposed to the Internet. Unfortunately perhaps, this dialogue distracts many from its more immediate and practical applications.

Perhaps more substantially, this brand of futurism has echoes of social reaction to many previous technologies. Everything from satellite communications, through to the Pill, radio, television, the telephone and the computer were all going to revolutionise society in the eyes of some commentators. In their own way, they often did, but never as fundamentally as was predicted.

A feature of the futurism associated with the Internet is the belief in a technology-enabled information society. Here, the freedom of creation, distribution and access to information is the mechanism through which many imagine the solution to a variety of perceived social ills. As with any group of people engaged in radical thinking, there are elements both of truth and wishful thinking here. Equally as likely, amongst the futurists, cyberspace will have been replaced in another decade by a new liberation technology.

16.4 The Internet as a commercial phenomenon

The growth of the public's interest in the Internet caught most computer and telecommunications companies by surprise. Communication has traditionally been the preserve of the telecommunications industry, and the market for information provision on home computers was going to be dominated by CD-ROM technology. Today the Internet is challenging the verities of what and how people should communicate, and we are unlikely to see these issues settled soon.

A variety of industries are now seeking to capitalise on the Internet. What makes this particular market so ripe for exploitation is that it is being fought over by so many separate industries, each today a giant in their own right. Telecommunications carriers, cable television companies, and personal computer companies for example, know that the Internet has the potential to transform their existing businesses. Equally, it also has the potential to wipe out much of that existing business.

There are four basic Internet 'businesses' - transport, connection, services, and content. **Transport** refers to the industries that provide the physical networks upon which the Internet is built, and across which the basic bits of information are moved. This 'bit shipping' is the domain of telecommunication companies and the cable and wireless network operators, and is fiercely competitive. As it becomes increasingly cheap to ship bits, these industries are forced to look to other more profitable kinds of Internet business to maintain their profitability.

Providing **connection** into the Internet is in itself a business. Increasingly service providers offer network connections to the Internet for individuals or groups who do not have the need, or cannot afford to build, their own networks. This is typically how most homes are presently connected to the Internet. Usually this involves signing a contract with a service provider who creates and maintains Internet accounts, and provides connection on some fee-for-service basis. Some of these service providers are well-established names like CompuServe and America Online, but they are being increasingly challenged by major computer companies who have also moved into the service-provision business. This is seen by many as an attempt by these computer companies to establish a foothold in the potentially even more profitable businesses of service and content provision.

For example, many diverse existing businesses can use the Internet to provide their **services** to a larger community of people. Customer information queries can now be satisfied by Web-based information sources, rather than needing to be handled by staff on the telephone. New means of advertising and marketing are also emerging. More fundamentally, the Internet provides businesses with new ways with which to interact with the public. These range from the ability to order pizza across the Internet through to browsing sales catalogues and placing orders, viewing homes with real estate agencies and to carrying out transactions with banks and other financial institutions.

Finally, the Internet has created a new demand for information. So-called **content** providers, be they traditional publishers, or companies that control other forms of information (for example mailing lists) are able to sell their information on the Internet. Consider the difference in costs for a publisher of an encyclopaedia between its traditional business and an Internet based one. Traditionally the public would be asked to buy a complete set of encyclopaedia volumes, representing a large personal investment by the family. Equally the company has to invest considerably in sales staff to sell the books. The Internet business model is completely different. Here the public accesses an electronic version of the encyclopaedia maintained by the company across the net. Every time a member of the public looks up information, a small charge is made by the encyclopaedia company. So, a business that relied on making relatively few but large sales using a local sales force, is transformed into a global company that makes a multitude of very small sales with no sales force. The implications of such business changes are substantial.

16.5 The Internet as an enterprise phenomenon

Although initially a global phenomenon, the Internet provides a new model for the way organisations can organise their internal communication and information systems. Most major academic institutions and corporations manage their own internal computer networks, fulfilling similar communication and information functions to the wider Internet. Perhaps unsurprisingly then, the technological advances that have driven the growth of the Web on the external Internet are just as applicable to these internal networks. The use of Internet technologies on an internal computer network creates what is termed an internal Internet, or **intranet**.

There are numerous benefits of an intranet model for large organisations. Firstly, at a technological level, their existing

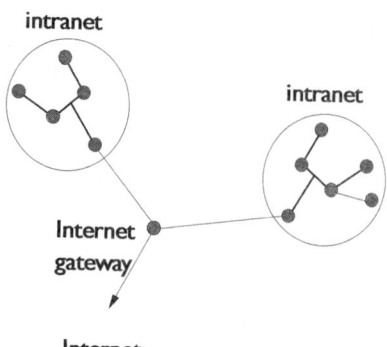

Figure 16.4:
Intranets are created from the computer networks within an organisation like a hospital or a company, use Internet technologies, and have the same benefits. They can also be connected by gateways to the open global Internet.

networks may consist of a mixture of systems running different communication protocols. Managing several different systems is complex, expensive and time-consuming. Using the Internet's IP allows a uniform protocol to be used across an enterprise's network. Just as attractively, the simplicity of the Web's multimedia and hypertext makes intranet systems much easier to use, and requires less specific training of staff.

Perhaps more importantly, the model of information publication and access offered by the Web is substantially different from the more traditional centralised corporate model. In the past, if an information service was to be made available, it would need to be created in conjunction with the organisation's Information Systems department. Because of the complexity of creating computer-based information resources, the necessary specialised expertise was concentrated here. If changes needed to be made to existing information resources, they also had to be funnelled through these same channels.

The end result of this model for large organisations was that their computer systems tended to become large and complicated over time, and increasingly difficult and expensive to maintain. Equally as critical, as the organisation and its information requirements changed, the centrally managed systems become increasingly out of date, since they could not change at the same rate.

The Web model allows workers across an organisation to create and locally maintain their own information services. For example, manuals and information packs can be placed on-line and updated without any central support being needed. In a hospital, the daily report on bed occupancy could be put on the Web and accessed by any machine on the hospital intranet.

Intranets can also be used by workers to share documents of mutual relevance. In this way, and in combination with other services like e-mail, the intranet starts to replace the functionality of more expensive and specialised Groupware software.

It also has the potential to change the model by which information is distributed. In the past it was common for the author of a document to have to arrange for its distribution to all those who had an interest in it, either in paper or electronic form. In the Web model, it is possible for the author of information to simply make it available on a network, and place the onus on those with an interest to retrieve it. Clearly the model of ownership of responsibility for information awareness must vary with circumstances. It would be inappropriate for example, for a hospital to place an urgent drug recall notice on its network and not notify medical staff. Equally it may be entirely appropriate for the minutes of a monthly meeting to be placed for viewing on a network without being announced.

16.6 Communication on the Internet

Now that the Internet has been described in broad terms, we can begin to look at more specific aspects of the way in which it is used. In this section, the specific communication methods available on the Internet will be explored.

There are a variety of ways in which individuals and groups can communicate on the Internet, starting with basic services like e-mail (see Chapter 13). These simple services can be combined to create more powerful services like private mailing lists and newsgroups. We can broadly characterise such services as either being **information push**, in which messages are pushed out at targeted individuals, or **information pull**, in which access is based on individuals seeking or being pulled toward information sources.

Mailing lists

An e-mail message is an example of a 'push' method and can be sent to multiple destinations. It is thus possible to draw up pre-defined distribution lists of people who should receive messages, much as one would do for internal memos, or circulars. This simple but

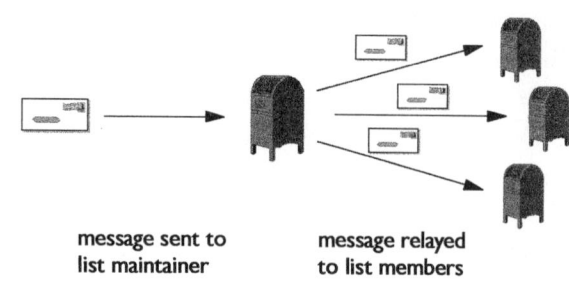

Figure 16.5: Mailing Lists. Before a message is received by all the members of a mailing list, it is sent to the maintainer of the list, who acts as a gatekeeper, possesses the addresses of all list members, and forwards on messages to them.

message sent to
list maintainer

message relayed
to list members

powerful feature of e-mail can be exploited to create mailing lists. Here a group of people can, for example, carry out an ongoing and private discussion by e-mail.

One or more individuals choose to maintain the list of names, and 'moderate' or referee the group interactions. People wishing to join the list send messages to the moderator, requesting that they be added to the list. People wishing to send a message to the group send the message to the moderator. The moderator vets the message for appropriateness, and then sends it out to the group for their consideration. The speed of message distribution is thus dependent on the rapidity with which the moderator forwards messages. Equally those in the moderator role have significant and sometimes absolute control over the discussion that takes place in the group.

There is nothing inherent in the way such groups can be constructed that makes it necessary that a single individual should control the list in an absolute way. For example, professional bodies may elect a moderator, draw up rules of conduct for message creation and distribution, or indeed have a panel of two or more individuals who collectively moderate messages.

Newsgroups and bulletin boards

In contrast to mailing lists, newsgroups are publicly accessible forums for discussion. Anyone with access to the Internet is able to access a wide variety of different discussion groups, read the messages placed in these groups, and respond to messages by e-mail. Newsgroups are thus an example of information 'pull' communication method. Message responses can be made public, by

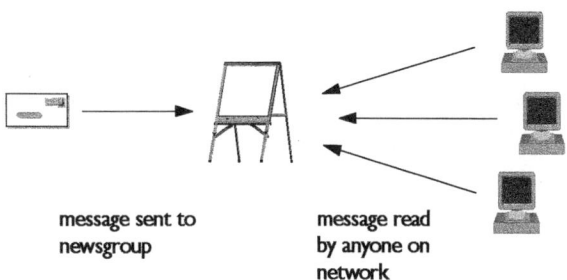

message sent to
newsgroup

message read
by anyone on
network

Figure 16.6:
Newsgroups and
bulletin boards are
maintained by a
moderator, who vets
messages that are
posted to the group.
Once posted there,
anyone with access to
the group is able to
read all current
messages.

posting back to the newsgroup, or private by posting back only to the originator of the message.

Newsgroups are usually classified systematically, according to the type of discussion that takes place in each group. The organisational structure is usually taxonomic, resulting in a family tree of newsgroups. Thus the newsgroup sci.med.informatics belongs to the overall sci group devoted to 'scientific' discussions, of which the med groups are in particular devoted to medical topics. Of the many medical newsgroups, the one in this example is devoted to discussions about informatics.

At present, there is a standard and relatively democratic process for the creation of new newsgroups. It begins when someone posts a call to existing groups, asking for a show of interest in the new group. This is followed by a period within which the public can vote for or against the creation of the group. With sufficient support, the group is given official status. The intention of the process is in part to prevent a proliferation of groups that have little support or transient appeal.

Even if newsgroups may have a 'professional' topic, access to the group is universal. Thus one is just as likely to find a member of the public, perhaps currently under treatment, posting a question about their therapy, as it is to find clinicians discussing treatment options amongst themselves. This means some readers might consider particular messages posted to a group to be inappropriate.

Since one of the problems with newsgroups is the time and effort needed to read the many messages posted every day, the privacy and relative security of a mailing list can be very attractive. When it works well, however, this mix of readership can be very powerful.

Box 16.2 - Fast Science and Cold Fusion

Some news stories are not handled well by traditional public broadcast media like radio and television. Newsgroups can carry out a vital role in such circumstances. For example, much of the first detailed technical information surrounding the 'discovery' of cold fusion in the mid-eighties was transmitted across the Internet.

After the initial announcement, scientists were able to pose questions quickly and get answers from colleagues in other nations in a way no other medium could have supported. Over the first few weeks of the cold fusion episode, physicists wrote and published numerous learned papers discussing the initial experiments, and the implications of their results. As scientists attempted to replicate the experiments, they published their interim results in newly created newsgroups specifically devoted to the subject.

The speed with which the scientific community was able to examine and respond to the implications of cold fusion was spectacular, made possible only by the Internet. Had the usual channels of peer-reviewed publications been used, it may have taken many years for the same scientific consensus to be reached about the validity of the original cold-fusion experiments.

Medical journals may be able to respond to similar scientific 'crises' in similar ways. Indeed some medical journals, such as the *Australian Medical Journal*, are already using a form of controlled rapid peer review using the Internet.

There are already examples of patients in geographically isolated countries posting questions about their symptoms to a newsgroup, and receiving a life-saving diagnosis from a specialist living in another country (M F Smith, 1996).

At its worst, people may post information that clinicians might consider ill-informed or dangerously incorrect. It is usually the nature of newsgroups that someone will quickly point out that information to the group, and explain why it is incorrect. Individual messages can have their impact moderated by the responses from others reading the newsgroup.

The effectiveness of newsgroups in disseminating information was one of the first pointers towards the wider potential of the Internet, prior to the introduction of the World Wide Web. Newsgroups have proved to be a powerful medium for rapidly conveying information

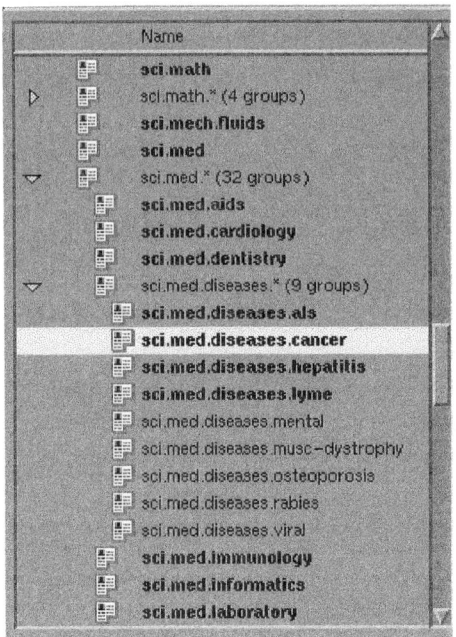

Figure 16.7:
Newsgroups are organised systematically, and classified according to subject. Messages appearing in a group are placed there by individuals who feel that their message will be appropriate to the group.

when other methods are inappropriate or restricted. For example, in areas of conflict or censorship, people have been able to send out information via the Internet, even when radio and television services in their own country have been shut down.

Along with the Internet newsgroups, many larger service providers will provide their own discussion forums and bulletin boards, available only to their subscribers. The content of some of the material that appears on these services is a current cause for concern. Some material that is posted onto bulletin boards contravenes the laws of various countries, either for security or moral reasons. Since by their very nature these systems are international, the legal implications of the material appearing on bulletin boards are still unclear. Some service providers initially chose to be very conservative in the discussion groups they supported. As a consequence, they closed down those that started to contain material breaking laws in any of the countries that their subscribers come from, even though the material may be acceptable in other countries.

Chapter summary

1. Essentially a network of networks, the Internet permits computers across the globe to communicate with each other. It evolved out of the Advanced Research Projects Network (ARPAnet) developed by the United States Department of Defence in the late 1960s.
2. Shaped by technological, social and economic forces, the Internet represents a complex conjunction of phenomena.
3. In economic terms, there are four basic Internet 'businesses' - transport, connection, services, and content.
4. Internet technologies permit new means for the publication and distribution of information without, and within organisations. The use of Internet technologies on an internal computer network creates what is termed an internal Internet, or **intranet**.
5. We can characterise communication services as either being **information push**, in which messages are pushed at targeted individuals, or **information pull**, in which access is based on individuals seeking out or being pulled information sources.
6. Several communication services are available on the Internet:
   - With mailing lists, an e-mail message is sent to multiple destinations. It is thus possible to draw up pre-defined distribution lists of people that should receive messages, much as one would do for internal memos, or circulars.
   - In contrast to Mailing lists, Newsgroups are publicly accessible forums for discussion. Anyone with Internet access is able to access a wide variety of different discussion groups, read the messages placed in these groups, and respond to messages by e-mail.
   - Work that began at the European Particle Physics Laboratory (CERN) in 1989 resulted in a set of communication standards and software that provided Internet users with a simple way of creating and accessing text, image and video documents. The standards they created were responsible for the appearance of an expanding global collection of interconnected information sources is known as the World Wide Web.

Chapter 17

The World Wide Web

The World Wide Web is perhaps the most important innovation to have occurred on the Internet in the last few years. The huge global computer network that forms the Internet, can at its simplest be thought of as an intricate transportation system for information. It provides the basic links between information sites, and the basic mechanisms for shipping information across those links. In the same way that fax services overlay the telephone system, the Web functions on top of the Internet's transport system. Its originators developed it 'to be a pool of human knowledge, which would allow collaborators in remote sites to share ideas and all aspects of a common project' (Bereners-Lee et al., 1994).

Conceptually the Web turns every computer on the Internet into a potential information source or library, and allows any other computer to look in onto these libraries and explore the information there. All these sources can further combine to create documents that exist on multiple computers and span the globe.

This expanding 'docuverse' is a new kind of library (Nelson, 1965), where information is created in one place and made immediately available everywhere. It is consequently almost infinitely flexible, allowing rapidly changing information to be both shared and updated quickly, in ways that traditional publishing is unable to achieve. Finally, because the Internet permits two-way transport, readers of documents can interact with and change them if the creators of the documents so desire. This kind of interaction of communication with information permits levels of collaboration that have previously not

Figure 17.1: The World Wide Web is overlaid on top of the Internet, and provides a standard way for creating, finding and accessing documents stored on computer, by any other computer connected to the network (IP - Internetworking Protocol, HTTP - HyperText Transfer Protocol - see Section 17.4).

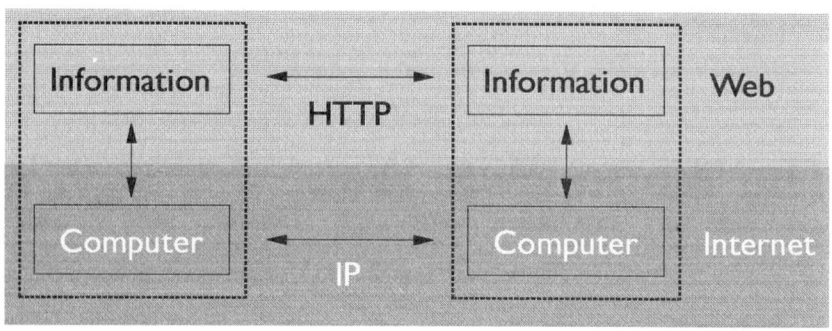

been possible. What is perhaps surprising is that the technologies underlying the Web are relatively simple. The establishment of the Web was achieved through the development and universal adoption of a set of software and software standards for operation over the Internet.

Healthcare is heavily reliant on collaboration and the sharing of information, and burdened by an ever growing body of research and clinical data, suffers because of this. The Web, because it is specifically designed to help in such circumstances, is thus shaping up to become a fundamental tool at all levels of healthcare, from research through to the clinic.

Given the importance of the Web for healthcare, this chapter will look at the ways in which information is created and accessed upon the Web. It will then take a particular look at each of the basic Web technologies, and explore their implications for the creation and dissemination of information.

17.1 Origins of the Web

As the Internet grew in the late eighties, it was beginning to be used in new ways. Most of the traffic across the network at that time was either email in the form of text, or consisted of data files. These data files were often themselves complicated documents - for example scientists commonly exchanged preliminary research papers in this way. There was no standard way that defined how these files should be created or viewed. The best available were standard printer languages like Postscript, which gave some guarantee that a file generated on one computer system could be printed on a different printing device at another site. Beyond fairly rudimentary file transfer protocols, there was also no easy way to exchange these more complicated documents on the computer system itself.

As we saw in the last chapter, research at the European Particle Physics Laboratory (CERN) began to look at this set of problems. A particular focus of the CERN work was to enable much richer documents to be created and exchanged. In particular, the document standard then created at CERN permitted the creation of multimedia documents that contained images, sound, or video (Figure 17.2).

One additional and critical part of these documents was that they could contain links within them, pointing to other documents. This type of document is known as hypertext, and permits a reader to select a link within a document and follow it outside the document. For example, if this chapter was written as hypertext, then a reference to a figure embedded within text could be active. Selecting that link would move the reader to the figure, wherever it might be. The notion of navigating around hypertext slowly evolved from the 60s onwards, as computer scientists tried to find ways of managing complex and rapidly changing information that was distributed across many locations (Lowe et al., 1996).

Hypertext document navigation is often characterised as being non-

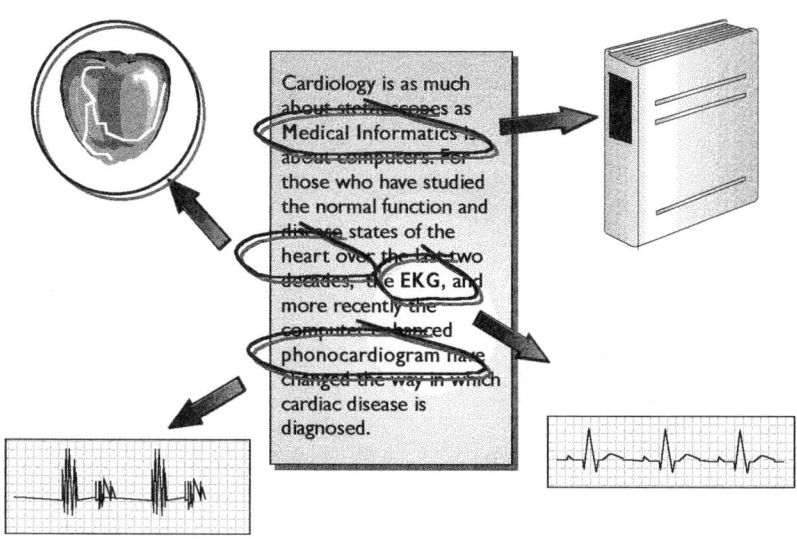

Figure 17.2:
Multimedia documents may contain text, still or moving images, and sound recordings. Hypertext systems permit such documents to be linked together, permitting the reader to follow links from one to another.

linear. One can jump across documents, following references that appear of interest to a particular reader. Consequently different readers will follow different 'paths' through the space of hypertext documents, based upon their needs. Links are not constrained to be local to a document, and could in principle point to other documents anywhere on a network.

The CERN vision of a world wide document pool meant that hypertext links permitted jumps to documents anywhere on the Internet (Figure 17.3). To make this happen, three technology standards had to be created:

- A standard way in which to create multimedia hypertext documents, called the HyperText Markup Language or HTML (see Box 17.1).
- A standard way to give each document an address on the Internet so that it could be located, called its Universal Resource Locator or URL (see Box 17.2).
- A standard way of transferring documents between computers, called the HyperText Transfer Protocol or HTTP (see Box 17.3).

17.2 Using the Web

For most users, their window onto the Web is provided by a program called a **browser**. This program runs on their computer, and provides

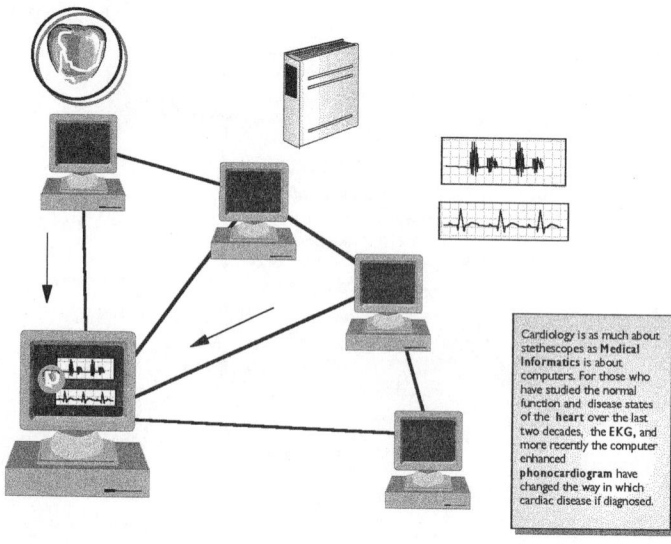

Figure 17.3: Web hypertext documents can be located on different computers, either on the same local computer network, or at distant Internet sites around the globe.

a means of interacting with the space of Web documents placed upon the Internet.

Only a few browsers are in widespread use and they share a common set of features. Typically, a browser has the following basic functions:

- It acts as a navigation tool for moving around the Web.
- It provides mechanisms for retrieving and storing documents that have been found on the Web.
- It acts as a viewing tool for these multimedia hypertext documents.
- It acts as a communication port, connecting for example with email systems.
- It may also incorporate methods for the creation of Web documents.

Finding a document

Once connected into the Web, there are several different ways in which one can search the information space. The method chosen ultimately depends on the type of information being searched, and the amount of information one has prior to commencing the search. At present, documents can be found in the following ways.

Specific address. If the location of a document is explicitly known, then specifying its address (known as a URL) will permit a browser to directly request a document from the computer it is stored upon.

Directories. Many directory services are offered on the Web, listing documents according to categories. The larger directory services are often privately run. These directories can be compiled in a number of ways. Initially it is usually possible in small subject areas for the creator of the directory to manually explore the Web, and list all sites that come within its scope. One can take advantage of the fact that most Web documents contain links to related documents, and follow a trail. Once directories have become established, they attain a certain amount of popularity, and document creators themselves will inform the directory maintainers about their document. For the document creator, this increases the visibility of new information once it is placed upon the Web.

Search engines. Given the large number of documents that exist on the Web, and their constant state of flux, it is inevitable that much of the information on the Web is not indexed in the larger directories. One solution to this problem is to create unstructured keyword indexes of as many documents as possible. Using these indexes, a user specifies the words that are likely to be associated with the topic of interest, much as one would when specifying search criteria for articles at a library. Agent programs or 'Web crawlers', automatically traverse the Web, following links from one document to the next. They look for new documents, and store relevant information about these documents in the index. Some indexes just store document titles and addresses, whilst others are far more ambitious and index all words that appear in a document, resulting in the creation of enormous databases.

Directories and search engines are powerful tools for exploring the information space of the Web. The problem of making the process of search tractable becomes ever harder as the number of documents on the Web grows. For example, using a search engine may result in many hundreds or even thousands of documents being identified with a set of keywords.

Developing appropriate strategies for using these tools thus becomes important. For example, starting with a few general words, it is often necessary to refine the search by making more specific searches with a larger number of keywords. The more information that is specified in a search, the fewer documents will be found to match.

The whole area of search mechanisms attracts considerable attention at present, and new ways for filtering and ranking search results are being developed. One potentially very promising avenue is for individuals to have a personal software agent. The agent might, for example, observe an individual's information search patterns, and see which type of documents tend to be retrieved. Using machine learning methods the program slowly builds up rules to identify documents that are likely to be appropriate in the future (see Chapter 19).

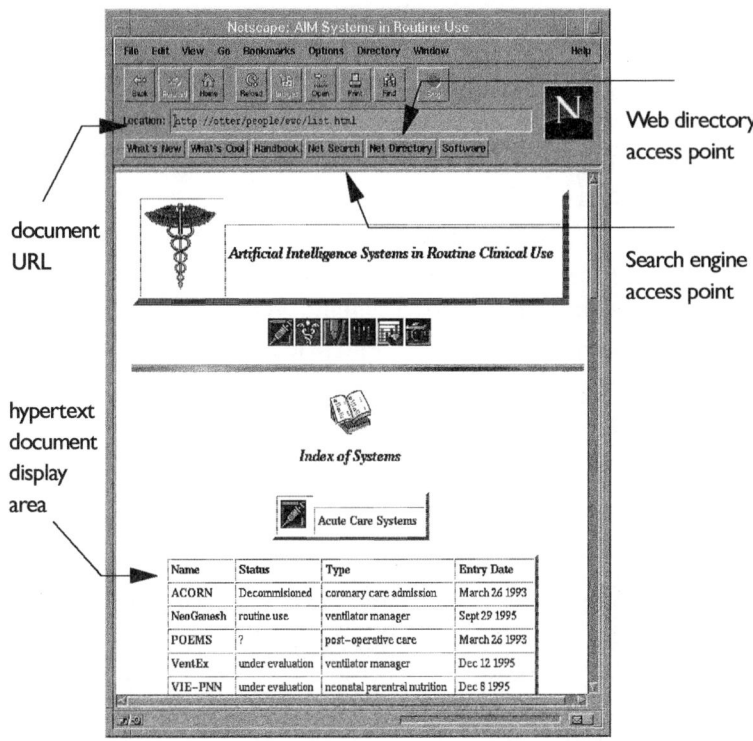

document URL

Web directory access point

Search engine access point

hypertext document display area

Figure 17.4: *Web browsers provide mechanisms for accessing hypertext documents on the Web, as well as search and directory services.*

17.3 Publishing on the Web

The Web established a simple standard for the way in which multimedia and hypertext documents are written. This standard is defined in the HyperText Markup Language or HTML. The practical consequence of having all documents written in HTML is that they can be universally read by anyone on the Internet possessing a browser that can interpret HTML.

This is important because previously creators of documents or software had to produce several different versions, each tailored to different computer systems. The acceptance of the HTML standard means that writers need not be concerned with the computer system upon which the document will appear.

As a consequence, document creation is now decoupled from the needs of specific computer systems. This burden is now shifted onto those who create browser software, which must be developed specifically for different computer operating systems and architectures. By creating a document according to the HTML standard, document creators need know nothing about this underlying complexity. They are guaranteed that their document will appear approximately as intended, as long as it is read by a browser that understands HTML.

This has meant that it is much easier for information to be created and placed upon the Web. This has contributed substantially to the explosion of information made available on the Web, as the barrier to creating and distributing electronic documents has been significantly lowered.

17.4 Retrieving information on the Web

The concept of a global information 'space' populated by information objects lies at the heart of the Web. These information objects might be documents but could in principle be any file type. They might, for example, be programs that exhibit complex behaviour. The idea is that anyone who accesses the Web is able to navigate around the information space and look at information objects wherever they might be.

As we saw earlier, this is made possible in part through the HTML standard, which guarantees that once an object is found, it can be examined by anyone who has an HTML browser. This, however, is insufficient to create the information space. The Web also needs to be structured in such a way that, when a computer looks into the information space, there is a standard way in which these information objects can be found and retrieved. Consequently, each object is given a Web 'address' or URL so that it can always be located from anywhere on the Internet.

Once an object has been found, it also needs to be copied and sent back to the computer that wants to look at it. This is accomplished by what is known as a computer network transport protocol. Such protocols define the way in which computers speak to each other, and how they exchange information. A specific protocol for HTML documents has been created for the Web, and is known as the HyperText Transport Protocol or HTTP.

Box 17.1: HTML: HyperText Markup Language

To allow hypertext documents to be created and read in a standard way, the researchers at CERN developed a language called HTML. This was a simplified subset of another standard called the Standard General Markup Language (SGML). HTML defines the way in which a document should be structured so that it can be universally viewed on the Web. It defines a set of tags or codes that appear throughout a document. These tags define how the document's contents should be interpreted. For example, there are standard tags used when text has to appear in emphasised fonts, or for text to be centred or justified. These tags also define where images, sounds and hypertext links are to be found on the Web, and how they should appear in a document.

Document viewing programs, or browsers, expect Web documents to be written in HTML. When they encounter the HTML codes in a document's text, they carry out its instructions to make the document appear as intended on the browser's system. This means that while computer system developers have to develop different browsers for different types of computer, document writers need not be concerned about the particular computer system on which their document will appear. There will be variations in the final appearance of a document based upon the viewing preferences of the reader.

There is presently a tension between the desire to enhance the richness of Web documents and the need to maintain a common standard so that the concept of universal accessibility is maintained. The initial HTML standard was relatively simple, but language developers are keen to see it improve, permitting more sophisticated documents to be created. For example, programming languages like Java have been developed commercially to allow other programs to be attached to HTML documents. This means that arbitrarily complex behaviours could in principle be attached to hypertext documents.

However, as HTML evolves, the result is a proliferation of slightly different standards. Older Web browsers are already unable to interpret documents created according to more recent standards. Consequently the universality inherent in the original vision will gradually erode. For this problem to be solved, there needs to be a way for all Web users to have access to browsers incorporating the latest HTML standard. There also needs to be a guarantee that documents written in older versions of HTML remain readable as the standard evolves.

Box 17.2: URL: Universal Resource Locator

In the same way that there are Web standards for the way in which documents should be created, there are protocols that define how they should be accessed across the network. Just as HTTP insulates document creators from the specifics of an individual computer, an object's Web address is separate from the underlying protocols that are needed to find and transport it between computers. The address system is based around what is termed a Universal Resource Locator (or URL).

There are several common ways in which files can be accessed. HTML documents are accessed according to the Hypertext Transport Protocol (or HTTP). Files that are written in other formats could be retrieved using the older File Transfer Protocol (or FTP).

The URL of an information object allows one to specify which protocol is to be used to access the object. So, for example, if one wanted to view an HTML document using HTTP, the URL would be of the form:

http://hostcomputername/objectname

If one wanted to copy the file across but not view it, the URL would be:

ftp://hostcomputername/objectname

Other protocols that are supported by the URL standard include Gopher, Telnet and Mailto. Mailto is used to indicate that an email is to be sent to the address specified in the second part of the URL. Thus the URL

mailto:"ewc@pobox.com"

will tell a browser that an email is to be sent to the address specified in the section enclosed in quotes.

17.5 Web publishing models

The consequence of having such standard protocols for the retrieval of information, along with standard methods of creating documents, is a change in the way information is published. Normally the creator of a paper document is also responsible for its distribution. In an organisation, for example, all the possible recipients of a document need to be identified, and the document copied and circulated to them (whether it be on paper or in electronic form).

The Web model of publishing allows a document creator to put the burden of information access onto the reader. A document is placed in a known location, and is simply made available to all those who might be interested in it. This is the same model that is adopted when a document is placed on a notice board, and is available to anyone who cares to stop and read it.

There are several clear advantages to this model. Firstly, there is no need to specifically identify the name and location of all the people for whom a document is intended. As a corollary, the readership of a document can be widened considerably. Secondly, the costs of distribution are eliminated. Finally, since only one copy of the document is kept on the computer system of the individuals responsible for creating the document, it can be quickly updated. Consequently, readers of the document can always have access to the most up-to-date version of any document.

There are also clearly cases in which this particular model of publication would be inappropriate. For example, if urgent information needs to be communicated, then it may be more appropriate to send out a notice to all those who need to be informed. In this case, one might prefer to use email for document

---

Box 17.3: HTTP: Hypertext Transport Protocol

The Web is built around a client-server network architecture. This means that documents are placed on a computer that acts as a server. Other computers on the network are able to be clients of the server, sending requests to it for information. Upon receipt of a request, the server responds by delivering the requested information - which on the Web might be a document written in HTML. The exchange of requests and responses between client and server are made according to a network protocol that both client and server understand. A protocol called HTTP has been developed for the Web, to allow the exchange of HTML documents. HTTP is thus designed to transfer a variety of different data formats, including plain text, hypertext, plain image, audio and video.

Network protocols are generally of two types. Connection-oriented protocols set up a synchronous link between computers, requiring that the 'line' stay open for the duration of the connection. This is how a telephone connection is made, for example. Packet-oriented approaches like HTTP are asynchronous, and are more like sending a letter (see Chapter 14). Here a request is sent as a 'packet' to the server. This requires one connection, followed immediately upon delivery of the packet, by disconnection. Once it has processed the information contained in the requesting packet, the server responds by sending back information to the requesting client in a similar fashion. HTTP adopts this approach to make more efficient use of the network.

Figure 17.5: Data,
models and views on
the Web. A Web
browser provides a
view onto the data in
a document, and
interprets how to
present it according
the model described
in HTML.

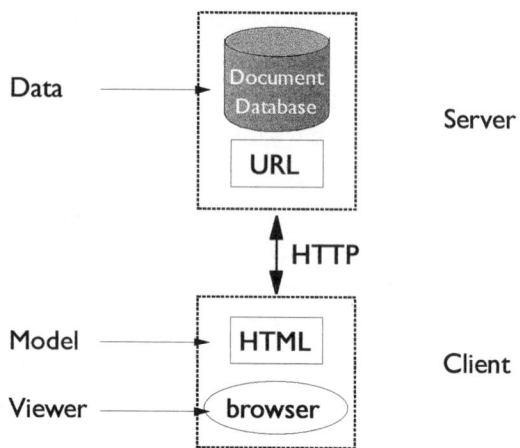

distribution in preference, or in addition, to updating a Web document.

17.6 Data, models and views

The information framework presented in Chapter 2 showed how every information system can be understood to comprise data, a set of data models, and data viewers. The Web cleanly exhibits this structure (Figure 17.5).

The documents scattered on computer servers across the Web are data files. These files are all constructed according to a standard model that is specified in HTML. Browser software, resident on a client computer, incorporates the HTML model within it. HTML therefore provides a model that permits these document files to be interpreted when they are retrieved from the server by the client.

17.7 Security on the Internet

The philosophy behind the Web is to provide open access to a global information space for everyone. It is this powerful vision, embodied in the open standards of Web technology, that has contributed so significantly to its growth.

There is an increasing need to use mechanisms that permit restrictions to be placed on the shipment of information. In particular, security measures that either limit access to documents or prevent documents being read may be required.

Such security restrictions are essential, for example, with electronic commerce. When a financial transaction is made across the Internet, information like credit card or bank account numbers may need to be shipped across the network. Since it is often possible to covertly intercept traffic across the network, sending such information without any form of protection is unsafe.

Security is also of fundamental importance in healthcare, where confidential patient data is involved. Not only is there often a need to restrict who has the right to access electronic patient data files, it is also clearly important to prevent that data being intercepted when it is being transported across the Internet.

There are thus two complementary ways that a degree of security can be ensured for data placed upon the Web. The first involves setting up barriers to accessing data files. For example an institution like a hospital may set up an internal network or intranet. Access to the intranet is dependent on users knowing passwords to authenticate that they are privileged to use the system. By controlling which computers can access the network, which users have accounts, and the complexity of the password system, intranets can be relatively closed and secure systems.

If a network is to be more open, for example using the Internet to allow access to documents, then the gateway between the Internet and the local system needs to be controlled. So-called **firewalls** are placed at the gateway to limit document access to appropriately authenticated users.

The second component of security is to prevent eavesdroppers outside a secure network. from intercepting information traffic. To prevent access to such confidential information, this data needs to be encrypted.

Encryption basically scrambles data according to a predefined method, and only someone with access to the encryption code used is able to decode the data. In information model terms, a new model is introduced into the system, and only those in possession of the model are able to interpret the data (Figure 17.6).

Figure 17.6: Once data (D) have been encrypted according to a code, they can be securely transported across a communication channel like the Internet. To be able to decode the data, one must posses a key or code that is the model (M) used to encrypt the data.

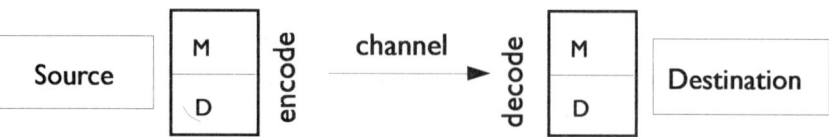

Encrypted data is secure as long as the encryption code is itself secure. Just as powerful encryption schemes are created, there are those who seek to develop methods to crack these codes. As a consequence, when it is absolutely essential that data remains secure, there is a constant pressure to adopt ever more powerful encryption mechanisms. For situations in which total security is not necessary, it is still reasonable to use codes that are in principle decodable, accepting that it is unlikely that most people would have the knowledge or desire to do so.

17.8 Future Web advances

There is now a good deal of experimentation occurring with new methods of interaction on the Internet. For example, there is active research into creating methods that allow interaction with others in virtual reality worlds across the Internet. In such worlds, people may be able to interact with each other through computer-rendered three dimensional scenes (Ragget et al., 1996). Such systems will no doubt produce newer interaction paradigms that will come into common use in the future.

One of the most immediate changes, the provision of voice telephony using Internet connections, is now becoming increasingly common. As the Internet develops the ability to deliver reliable and high quality connections, comparable to existing telecommunication services, it is likely that there will be significant opportunities to develop richer ways of providing computer-supported telephone services. Equally, there should be some major changes in the nature of the telecommunications market place.

Chapter summary

1. The Web has been created on top of the Internet's transport system. Conceptually the Web turns every computer on the Internet into a potential information source, and allows other computers to look in on it and explore the information there. All these sources can further combine to create documents that exist on multiple computers and span the globe.

2. To make this happen, three technology standards had to be created:
   - A standard way in which to create multimedia hypertext documents, called HTML (HyperText Markup Language).
   - A standard way to give each document an address on the Internet so that it could be located, called its URL (Universal Resource Locator).
   - A standard way of transferring documents between computers, called HTTP (HyperText Transfer Protocol).

3. The features of the HTML publishing model on the Web are:
   - A document written in HTML can be read on any computer that possesses an HTML browser.
   - Document authors need not know anything about the specifics of different computer systems when creating documents.
   - Specific versions of HTML browsers need to be developed for different computer operating systems and architectures.

4. The features of the URL and HTTP access model on the Web are:
   - Each information object has a unique address or URL.
   - The URL is independent of any specific network protocol, and allows a desired protocol to be specified along with the information object itself.
   - The protocol specified in HTTP is used for accessing HTML documents, and being packet-oriented, makes efficient use of network capacity.

Chapter 18

The Internet, the Web and healthcare

Healthcare is an information dependent enterprise, and the Internet and the Web represent one of the most powerful instruments for the creation and dissemination of information yet created. The rapid rate with which different sectors of healthcare have adopted these technologies is as much evidence of a large unmet need as it is of the technologies' ability to satisfy that need.

The number of medical sites joining the Internet increases monthly, as does the number of information resources available upon it. Indeed, it would require a lengthy book to simply enumerate what health-related information resources are currently available on the Web and that listing would be out of date well before it appeared in print. The best place to put a list of healthcare Web resources is actually on the Web. No other publication medium is able to cope with the rapidity of change of such material. Many such listings now exist.

This chapter concludes the part on the Internet by looking specifically at the ways in which healthcare can benefit from Web technologies and the growing Internet supporting it. In particular, the way information can be published, distributed, and accessed will all be examined in detail. The chapter will conclude with an examination of the role of the Internet in evidence-based clinical practice, and look ahead to some challenges that the growth of the Internet poses for healthcare.

18.1 Publication, distribution and access

The different flows of information associated with the care process were presented in Chapter 4. In particular, the three loop model was used to describe the way knowledge is created, applied and evaluated.

In practical terms, these loops require information to be first published by its creators, then distributed, and finally accessed by those who intend to use the information (Figure 18.1). This is the case whether one is 'publishing' information about a particular patient as part of the medical record, or whether the information is being published as a technical contribution. In either case, the authors of the information are creating a document that will be stored for future use by others, and that will need to be in a form that can be easily accessed.

It should be clear from the preceding chapters that many of the assumptions about how information is created, distributed and communicated are gradually being broken down. The Internet should be capable of providing a powerful distribution infrastructure over which healthcare organisations can move information. Further, the technical innovations associated with the Web provide tools for accessing and publishing that information.

Indeed, it is because the Internet and Web are able to meet many of the information needs in healthcare, that they have been adopted so rapidly. This contrasts starkly with earlier, and arguably more complex, information technology, which has generated far less enthusiasm within healthcare.

18.2 Publishing knowledge

In the past, the notion of publishing information was associated with formal processes of manuscript preparation, and physical publication of the work by a publishing house or learned journal. As information technology has become more pervasive, the physical aspects of publication have become easier to control, and have shifted some of the act of publication closer to the creator of the original information. It is now accepted for example, that anyone with word-processing

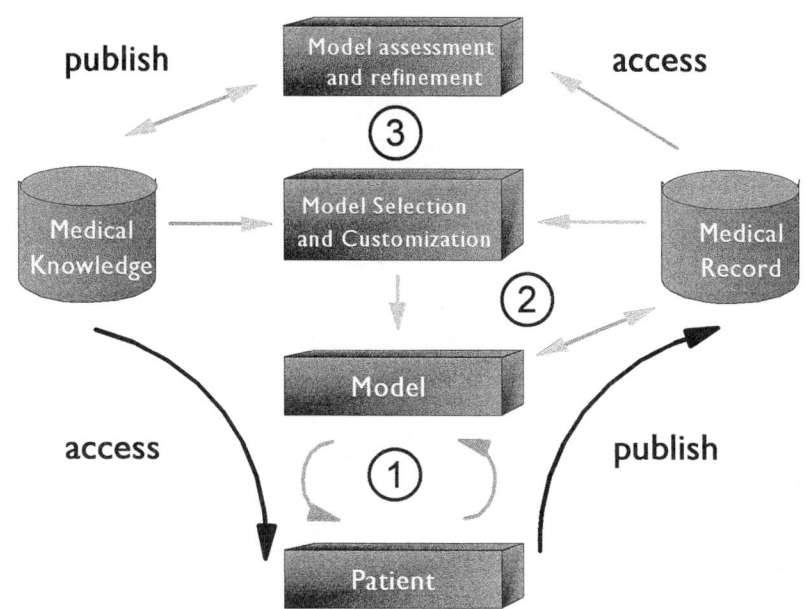

Figure 18.1:
Information flows through the three loops are based upon the publication and access of information. Underlying both of these processes are mechanisms for the distribution of the information.

and local printing facilities can create and distribute their own documents, either electronically or on paper. In such circumstances, it is still the case however, that for 'formal' publication to a public audience, an intermediary like a publisher is necessary. By using the Web however, an author can become not just publisher, but also the distributor of their work. As we shall see below, this brings considerable advantages, and some risks, for the practice of healthcare.

Another important phenomenon on the Web is that the permanence of information begins to eroded. Traditionally, with formal publication in an archival journal, the author of the work is making some commitment to the long-term stability of the work. Patient records fall into a similar category, since they too are created with the intent that they will enter a permanent archive. However, work that is incomplete, or in its early stages can be just as easily distributed using the Internet. For such less stable work, the process of early distribution can allow widespread commentary and interaction with the work, to improve it prior to 'final' publication. With this change to the model of publication, the degree of commitment needed prior to publishing information is decreased. Consequently, the process of examination and refinement of knowledge, as embodied in the three loop model, can be vastly accelerated.

A perhaps more subtle, but equally important consequence of increasing informality in publication may be a shift in our perception of medical information. It is likely that knowledge will start to be more widely recognised for its transitory nature. When the cost of updating theories is high, theories become verities. Thus, although the scientific method has always been emphasised in medicine, it has not always been practical to carry this point of view over into daily practice. Clinicians, hard pressed to keep up with advances in medicine, have seen their clinical knowledge become relatively fixed over time, and fixed knowledge decays.

This is not a process unique to medicine, but rather is fundamental to all knowledge. All our models of the world are prone to decay in accuracy and relevance with time (see Chapter 6). The ongoing process of knowledge refinement ensures that the view of the world captured in a piece of knowledge is gradually superseded. Thus, all the generalisations that are contained within our models of the world decay with the passage of time (Hogarth, 1986). In a world where the most recent clinical practice information is easily available and is constantly refreshed through a public process of critique, the transitional nature of knowledge might be harnessed rather than being a liability.

Peer-reviewed archival knowledge

Tradition places biomedical journals at the pinnacle of the medical publication process. Their role is to solicit, scrutinise, and then distribute the best scientific research. Yet the rigour of the review process places a significant delay between submission of material to be published, and final publication. Once published, such material enters the archive, or long term memory of medical knowledge.

Up until recently this was a successful process. Now, however, the delays in publication are leading to delays in the institution of appropriate treatments. Worse, the amount of information now being published weekly, in many thousands of journals, makes accessing that archive problematic.

As a result there has been a shift to journal publication over the Web. Major journals appear on the Web, sometimes in preference to, or in advance of print. For example the *British Medical Journal, The New England Journal of Medicine*, the *Lancet* and *JAMA* are published in paper and Internet versions.

For such journals, publication on the Internet has the following advantages:

Speed of publication. Eliminating the need to physically print journals, and then distribute them through a postal system, reduces the time between publication and appearance of a journal. Once placed in electronic form on the Web, journals are immediately accessible.

Cost of publication, distribution and access. The elimination of printing and distribution stages also makes the publication process potentially cheaper. Indeed, most Internet-based journals charge no fee for access, even though it may not represent the full journal contents. For healthcare workers in some nations, particularly in the developing world, paper-based journals are not affordable, and the Internet may be the only means they have to keep abreast fully of the latest research.

Form of publication. The multimedia and hypertext capacity for Web documents means that research appearing on the Web can appear in far richer forms than is possible on paper. For fields like clinical imaging, the Web thus adds an extra dimension to published research. One can create papers that contain text, graphics, sound, and moving images.

Content of publication. The Internet's data capacity has significant implications for the way in which clinical research can be communicated. When clinical research is published on paper, it is usually only possible to provide summaries of the study data. Readers can examine the statistical methods used upon the data, but have no recourse to the raw data itself. When research is published on the Internet, no such restrictions exist. A research paper can include all the data obtained during the investigation, and make this available to readers and other researchers (Delamothe, 1996). This has an immediate benefit, allowing the validity of the study data to be reviewed. Many examples of scientific fraud are only detected when other researchers have eventually been permitted to examine the raw data, which is then discovered to be fraudulent. Secondly, and more positively, the published data can now be used by subsequent researchers. They may wish to reanalyse the data, either to check the conclusions reached, or to contribute to further research. This means that the life of a piece of medical research no longer needs to end upon publication. It can enter a living pool of data that contributes to ongoing research for many years to come.

Method of interaction. The relationship of reader to text is changed on the Web, because of the potential for significant interaction between publisher and reader. Some journals, like the *Medical Journal of Australia*, have taken advantage of the two-way communication afforded by Internet-publication to open up the peer-review process of articles to the journal's readership.

These changes have lead some to predict the 'death of biomedical journals' in their present form (LaPorte et al., 1995). It is more likely that, freed from the limitations of paper, and taking advantage of the communication powers of the Internet, journals will change the role that they play. There will always be a need for an archival store of research, where important new ideas and experiences are recorded, and where necessary, priority of invention is established. The ways in which this archival store will be accessed, as discussed below, will be vastly different.

Peer-reviewed transitional knowledge

Journals have traditionally also been the place in which reviews of best clinical practice are distributed. These are intended to directly influence clinical practice, and represent the current understanding of the best approaches to management of disease, based on some form of considered expert consensus.

In a very real sense, if archival research represents the raw data, then guidelines represent condensed interpretations of that data. While research data remains a part of the basic pool of medical knowledge, interpretations are subject to change. As such, guidelines are a qualitatively different form of knowledge to the archival records of medical research.

The move to evidence-based medicine makes the publication of guidelines central to defining and controlling the process of care, and to ensuring optimal clinical outcomes. The more transitional nature of guidelines means that they have a short 'shelf-life' on paper. It is not surprising then that best practice guidelines are increasingly being placed upon the Internet by medical bodies, in preference to other publication models (see Section 9.3).

There is a mismatch between the speed with which information about new treatments can appear on the Internet, and the time it takes to accumulate the evidence needed to disseminate a practice guideline. Indeed this is a problem for the scientific community in general. There is a substantial difference between the rapidity with which new scientific results can be disseminated, and the length of time required for careful peer review. It may yet be possible, through innovative approaches to scientific publishing, to use the Internet itself to redress this imbalance (LaPorte et al., 1995).

The medical record

In volume, the medical record must represent one of the largest components of published medical knowledge. In contrast to journal and textbook material, the medical record has traditionally been written once but not duplicated. Access to it in archival form can thus be difficult, and once a record is lost it may not be replaceable.

This situation has long been tolerated because it has been unlikely that a patient's records will, on average, need to exist in more than one copy. However, there is a growing distribution of responsibility for patient care, whether a patient is being attended to in a primary care or hospital setting. It is thus now likely that many people will share in an individual's care. As a consequence the need to publish and distribute portions of a patient record to all those involved in care, wherever they may be, is now an unavoidable consequence of the way in which healthcare is practised.

The solution to this problem has been to begin to move the medical record across to computer-based information systems. Once a healthcare worker enters information in the electronic record, the intent is that it can be distributed to and accessed by others.

As we saw in Chapter 4, this sharing of patient information amongst colleagues occurs in loops 1 and 2 of the three information loops (Figure 18.1). The need for regulatory and financial bodies to track the overall performance of health systems means that they need to pool this data, and examine it from a broader population perspective, comparing trends. This occurs as part of loop 3. The need to perform such regulatory analysis has often been at least as strong a driver, if not more so, for the creation of electronic medical records. The result has sometimes been that systems have been designed primarily for data collection, rather than use by healthcare workers in daily clinical practice. Unsurprisingly, this approach creates systems that tend to be poorly regarded by those who use them for clinical purposes.

Unlike more highly 'designed' systems (see Chapter 4) Web based systems make little or no demands on the structure of knowledge, and emphasise ease of publication, distribution and access to information. As a consequence, many now consider that Web-based systems represent the ideal tool with which to build electronic medical records. This reverses the traditional strategy that starts out designing clinical systems to collect data for administrative purposes, and then refines them to more closely meet clinical needs. Web based systems can start by permitting clinical users to share the information needed to carry out patient care and, over time, can be structured and refined to collect population data.

One constant in the development of the electronic medical record has been the running battle with obsolescence of the functional specification of these systems. Once a system has been designed, it can prove very difficult to introduce a radically different functionality into it without a major rewriting of the system software. For example, a system designed to carry out order entry and results reporting is unlikely to be easily modified to allow viewing of clinical images, or browsing electronic documents from a library.

Because the basic Web technology makes very little specification about how it is to be used, it is relatively open. A Web browser is just as able to examine a document containing notes of a patient's progress, a form for ordering a laboratory test, or a multimedia document from an electronic textbook. This ability to introduce radically new functionality easily into an existing system is a powerful argument for adopting Web technologies over existing methods.

Since a Web-based electronic record can be built around a local Intranet, there is no inherent increase in security risk over traditional computer-based solutions. As we saw in the previous chapter, the security risks increase considerably when local information is distributed using the open and public Internet.

Local knowledge

One of the clear effects of the Web has been an increase in the population of those who publish information. Much of this information is for local consumption but by using the Internet, it becomes globally accessible.

For example, local variations in disease incidence, resources and skills may mean that clinical guidelines generally appropriate for the population at large do not apply locally. In such circumstances local guidelines can appear on the Internet. One would for example, not expect a guideline written in Boston to manage and diagnose abdominal pain to apply in Somalia or Indonesia.

As a side effect of supporting regional publication of information, however, there comes the possibility of sharing such information wherever the need applies. Some uses of local knowledge are trivial. For example, prior to travelling to a hospital overseas, it is sometimes easier to interrogate the hospital's Web site to retrieve maps and other local information than it is to ask people to provide that information. More critically, were a patient to return from a foreign country with an infectious disease, the Web might be the best place to first look for local information about likely pathogens, diagnostic tests, and treatment.

18.3 Accessing knowledge

Information, no matter how easily created, is useless if it cannot be accessed when it is needed. It is the combination of powerful communication-based access mechanisms, as well as information creation mechanisms that characterise the Web and Internet.

In many ways, healthcare has always been information rich, but has severely been hampered by mechanisms for distribution and access to that information. As a consequence, one of the most tangible changes that comes from putting information on intranets, or the Internet, is a major improvement in information distribution and access.

For clinical workers, researchers and students, information access should be improved in the following ways.

Amount of information. With the cost of publication on the Internet being so low, and the ease of publication being so high, many people have been encouraged to publish information that is clinically valuable, but that might not otherwise have an appropriate vehicle for publication. There is unsurprisingly a large amount of material available on the net that is unavailable elsewhere. This extends from educational material that is created for local use, but is also made available to anyone who might be interested. It also includes specialised research data. There is for example an enormous amount of information about the Human Genome project available on the Internet that would in the past have been available to only those closely associated with the project (Hochstrasser et al., 1995). For local intranets, the situation is much the same. The potential exists to make a large amount of information from drug interaction data through to image libraries available throughout an organisation.

Speed of appearance. The rapidity with which changes in Web-based information can be made available to its readers cannot be matched by non-electronic distribution mechanisms.

Timeliness. A corollary of the speed of publication is the rapidity with which information is now able or permitted to change. Information is potentially always up-to-date, which is valuable for time-critical information needs. It is common for information sites on the Web to be updated regularly, often in response to feedback from those accessing the information.

Version control. In contrast to other forms of publication, where multiple editions may exist (for example a clinical guideline), there is only one access point for a Web document, and it is always the current version. There are clear advantages here not just in just in timeliness, but in elimination of possible confusion between editions of an information source. Where older editions need to be kept, some Web sites maintain archives that can be accessed if needed.

Types of information. Many medical publications take full advantage of the multimedia and hypertext facilities offered on the Web, to create publications that could not have previously been possible. Indeed the quality of Web documents are now so high that they are used by many medical educational institutions. The University of Utah, for example, has an extensive library of anatomical pathology images called WebPath for its students. At the University of Iowa a set of teaching materials is assembled in their Virtual Hospital. The National Library of Medicine's Visible Human project aims to create a complete, anatomically detailed, three-dimensional representations of the male and female human body and to make this available on the Internet. The project is collecting transverse CAT, MRI and cryosection images of male and female cadavers at one millimetre intervals.

Manner of interaction. Web resources are not necessarily passive information repositories. They can be constructed to solicit input form the reader. It is this capacity which allows electronic patient records to be created on the Web. From an educational point of view, the possibility for structured interaction with teaching materials on the Web is an exciting development. Web based resources permit structured browsing, and problem exploration behaviours. One can now find Web sites that allow diagnostic problems to be posed for students, who are then able to search interactively for appropriate information amongst the patient data presented. Once the student submits answers to the problem set, they can then be assessed as necessary.

Searching. While it has been commonplace to search for material published in journals, for example through a library, other information has not been so accessible. One of the advantages of the Web is that, through the search engines and indexes that now exist, one can perform the same type of search on other kinds of information. For example, it is increasingly common for medical organisations to create their own sites on the Web. Here one can discover the activities of the group, their interests, and their staff. It is often possible to e-mail individuals directly in this manner. As a consequence, one can now search for, find, and communicate with individuals who have specialised expertise globally, in a manner that previously was not been possible, even locally.

18.4 Distributing knowledge

While publishing using Web technologies is a powerful way to disseminate information, it is dependent on individuals actively seeking that information. In this sense it is a passive broadcast medium. In many circumstances in healthcare, this model is inadequate. This is especially the case when it is necessary to make sure defined individuals receive critical information in a timely fashion. For example, a laboratory might wish to alert a clinician about a patient's test results. In this case, some form of peer to peer communication is more appropriate. If a government regulatory authority needs to issue an urgent bulletin informing healthcare workers about a public health warning, than a 'narrowcast' method may be more appropriate.

The Internet changes the way an organisation is able to communicate through the distribution of information. In Chapter 16 the basic mechanisms of e-mail , mailing lists and newsgroups were described. Such facilities can in principle be created on any computer network, whether local or global, and are able to satisfy a variety of different communication tasks (Table 18.1).

Table 18.1: Types of communication distribution task, and some methods suited to these tasks.

Communication Task	Communication Method
Peer to Peer	Email, Fax
Narrowcast	Email, Fax lists
Broadcast	Web, Newsgroups

It is often the case with publicly sensitive information that healthcare workers need to be notified in advance of the public, so that they can be prepared to deal with the consequences of such announcements. A recent example in the UK arose when the public was informed of the withdrawal of certain forms of the oral contraceptive pill, but many general practitioners were not informed in advance of the announcement. (Coiera, 1996a). Unsurprisingly, much anxiety and confusion resulted. In such cases, what is needed is a targeted narrowcast to healthcare workers, in advance of the broadcast to the general public.

Some rudimentary systems have already been put in place to communicate urgent public health information. Through a combination of fax, paging and e-mail technologies, it is possible to contact most people in western countries. To solve the problem posed by the sheer number of individuals that need to be contacted, some authorities (e.g. in the UK) use a cascade communication system. Here, a message is passed on to a small group, who in turn relay it to their own regions according to locally maintained lists of names. Several cascade steps may be needed to get the multiplication effect needed to ensure that everyone is contacted within an appropriate time.

Contrast the complexity of this cascade system with one based on e-mail and computer generated faxes, where a message can be sent once without any necessary intermediate steps. Lists of names can be maintained locally, to ensure accuracy, but can be made available on the Web to the organisations that need to access them. These lists can contain e-mail addresses, telephone fax numbers, or whatever contact medium is most appropriate for different individuals. Once sent, the communication system is able to generate the message in the form appropriate to the facilities available for different individuals. Certainly, as more healthcare workers obtain routine Internet access, even this technical complexity can be side-stepped in favour of pure e-mail -based messaging.

18.5 Collaboration

It is now common for healthcare to be delivered by teams whose members have differing skills, and who might be geographically quite distributed. This is as true for primary care workers, as it is for workers in larger healthcare organisations. It is also very much the case for medical research, where collaborations often extend across the world.

A feature of collaboration is the need to create and exchange information amongst members of such teams. In Chapters 4 and 13, the basic needs for exchanging informal information amongst healthcare workers was presented, and the role that communication technologies have to play established.

For some time, the notion of **groupware** has been explored within the information sciences. It emphasises the capture and exchange of information amongst group members, and facilitating collaboration on common documents using shared information spaces on a network. The Web is more permissive than many early groupware offerings in this respect, since it allows individuals to create and distribute information with little regard to its structure. Increasingly it is being suggested that the Web intrinsically is a groupware platform, since it naturally facilitates common access to files in a distributed environment.

Combining the Web's powerful information management tools, with more basic Internet communication facilities like e-mail can thus contribute significantly to collaboration when individuals are separated by time or distance.

18.6 Internet healthcare services

Up until now, the type of Internet uses that have been described represent extensions of existing processes. Although still relatively immature, there is a clear desire by many to see entirely new ways of delivering care created. That desire is not unique to healthcare, but exists across the board from financial institutions to sales and public service sectors. This is in part due to a much bigger market that exists on the Web. From a commercial point of view this means that highly specialised services that would not be sustainable in a local region may now be able to survive on the Internet.

Examples of some new medical services that have appeared on the Internet include.

Brokering. Healthcare specialists offering to give advice to patients can register with a brokering service, which creates a list of specialists in different categories. Patients approach the brokering service and are put in contact with the specialist that is most suitable, perhaps because of experience, interests, or because of geography. Such brokering services transcend state and national boundaries, and their implications are yet to be fully examined (see Section 18.7).

Consultation by e-mail. Whether via a broker, or by searching the Web for a specialist's own Web pages, patients are able to set up their consultations over the Internet. Such consultations may be carried out entirely by e-mail , or may in the future be a prelude to consultation taking place across a video-link. Many of these services are seen by some groups as potentially powerful ways of generating revenue. For example, some internationally renowned centres of medical excellence now sell their expertise via telemedical video-links. As the need for specialised links for video consultation diminish over the next decade, these services will potentially be provided by anyone with access to standard communication systems. *Critical incident reporting.* Governmental bodies usually have well developed systems for reporting adverse drug reactions, permitting the performance of newly licensed substances to be monitored. Such reporting can be occur over an Internet service. The type of incident reported need not be limited to drug reactions, however. For example, critical incidents during anaesthesia might relate to human error or device malfunction. Adverse or critical incidents during other types of procedure can also be submitted, possibly anonymously, to enhance the likelihood of obtaining reports (Staender et al., 1996).

18.7 The Internet's challenges to healthcare

There are significant challenges in developing Web and Internet technology, and their application to healthcare. There are also challenges arising from the growth of the Internet that are external to the formal delivery of healthcare, but that may have a major impact on it. Some of these will increase in importance over the next few years.

Patient access to healthcare information

It is clear that access to healthcare information on the Internet will be of major benefit to patients. There are already numerous electronic discussion groups in which patients may ask questions and share experience. Some health-related Internet sites offer e-mail advice on a fee for service basis. Others provide free access to information. It is important to realise that information on the Internet is accessible from most parts of the globe, and that once made public, information access and dissemination is largely uncontrolled, and uncontrollable.

There is an information mass market developing on the Internet, where the general public has access to a wide variety of health-related material, often of variable quality or relevance (Bower, 1996). The proportion of patients who have access to this information source will continue to grow over the next few years, as will the quantity of information placed upon the Internet. It may even be the case at present that a higher percentage of patients in some territories have access to the Internet than their GPs.

For health care systems in which patients are free to participate in their choice of treatment, the Internet provides a rich source of information on treatment options. Since such information may potentially vary from the most up-to-date practice guidelines from leading clinical centres, to out-of-date or inaccurate recommendations, managing patient expectations and requests may represent a greater challenge that it is at present.

In countries in which healthcare provision is more centrally managed, even greater challenges exist. We must assume that patients will soon have access to information on best practice from a variety of sources on the Internet and will demand it when it is known.

However the health service is resource bound, and must attempt to ration treatment (Klein, 1995). Treatments that are the most cost-effective over a population may be favoured over treatments that are best in class. This will lead to a conflict between the informed desire of patients to obtain the best treatment for themselves as individuals, and the system's ability to deliver. Will individuals who have an almost limited access to information, but limited access to healthcare resource, tolerate sub-optimal care? The Child B case in the UK is a prime example of the type of conflicts that will arise between a free market in information and a controlled market in healthcare (Ham, 1995).

Legal implications

Worryingly for practitioners, they may also be exposed to increased legal challenge. While patients may be motivated to seek out the most recent literature for their condition, and can invest considerable effort in that search, most practising clinicians cannot. The Bolam principle, established in the UK in 1957, protects a doctor against a claim of negligence if other colleagues would have acted in the same manner (Bolam, 1957).

The Bolam principle was overturned in an Australian court in 1995, and the same may happen in other countries where it applies, like the UK (Economist, 1995). Similarly in the US, some states have begun the move towards protecting healthcare workers against litigation if they treat a patient according to recognised guidelines. If the law were to judge a clinician negligent for failure to institute recognised best practice, then an informed patient population and an over-worked clinical community provides a recipe for increasing litigation.

Thankfully, this problem has been recognised in part by the move towards evidence-based medical practice. The role of bodies like the Cochrane Collaboration in providing best practice advice thus becomes pivotal, as does the development of clinical tools for rapid and accurate access to such information across the Internet. Not only will the creation of pooled practice guidelines be a resource for clinicians, but in all probability, they will necessarily be a resource for patients too. Patients will be faced with an enormous quantity of information of variable quality, and are ill-equipped in general to separate the wheat from the chaff. The opportunity to access guidelines 'certified' by recognised medical bodies would no doubt be readily taken up.

Another area of legal uncertainty surrounds the delivery of healthcare services across the Internet. This, along with other communication-based services like telemedicine, allows practitioners to deliver care beyond state and national boundaries. Unfortunately most of the legal machinery developed to protect both patients and practitioners is based upon the assumption that care takes place within tight geographic bounds, where particular laws have jurisdiction. It is difficult at present to know how one would take legal action for care delivered across national boundaries. Further, it is not clear how one would obtain reimbursement for such services, given that many patients would seek to recover costs from state funds or private health insurance schemes.

Chapter summary

1. The Internet should be capable of providing a powerful distribution infrastructure over which healthcare organisations can move information. Further, the technical innovations associated with the Web provide tools for accessing and publishing that information.
2. Peer-reviewed medical journals appearing on the Internet are able to publish more quickly and cheaply than paper editions, can utilise multimedia, allow readers to interact directly and deliver feedback, and make supporting data available when research papers are published.
3. Unlike more highly 'designed' systems, Web based electronic medical record systems make little or no demands on the structure of knowledge, and emphasise ease of publication, distribution and access to information. As a consequence, many now consider that Web-based systems represent the ideal tool with which to build electronic medical records.
4. One of the effects of the Web is a widening of the population of those who publish information. Much of this is for local consumption but it becomes globally accessible. For example, local variations in disease incidence, resources and skills may mean that clinical guidelines generally appropriate for the population at large do not apply locally. In such circumstances local guidelines can appear on the Internet.
5. The Internet changes the way an organisation is able to communicate through the distribution of information. For example, it permits broad and narrow-casting of information and it facilitates collaboration between colleagues
6. The Internet makes a wide variety of material, both appropriate and inappropriate, available to patients. With patients having ready access to material on clinical best-practice, there may be legal implications if clinicians are not similarly equipped.

Part Seven

Intelligent Clinical Decision Support

Chapter 19

Artificial intelligence in medicine

From the very earliest moments in the modern history of the computer, scientists have dreamed of creating an 'electronic brain'. Of all the modern technological quests, this search to create artificially intelligent (AI) computer systems has been one of the most ambitious and, not surprisingly, controversial.

It also seems that very early on, scientists and doctors alike were captivated by the potential such a technology might have in medicine (e.g. Ledley and Lusted, 1959). With intelligent computers able to store and process vast stores of knowledge, the hope was that they would become perfect 'doctors in a box', assisting or surpassing clinicians with tasks like diagnosis.

With such motivations, a small but talented community of computer scientists and healthcare professionals set about shaping a research program for a new discipline called Artificial Intelligence in Medicine (AIM). These researchers had a bold vision of the way AIM would revolutionise medicine, and push forward the frontiers of technology.

AI in medicine at that time was a largely US-based research community. Work originated out of a number of campuses, including MIT-Tufts, Pittsburgh, Stanford and Rutgers (e.g. Szolovits, 1982; Clancey and Shortliffe, 1984; Miller, 1988). The field attracted many of the best computer scientists and, by any measure, their output in the first decade of the field remains a remarkable achievement.

In reviewing this new field in 1984, Clancey and Shortliffe provided the following definition:

> 'Medical artificial intelligence is primarily concerned with the construction of AI programs that perform diagnosis and make

therapy recommendations. Unlike medical applications based on other programming methods, such as purely statistical and probabilistic methods, medical AI programs are based on symbolic models of disease entities and their relationship to patient factors and clinical manifestations.'

Much has changed since then, and today this definition would be considered narrow in scope and vision. Today, the importance of diagnosis as a task requiring computer support in routine clinical situations receives much less emphasis (Durinck et al., 1994). So, despite the focus of much early research on understanding and supporting the clinical encounter, expert systems today are more likely to be found used in clinical laboratories and educational settings, for clinical surveillance, or in data-rich areas like the intensive care setting. For its day, however, the vision captured in this definition of AIM was revolutionary.

After the first euphoria surrounding the promise of artificially intelligent diagnostic programmes, the last decade has seen increasing disillusion amongst many with the potential for such systems. Yet, while there certainly have been ongoing challenges in developing such systems, they actually have proven their reliability and accuracy on repeated occasions (Shortliffe, 1987).

Much of the difficulty has been the poor way in which they have fitted into clinical practice, either solving problems that were not perceived to be an issue, or imposing changes in the way clinicians worked. What is now being realised is that when they fill an appropriately role, intelligent programmes do indeed offer significant benefits. One of the most important tasks now facing developers of AI-based systems is to characterise accurately those aspects of medical practice that are best suited to the introduction of artificial intelligence systems.

In the remainder of this chapter, the initial focus will thus remain on the different roles AIM systems can play in clinical practice, looking particularly to see where clear successes can be identified, as well as looking to the future. The next chapter will take a more technological focus, and look at the way AIM systems are built. A variety of technologies including expert systems and neural networks will be discussed. The final chapter in this section on intelligent decision support will look at the way AIM can support the interpretation of patient signals that come off clinical monitoring devices.

19.1 AI can support both the creation and the use of medical knowledge

Human cognition is a complex set of phenomena, and AI systems can relate to it in two very different ways. Proponents of so-called 'strong' AI are interested in creating computer systems whose behaviour is at some level indistinguishable from humans (see Box 19.1). Success in strong AI would result in computer minds that might reside in autonomous physical beings like robots, or perhaps live in 'virtual' worlds like the information space created by something like the Internet.

An alternative approach to strong AI is to look at human cognition and decide how it can be supported in complex or difficult situations. For example, a fighter pilot may need the help of intelligent systems to assist in flying an aircraft that is too complex for a human to operate on their own. These 'weak' AI systems are not intended to have an independent existence, but are a form of 'cognitive prosthesis' that supports a human in a variety of tasks.

AIM systems are by and large intended to support healthcare workers in the normal course of their duties, assisting with tasks that rely on the manipulation of data and knowledge. An AI system could be running within an electronic medical record system, for example, and alert a clinician when it detects a contraindication to a planned treatment. It could also alert the clinician when it detected patterns in clinical data that suggested significant changes in a patient's condition.

Along with tasks that require reasoning with medical knowledge, AI systems also have a very different role to play in the process of scientific research. In particular, AI systems have the capacity to learn, leading to the discovery of new phenomena and the creation of medical knowledge. For example, a computer system can be used to analyse large amounts of data, looking for complex patterns within it that suggest previously unexpected associations. Equally, with enough of a model of existing medical knowledge, an AI system can be used to show how a new set of experimental observations conflict

Box 19.1 - The Turing test

How will we know when a computer program has achieved an equivalent intelligence to a human? Is there some set of objective measures that can be assembled against which a computer program can be tested? Alan Turing was one of the founders of modern computer science and AI, whose intellectual achievements to this day remain astonishing in their breadth and importance. When he came to ponder this question, he brilliantly side-stepped the problem almost entirely.

In his opinion, there were no ultimately useful measures of intelligence. It was sufficient that an objective observer could not tell the difference in conversation between a human and a computer for us to conclude that the computer was intelligent. To cancel out any potential observer biases, Turing's test put the observer in a room, equipped with a computer keyboard and screen, and made the observer talk to the test subjects only using these. The observer would engage in a discussion with the test subjects using the printed word, much as one would today by exchanging e-mail with a remote colleague. If a set of observers could not distinguish the computer from another human in over 50% of cases, then Turing felt that one had to accept that the computer was intelligent.

Another consequence of the Turing test is that it says nothing about how one builds an intelligent artefact, thus neatly avoiding discussions about whether the artefact needed to in anyway mimic the structure of the human brain or our cognitive processes. It really didn't matter how the system was built in Turing's mind. Its intelligence should only to be assessed based upon its overt behaviour.

There have been attempts to build systems that can pass Turing's test in recent years. Some have managed to convince at least some humans in a panel of judges that they too are human, but none have yet passed the mark set by Turing.

with the existing theories. We shall now examine such capabilities in more detail.

19.2 Reasoning with medical knowledge

Expert or knowledge-based systems are the commonest type of AIM system in routine clinical use. They contain medical knowledge, usually about a very specifically defined task, and are able to reason with data from individual patients to come up with reasoned conclusions. Although there are many variations, the knowledge within an expert system is typically represented in the form of a set of rules.

There are many different types of clinical task to which expert systems can be applied.

Generating alerts and reminders. In so-called real-time situations, an expert system attached to a monitor can warn of changes in a patient's condition. In less acute circumstances, it might scan laboratory test results or drug orders and send reminders or warnings through an e-mail system.

Diagnostic assistance. When a patient's case is complex, rare or the person making the diagnosis is simply inexperienced, an expert system can help come up with likely diagnoses based on patient data.

Therapy critiquing and planning. Systems can either look for inconsistencies, errors and omissions in an existing treatment plan, or can be used to formulate a treatment based upon a patient's specific condition and accepted treatment guidelines.

Agents for information retrieval. Software 'agents' can be sent to search for and retrieve information, for example on the Internet, that is considered relevant to a particular problem. The agent contains knowledge about its user's preferences and needs, and may also need to have medical knowledge to be able to assess the importance and utility of what it finds.

Image recognition and interpretation. Many medical images can now be automatically interpreted, from plane X-rays through to more complex images like angiograms, CT and MRI scans. This is of value in mass-screenings, for example, when the system can flag potentially abnormal images for detailed human attention.

There are numerous reasons why more expert systems are not in routine use (Coiera, 1994). Some require the existence of an electronic medical record system to supply their data, and most institutions and practices do not yet have all their working data available electronically. Others suffer from poor human interface design and so do not get used even if they are of benefit.

Much of the reluctance to use systems simply arose because expert systems did not fit naturally into the process of care, and as a result using them required additional effort from already busy individuals.

It is also true, but perhaps dangerous, to ascribe some of the reluctance to use early systems upon the technophobia or computer illiteracy of healthcare workers. If a system is perceived by those using it to be beneficial, then it will be used. If not, independent of its true value, it will probably be rejected.

Happily, there are today very many systems that have made it into clinical use (Table 19.1). Many of these are small, but nevertheless make positive contributions to care. In the next two sections, we will examine some of the more successful examples of knowledge-based clinical systems, in an effort to understand the reasons behind their success, and the role they can play.

Diagnostic and educational systems

In the first decade of AIM, most research systems were developed to assist clinicians in the process of diagnosis, typically with the intention that it would be used during a clinical encounter with a patient. Most of these early systems did not develop further than the research laboratory, partly because they did not gain sufficient support from clinicians to permit their routine introduction.

It is clear that some of the psychological basis for developing this type of support is now considered less compelling, given that situation assessment seems to be a bigger issue than diagnostic formulation (Section 6.2). Some of these systems have continued to develop, however, and have transformed in part into educational systems.

DXplain is an example of one of these clinical decision support systems, developed at the Massachusetts General Hospital (Barnett et al., 1987). It is used to assist in the process of diagnosis, taking a set of clinical findings including signs, symptoms, laboratory data and then produces a ranked list of diagnoses. It provides justification for each of differential diagnosis, and suggests further investigations. The system contains a data base of crude probabilities for over 4,500 clinical manifestations that are associated with over 2,000 different diseases.

SYSTEM	DESCRIPTION
ACUTE CARE SYSTEMS	
ACORN (Wyatt, 1989)	Chest pain triage advisor for CCU
POEMS (Sawar et al., 1992)	Post-operative care decision support
VIE-PNN (Miksch et al., 1993)	Parenteral nutrition planning for neonatal ICU
NéoGanesh (Dojat et al., 1996)	ICU ventilator management
SETH (Darmoni, 1993)	Clinical toxicology advisor
LABORATORY SYSTEMS	
GERMWATCHER (Kahn et al.,1993)	Analysis of nosocomial infections
HEPAXPERT I, II (Adlassnig et al., 1991)	Interprets tests for hepatitis A and B
Acid-base expert system (Pince, et al., 1990)	Interpretation of acid-base disorders
MICROBIOLOGY/PHARMACY (Morrell et al., 1993)	Monitors renal active antibiotic dosing
PEIRS (Edwards et al., 1993)	Chemical pathology expert system
PUFF (Snow et al., 1988)	Interprets pulmonary function tests
Pro.M.D.- CSF Diagnostics (Trendelenburg, 1994)	Interpretation of CSF findings
EDUCATIONAL SYSTEMS	
DXPLAIN (Barnett et al., 1987)	Internal medicine expert system
ILLIAD (Warner et al., 1988)	Internal medicine expert system
HELP (Kuperman et al., 1991)	Knowledge-based hospital information system
QUALITY ASSURANCE AND ADMINISTRATION	
COLORADO MEDICAID UTILIZATION REVIEW SYSTEM	Quality review of drug prescribing practices
MANAGED SECOND SURGICAL OPINION SYSTEM	Aetna Life and Casualty assessor system
MEDICAL IMAGING	
PERFEX (Ezquerra et al., 1992)	Interprets cardiac SPECT data
PHOENIX (Kahn, 1991).	Selects most appropriate radiological procedures

Table 19.1: A wide variety of expert systems have been placed into routine clinical use. These systems are typical examples.

DXplain is in routine use at a number of hospitals and medical schools, mostly for clinical education purposes, but is also available for clinical consultation. It also has a role as an electronic medical textbook. It is able to provide a description of over 2,000 different diseases, emphasising the signs and symptoms that occur in each disease and provides recent references appropriate for each specific disease.

Decision support systems need not be 'stand alone' but can be deeply integrated into an electronic medical record system. Indeed, such integration reduces the barriers to using such a system, by crafting them more closely into clinical working processes, rather than expecting workers to create new processes to use them.

The HELP system is an example of this type of knowledge-based hospital information system, which began operation in 1980 (Kuperman et al., 1990; Kuperman et al., 1991). It not only supports the routine applications of a hospital information system (HIS) including management of admissions and discharges and order entry, but also provides a decision support function. The decision support system has been actively incorporated into the functions of the routine HIS applications. Decision support provide clinicians with alerts and reminders, data interpretation and patient diagnosis facilities, patient management suggestions and clinical protocols. Activation of the decision support is provided within the applications but can also be triggered automatically as clinical data is entered into the patient's computerised medical record.

Expert laboratory information systems

One of the most successful areas in which expert systems are applied is in the clinical laboratory. Practitioners may be unaware that while the printed report they receive from a laboratory was checked by a pathologist, the whole report may now have been generated by a computer system that has automatically interpreted the test results. Examples of such systems include the following.

- The PUFF system for automatic interpretation of pulmonary function tests has been sold in its commercial form to hundreds of sites world-wide (Snow et al., 1988). PUFF went into production at Pacific Presbyterian Medical Centre in San Francisco in 1977, making it one of the very earliest medical expert systems in use. Many thousands of cases later, it is still in routine use.

- GermWatcher checks for hospital-acquired (nosocomial) infections, which represent a significant cause of prolonged inpatient days and additional hospital charges (Kahn et al.,1993). Microbiology culture data from the hospital's laboratory system are monitored by GermWatcher, using a rule-base containing a combination of national criteria and local hospital infection control policy.

- A more general example of this type of system is PEIRS (Pathology Expert Interpretative Reporting System) (Edwards et al., 1993). During it period of operation, PEIRS interpreted about 80-100 reports a day with a diagnostic accuracy of about 95%. It accounted for about which 20% of all the reports generated by the hospital's Chemical Pathology Department. PEIRS reported on thyroid function tests, arterial blood gases, urine and plasma catecholamines, hCG (human chorionic gonadotrophin) and AFP (alpha fetoprotein), glucose tolerance tests, cortisol, gastrin, cholinesterase phenotypes and parathyroid hormone related peptide (PTH-RP).

Laboratory expert systems usually do not intrude into clinical practice. Rather, they are embedded within the process of care, and with the exception of laboratory staff, clinicians working with patients do not need to interact with them. For the ordering clinician, the system prints a report with a diagnostic hypothesis for consideration, but does not remove responsibility for information gathering, examination, assessment and treatment. For the pathologist, the system cuts down the workload of generating reports, without removing the need to check and correct reports.

19.3 Machine learning systems can create new medical knowledge

Learning is seen to be the quintessential characteristic of an intelligent being. Consequently, one of the driving ambitions of AI has been to develop computers that can learn from experience. The resulting developments in the AI sub-field of **machine learning** have resulted in a set of techniques which have the potential to alter the way in which knowledge is created.

All scientists are familiar with the statistical approach to data analysis. Given a particular hypothesis, statistical tests are applied to data to see if any relationships can be found between different parameters. Machine learning systems can go much further. They look at raw data and then attempt to hypothesise relationships within the data, and newer learning systems are able to produce quite complex characterisations of those relationships. In other words they attempt to discover humanly understandable concepts.

Learning techniques include neural networks, but encompass a large variety of other methods as well, each with their own particular characteristic benefits and difficulties. For example, some systems are able to learn decision trees from examples taken from data (Quinlan, 1986). These trees look much like the classification hierarchies discussed in Chapter 10, and can be used to help in diagnosis.

Medicine has formed a rich test-bed for machine learning experiments in the past, allowing scientists to develop complex and powerful learning systems. While there has been much practical use of expert systems in routine clinical settings, at present machine learning systems still seem to be used in a more experimental way. There are, however, many situations in which they can make a significant contribution.

- Machine learning systems can be used to develop the knowledge bases used by expert systems. Given a set of clinical cases that act as examples, a machine learning system can produce a systematic description of those clinical features that uniquely characterise the clinical conditions. This knowledge can be expressed in the form of simple rules, or often as a decision tree. A classic example of this type of system is KARDIO, which was developed to interpret ECGs (Bratko et al., 1989).

- This approach can be extended to explore poorly understood areas of medicine, and people now talk of the process of 'data mining' and of 'knowledge discovery' systems. For example, it is possible, using patient data, to automatically construct pathophysiological models that describe the functional relationships between the various measurements. For example, Hau and Coiera (1997) describe a learning system that takes real-time patient data obtained during cardiac bypass surgery, and then creates models of normal and abnormal cardiac physiology. These models might be used to look for changes in a patient's condition if used at the time they are created. Alternatively, if used in a research setting, these models can serve as initial hypotheses that can drive further experimentation.

- One particularly exciting development has been the use of learning systems to discover new drugs. The learning system is given examples of one or more drugs that weakly exhibit a particular activity, and based upon a description of the chemical structure of those compounds, the learning system suggests which of the chemical attributes are necessary for that pharmacological activity. Based upon the new characterisation of chemical structure produced by the learning system, drug designers can try to design a new compound that has those characteristics. Currently, drug designers synthesis a number of analogues of the drug they wish to improve upon, and experiment with these to determine which exhibits the desired activity. By boot-strapping the process using the machine learning approach, the development of new drugs can be speeded up, and the costs significantly reduced. At present statistical analyses of activity are used to assist with analogue development, and machine learning techniques have been shown to at least equal if not outperform them, as well as having the benefit of generating knowledge in a form that is more easily understood by chemists (King et al., 1992). Since such learning experiments are still in their infancy, significant developments can be expected here in the next few years.

- Machine learning has a potential role to play in the development of clinical guidelines. It is often the case that there are several alternate treatments for a given condition, with slightly different outcomes. It may not be clear however, what features of one particular treatment method are responsible for the better results. If databases are kept of the outcomes of competing treatments, then machine learning systems can be used to identify features that are responsible for different outcomes.

Chapter summary

1. Artificial intelligence (AI) systems are intended to support healthcare workers in the normal course of their duties, assisting with tasks that rely on the manipulation of data and knowledge.

2. Expert systems are the commonest type of AIM system in routine clinical use. They contain medical knowledge, usually about a very specifically defined task, and are able to reason with data from individual patients to come up with reasoned conclusions. Their uses include:
   - generating alerts and reminders,
   - diagnostic assistance,
   - therapy critiquing and planning,
   - agents for information retrieval,
   - image recognition and interpretation.

3. Reasons for the failure of many expert systems to be used clinically include:
   - dependence on an electronic medical record system to supply their data,
   - poor human interface design,
   - failure to fit naturally into the routine process of care,
   - reluctance or computer illiteracy of some healthcare workers.

4. Many expert systems are now in routine use in acute care settings, clinical laboratories, educational institutions, and incorporated into electronic medical record systems.

5. Some AI systems have the capacity to learn, leading to the discovery of new phenomena and the creation of medical knowledge. These machine learning systems can be used to:
   - develop the knowledge bases used by expert systems,
   - assist in the design of new drugs,
   - advance research in the development of pathophysiological models from experimental data.

Chapter 20

Intelligent Systems

The field of artificial intelligence has over the years explored many different avenues in its quest to develop computational intelligence. Despite the many debates over whether one should build or 'evolve' intelligent behaviour, or whether we should replicate or merely simulate human cognitive processes, there has been much common ground amongst scientists. All probably agree for example, that for the behaviour we call 'intelligence' to be recreated in human-built artefacts, we need to develop methods that somehow capture knowledge about the world, and then manipulate that knowledge.

There is much ongoing discussion on just how explicit or detailed such knowledge needs to be. At one extreme we find a camp that feels that intelligence often emerges from the interaction of simple reasoning agents and their environment. These workers in the field of 'artificial life' are inspired by biology, citing for example the way a colony of ants can exhibit intelligent behaviour despite each ant being a relatively simple creature. As a consequence, they see little need to fill AI systems with detailed knowledge about the world (Steels and Brooks, 1995).

At the other extreme sit those researchers that believe an AI system needs to have its intelligence pre-programmed (e.g. Genesereth and Nilsson, 1988). These researchers feel that an AI should contain large amounts of knowledge about the world. This knowledge might need to cover everything from what most of us would call common sense through to complex technical knowledge that might come from a textbook.

From the point of AI in medicine, we are interested in these debates from a practical level, in so far as they can provide us techniques that can be applied to healthcare. As we saw in the last chapter, AI offers medicine methods for constructing computer systems that can carry out tasks that require some understanding of the world for their execution. In other words, intelligent systems have some capacity to capture, and then reason with, medical knowledge.

Given the richness and technical complexity of AI, it would be impossible to cover the breadth of issues involved in constructing intelligent systems here. This chapter will simply attempt to sketch the broad issues involved in developing the sort of AI system that is likely to be encountered in medical practice over the next decade. More comprehensive and specialised texts deal with this subject in far greater depth (e.g., Charniak and McDermott, 1985; Stefik, 1995; Winston, 1984).

20.1 Before reasoning about the world, knowledge must be captured and represented

We saw in the previous chapter that AI systems can have two quite distinct capabilities. Some are able to take medical knowledge and use it to reason from data. Other learning systems are able to take data, and help convert the relationships that might exist amongst different data elements to create new knowledge.

At a very abstract level, we can consider these AI systems either helping to generate models, or using these models to come up with some inference. In this way, they fit very well with the description of models, systems and information developed in the first section of this book (Figure 20.1).

It follows then that the designer of an AI program has several distinct problems to consider.

On what task will the AI system be used? A recurring theme throughout this book has been that the characteristics of a task determines the characteristics of the technology applied to it. This is just as true with complex AI systems. In particular, different **reasoning tasks** like diagnosis, planning or learning need very different types of AI system. Consequently, a system designed to assist in the planning of chemotherapy is technically very different to one intended to detect malignant patterns in a mammogram.

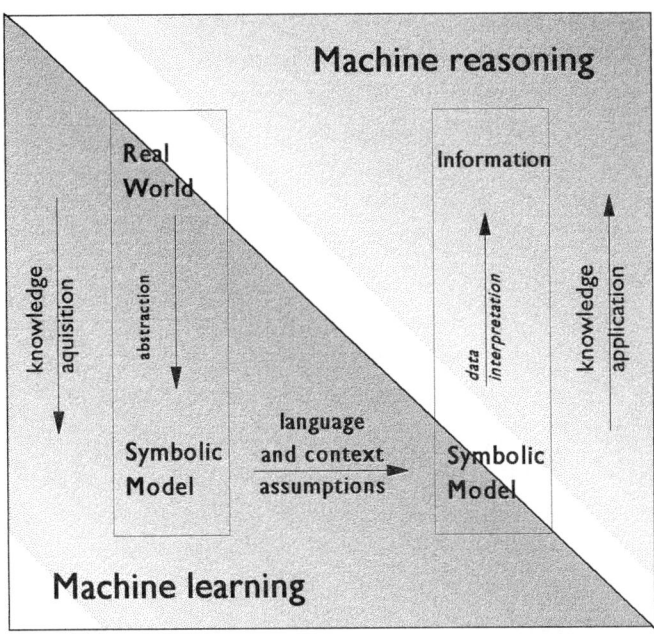

Figure 20.1:
Machine learning programs can help acquire knowledge. AI programs like expert systems can apply that knowledge to reason about the world.

In what circumstances will the task be executed? The resources, skills and needs of individual workers, patients and institutions vary considerably. Consequently they will have very different requirements of a system, even if it apparently executes the same task. The amount of time available, the degree of accuracy expected of a decision, and the skill and training of the individual who might be using the system can all affect the way one designs a system. For example, a program designed to suggest diagnoses will need to perform very differently in different situations. If it is used to help with triage in a battlefield hospital, then it may need to focus on life-threatening conditions than can be actively managed. If it is used by a medical student in training, then it might suggest a long list of differential diagnoses and supply background reading and pathophysiological explanations.

What knowledge will the system have? Human knowledge varies considerably in its level of detail and form. Some aspects of the world are very well defined, and could be expressed for example as a set of detailed mathematical equations. The designs of ventilator machines or the descriptions of some aspects of cardiovascular

*A 'rule of thumb' is also known as a **heuristic**.*

physiology fall into this group. When detailed models exist, they permit some form of explanation about why something occurs. In other areas, our knowledge is much slimmer. It might only be based on experience, and be captured as a set of aphorisms or rules of thumb. In this case, we are only able to say 'this is how it has been in my experience'. Thus, the quality of knowledge available has significant impact on how it can be use by an AI system. We would not expect an expert system, for example, to be able to generate explanations for a set of differential diagnoses if its knowledge only consisted of very simple rules of thumb.

How will that knowledge be presented to the computer? Once it is clear just how much knowledge is available for a particular task, then a choice can be made about the best **knowledge representation** to use within the program. We saw, for example, in Chapter 8 that clinical guidelines could be represented in many different ways, and that the choice of representation depended upon the way the guideline knowledge would be used. Similarly, for an expert system, it might be most appropriate to use a simple set of rules, rather than a complex set of simultaneous differential equations to make a diagnosis, even though both are available. This might be because the equations take too long to solve, require too much data to be provided by the human user, or simply because the accuracy of the answer need only be approximate given the circumstances.

20.2 An AI system designer makes specific choices about reasoning and representation

Amongst the issues discussed in the previous section, two in particular have significant technical implication in the design of an AI system. Once a task has been identified, the designer of the system needs to consider which reasoning method and which knowledge representation will be used.

For example, the different reasoning methods one could use in arriving at a diagnosis might be to use statistics, rules of thumb, neural networks, comparison to past cases and so forth. The knowledge representation chosen is closely related to the reasoning method. For example, one would clearly need to use a model of disease based upon probabilities to support a statistical reasoning method.

It is not possible here to cover the many different approaches to reasoning and representation devised by AI researchers. However, two of the most enduring and successful will methodologies, rule-based expert systems and neural networks, will be described, along with the more complex model-based approach. Since they represent quite different approaches to the problems of reasoning and representation, contrasting them will help to demonstrate the complex issues behind attempts to devise intelligent systems.

20.3 Rule-based expert systems

An expert system is a program that captures elements of human expertise and performs reasoning tasks that normally rely on specialist knowledge. Examples include programmes that can diagnose the cause of abdominal or chest pain, based on clinical observations fed to the programme.

Expert systems perform best in straightforward tasks, which have a predefined and relatively narrow scope, and perform poorly on ill-defined tasks that rely on general or common-sense knowledge (Coiera, 1992a).

In an expert system, the knowledge is usually represented as a set of rules. The reasoning method is usually either logical or probabilistic.

An expert system consists of three basic components.

- A **knowledge base** which contains the rules necessary for the completion of its task.
- A **working memory** in which data and conclusions can be stored.
- An **inference engine** which matches rules to data to derive its conclusions

For a task like interpreting an ECG, an example of a rule which could be used to detect asystole might be:

> RuleASY1:
>   If heart rate = 0
>   then conclude asystole

Box 20.1 - The rules of logical inference

If asked, most clinicians would say that the logical process of diagnosis is most like the **deduction** of Sherlock Holmes. In fact, diagnoses (and most of Mr. Holmes' conclusions) are obtained by using a logical rule called **abduction**. Along with **induction**, these three together form the basic rules of logical inference.

The difference between these logical rules can be understood very simply. We start by assuming there is a **cause and effect** statement about the world which we know to be true. For example, assume that 'pneumonia causes fever' is always true. Pneumonia in this case is the cause, and fever is the effect. Another true statement might be that 'septicaemia causes fever'.

For the process of deduction, we are told that some cause is true, and then infer all the effects that arise naturally as a consequence. In this example, having been told a patient has pneumonia, deduction will tell us that the patient will therefore develop a fever.

In contrast, abduction takes the cause and effect statements we know, and given an observed effect, generates all known causes. In this case, we might be told a patient has fever. Abduction would say that pneumonia or septicaemia are both possible causes. Note that while deduction produces statements of certainty, abduction produces statements of possibility. To choose between the options generated by abduction, one may need to turn to other information, such as statements of probability. If the probability that a feverish patient has pneumonia is greater than for septicaemia, one might conclude on balance that the patient probably has pneumonia.

In contrast to the previous rules of logic which use cause and effect statements, the role of induction is to actually create these statements from observations. For example, a doctor may have observed many patients who have had fevers. Some of these die, and post-mortem examination shows they all have an infection of the lung which the doctor labels 'pneumonia'. The doctor then might decide that 'fever causes pneumonia'.

Unlike the other rules of logic, induction is unsound. In other words, it may lead to false conclusions. Thus, when our doctor finds a feverish patient that does not have pneumonia on autopsy, the original conclusion becomes invalid. Perhaps then, the doctor reuses induction to hypothesise this time the reverse statement 'pneumonia causes fever'. Induction then, is the process of generalisation which creates our models of the world.

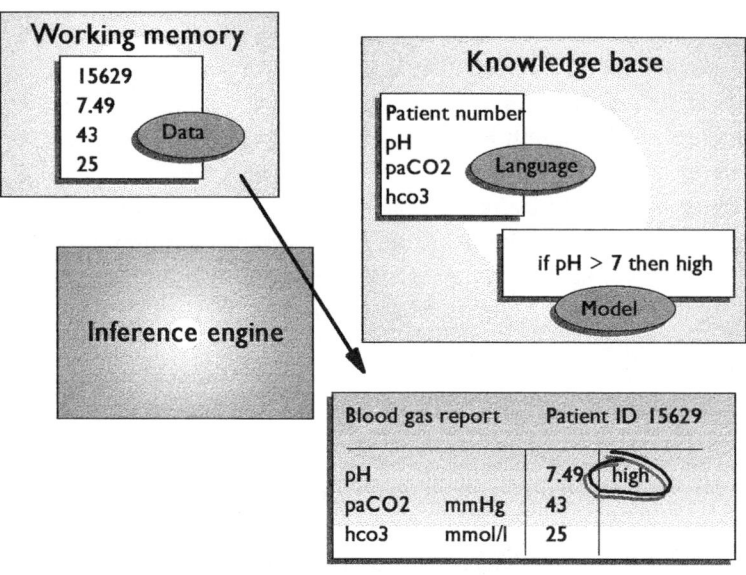

Figure 20.2: *An expert system has three components responsible for modelling knowledge, storing data, and carrying out reasoning procedures.*

If the expert system was attached to a patient monitor then a second rule whose role was to filter out false asystole alarms in the presence of a normal arterial waveform might be:

>   Rule ASY2:
>   If asystole
>   and (ABP is pulsatile and in the normal range)
>   then retract asystole

In the presence of a zero heart rate, the expert system would first match rule ASY1 and conclude that asystole was present. However, if it next succeeded in matching all the conditions in rule ASY2, then it would fire this second rule, which would effectively filter out the previous asystole alarm. If rule ASY2 could not be fired because the arterial pressure was abnormal, then the initial conclusion that asystole was present would remain.

Rules tend to become much more complicated than the simple examples presented here, and the process of manual knowledge acquisition from human experts can become a drawn out affair. To counter this problem, much machine learning research has gone into developing techniques to automate the acquisition of knowledge in

---

Box 20.2 - Bayes' theorem

How likely is it that a patient has a disease, given a certain symptom? This is the question Bayes' theorem sets out to answer, using other statistical data that might be more easily obtainable from a population of individuals.

The theorem states that the probability of a disease given a symptom $P(d|s)$ is dependent on the probability that anyone in the population has the disease $P(d)$, has the symptom $P(s)$, and the likelihood that given the disease, the symptom might develop $P(s|d)$ i.e.:

$$P(d|s) = \frac{P(d)P(s|d)}{P(s)}$$

More complex formulations of the theorem are possible for multiple symptoms, which usually rely on assumptions that individual symptoms are statistically independent of one another.

---

the form of rules or decision trees from databases of cases (e.g. Quinlan, 1986).

For the rules in the previous example, reasoning was based on the application of simple logical rules of inference (see Box 20.1). If the knowledge available to manage a problem was less certain, then the rules could use probabilities. For example:

> RuleASYI:
> If heart rate = 0
> then conclude asystole with probability (0.8)
>
> RuleASY2:
> If heart rate = 0
> then conclude 'ECG leads fallen off' with probability (0.2)

In this case, the inference engine would be designed to come up with the most probable conclusion, based upon an assessment of the data and the known probabilities. One of the commonest probabilistic inference rules used in expert systems is the classic Bayes' theorem (Box 20.2).

20.4 Model-based systems

One of the important contributions of AI has been a growing understanding of the ways in which knowledge can be represented and manipulated. Rule-based representations of knowledge, as we have seen, are only appropriate for narrowly defined problems like diagnosing chest pain. Humans deal with a broader class of problems by invoking other types of knowledge than the rules-of-thumb that are typically stored in an expert system.

Especially with difficult or rare problems, humans may attempt to reason from first principles, using models of pathophysiology or biochemistry to explain a set of clinical manifestations. For example, when several diseases are present at one time, it may only be possible to unravel the constellation of symptoms and signs by recourse to disease models. This contrasts with the simple structure of rules which record commonly seen patterns of disease, and which can only deal with interactions by explicitly enumerating them. The vast number of possible interactions makes such an enumeration of rules impractical (Coiera, 1990).

Model-based systems (sometimes called second-generation expert systems) are designed to utilise disease models in the hope that they will be able to cover a broader set of clinical problems than possible with rules (Uckun, 1992). These models might be constructed from a variety of different representations including mathematical models of physiological relationships, compartmental system models, or indeed statistical models.

As is often the case in medicine, formal models of disease phenomena are often not available or poorly formalised. In such cases, there is evidence that clinicians carry around looser models, expressible in non-numeric or qualitative terms (Kuipers and Kassirer, 1984). Such qualitative representations of medical knowledge have now been formalised, and can be used to capture useful portions of medical knowledge (Coiera, 1992a). These representations have actually proved to be useful in diagnosis (e.g. Ironi et al., 1990), and patient monitoring (e.g. Coiera, 1990; Widman, 1992; Uckun et al., 1993).

Model-based systems are perceived as being better at explanation than 'shallower' rule-based systems, and better at dealing with novel or complex problems. They are also, however, more computationally

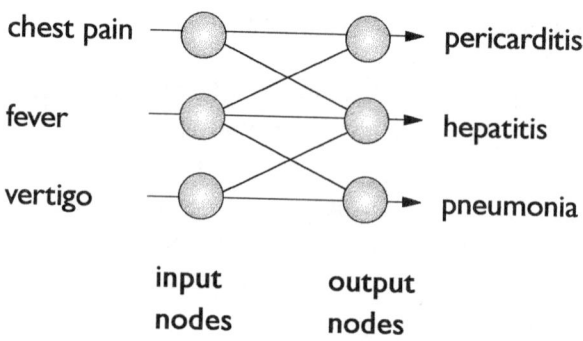

Figure 20.3: *A two layer neural network. Input nodes on the left receive a pattern to be classified, and output nodes on the right are triggered to produce a classification. The sum of the signals received at an output node determine whether or not it will fire.*

expensive to run. In other words, it takes longer to solve a problem using these systems, (although for most common problems, the difference is probably not going to be appreciable). This is because it takes longer to reason a problem out from first principles than it does to simply recognise it from previous experience. Thus there is a move amongst researchers to build systems which combine the two sorts of system, having on the one hand the facility to invoke deep pathophysiological models should they be needed, but also being able to rely on efficient rules whenever they are applicable.

20.5 Neural networks

Neural networks are computer programs whose internal function is based upon a simple model of the neurone (Kohonen, 1988). Networks are composed of layers of neurones (or nodes) with interconnections between the nodes in each layer (Figure 20.3).

For example, a network might be built to connect a set of observations with a set of diagnoses. Each input node would be assigned to a different datum. Each output node would similarly have a corresponding diagnosis assigned to it. The network is then told which observations have been detected, and the output node that has been most 'stimulated' by the input data is then preferential fired, thus producing a diagnosis.

The knowledge associating combinations of observations and diagnoses are stored within the connections of the network. The strength of the connections between different nodes is modelled as a weight on that connection. The stronger the connection between nodes, the greater the assigned weight. Thus, in contrast to an expert system, knowledge in a network is captured in a way that is not easily understood when inspected.

The reasoning procedure is similarly inspired by the way neurones fire once a certain level of activation has been reached. A node in the network fires when the sum of its inputs exceeds a predetermined threshold. These inputs are determined by the number of input connections that have been fired, and the weights upon those connections. Thus, when a net is presented with a pattern on its input nodes, it will output a recognition pattern determined by the weights on the connections between layers.

These weights in a network are obtained by a period of training. A raw network is presented with examples of the data patterns it is intended to recognise, and the weights in the net are slowly adjusted until it achieves the desired output. A neural network thus actually encodes within its weights a discriminating function that is optimised to distinguish the different classes present within its training set.

In theory, any such discriminant function can be approximated by a network (Stinchombe and White, 1989). Despite initial claims of uniqueness for the computational properties of neural nets, it is becoming clear that they have clear and important relationships with a number of more traditional discrimination methods including markov models (Bourland and Wellekens, 1990), Bayesian networks, and decision trees.

The properties of neural networks make them useful both for pattern recognition tasks and real-time signal interpretation. Neural networks have been used to recognise ECG patterns (Pietka, 1989), identify artefacts in arterial blood pressure signals (Sebald, 1989), image recognition (e.g. ultrasound Nikoonahad, 1990) and in the development of clinical diagnostic systems (Hart and Wyatt, 1989).

While the interpretative facility of nets has found numerous applications, it is limited by its inability to explain its conclusions. The reasoning by which a net selects a class is hidden within the distributed weights, and is unintelligible as an explanation. Nets are thus limited to interpreting patterns where no explanation or justification for selecting a conclusion is necessary. Since the need to justify a clinical diagnosis is recognised as an important part of the process of decision support, this limits the application of nets in such tasks.

20.6 The choice of reasoning and representation methods should be based upon the needs of the task

It is still not uncommon to find individuals advocating that one method of reasoning is generally superior to another. In the early days of AIM, there was an extended discussion over the comparative value of probabilistic reasoning and heuristic (or rule of thumb) systems. This was superseded by those who argued for the inherent superiority of brain-inspired neural networks. In their turn, proponents for fuzzy systems, evolutionary computing and genetic algorithms have all made similar claims.

In truth, there is now sufficient understanding of the strengths and weakness of each of these competing reasoning and representation schemes to permit some rational choices to be made. As a system designer, one can thus imagine a toolbox of different techniques being available. Depending on the particular problem to be solved, the most appropriate method can be selected.

20.7 Limitations to interpretation

While expert systems and neural networks can perform at clinically acceptable levels, as with humans there are inherent difficulties in the reasoning process. These limitations need to be made explicit, and should be borne in mind by clinicians who use automated interpretation systems.

Data

Interpretative systems do not have eyes or ears, but are limited to accessing data provided to them electronically. While this constitutes a potentially enormous amount of data to work with, it does mean that critical pieces of contextual information may be unavailable. Thus interpretations need to be judged partly on the data available to the system when making its decision. This highlights the importance of designing an explanatory facility into expert systems, so that clinicians can understand the reasoning behind a particular recommendation by tracing the pieces of data that were used in its formulation.

The task of validating data may have to be one of the first tasks that an interpretative system undertakes. While there are many clues available to suggest whether a datum represents a real measurement or is an error, this is not always decidable based solely on the electronic evidence. There may be no way for a machine to decide that a transducer is incorrectly positioned, or that blood specimens have been mixed up. Clinicians will always need to be wary of the quality of the data upon which interpretations have been made.

Knowledge

Knowledge is often incomplete, and this is an everyday reality in the practice of medicine. Clinicians deal with physiological systems they only incompletely understand, and have evolved techniques for dealing with this uncertainty. While a clinician is able to acknowledge that he or she is performing at the edge of their expertise, and adjust their methods of handling a problem accordingly, it is much harder to incorporate such a facility in a computer system.

Computers at present treat all knowledge equally. While they are able to weigh up probabilities that a set of findings represent a particular condition, they do not take into account they likelihood that some pieces of knowledge are less reliable than others.

Further, most present day systems are forced to utilise a static knowledge base. While there are many techniques which can be used to update knowledge bases, it will not be the case that a system necessarily incorporates the latest knowledge on a subject.

The technical problems associated with the process of knowledge acquisition mean that there are always potential mistakes in the system. Just as a normal computer program can contain 'bugs', so a knowledge base can contain errors, since it is simply another form of program. Wherever possible, the explanation offered by a system should be examined, to ensure that the logical flow of argument reflects current clinical understanding.

Chapter summary

1. Once a task has been identified, the designer of an AI system needs to consider which **reasoning method** and which **knowledge representation** will be used. For example, the different reasoning methods one could use in arriving at a diagnosis might be to use statistics, rules of thumb, neural networks, and comparison with past cases. The knowledge representation chosen is closely related to the reasoning method.

2. An expert system is a program that captures elements of human expertise and performs reasoning tasks that normally rely on specialist knowledge. Expert systems perform best in straightforward tasks, which have a predefined and relatively narrow scope, and perform poorly on ill-defined tasks that rely on general or common-sense knowledge.

3. An expert system consists of three basic components.
   - A **knowledge base** which contains the rules necessary for the completion of its task.
   - A **working memory** in which data and conclusions can be stored.
   - An **inference engine** which matches rules to data to derive its conclusions.

4. Model-based systems (sometimes called second-generation expert systems) are designed to utilise disease models in the hope that they will be able to cover a broader set of clinical problems than possible with rules. These models might be constructed from a variety of different representations including mathematical models of physiological relationships, compartmental system models, or indeed statistical models.

5. Neural networks are computer programs whose internal function is based upon a simple model of the neurone. Networks are composed of layers of neurones (or nodes) with interconnections between the nodes in each layer.

6. AI systems are limited by the data they have access to, and the quality of the knowledge captured within their knowledge base.

Chapter 21

Intelligent monitoring and control

Advances in patient monitoring are usually associated with the development of new clinical measurements, or improvements in the processing of existing ones. Through the introduction of advanced computer techniques, it is now possible to develop monitoring systems that automatically interpret patient signals (Coiera, 1993). Rather than simply displaying measurements for clinicians to interpret, these intelligent monitoring devices can assist clinicians in the task of interpretation itself.

Similar techniques can be used to design intelligent therapeutic devices like patient ventilators or drug delivery systems. These devices are able to monitor patient status to control the delivery of therapy to a patient automatically. Such advances are made possible through developments in the fields of signal processing, pattern recognition and artificial intelligence.

This chapter will look at the role intelligent monitoring and control systems have to play in medicine. The various levels of possible interpretation will be described, along with an introduction to the techniques that are used to create these interpretations.

21.1 The need for automated interpretation and control

The motivations for automating the interpretation of patient measurements and the control of patient systems are numerous. The most pressing arise from the difficulties clinicians face when they continuously monitor patient data, and of themselves are not unique to medicine. They are also an issue for example, in the design of systems used by airline pilots and nuclear power plant operators. These human factors include the problems of cognitive overload, varying expertise, and human error (Wickens, 1992).

Cognitive overload

It should come as no surprise that clinicians may have difficulty in interpreting information presented to them on current patient monitoring systems (Weigner and Englund, 1990). There are finite limits to the cognitive resources that humans can devote to reasoning. These resources can be overloaded by some activities at the cost of others. This cognitive overloading can result in critical patient information being missed or misinterpreted. There are several major mechanisms that contribute to this phenomenon in the clinical environment.

Firstly, the amount of information available on some monitoring systems may be greater than can be assimilated by an individual at one time. This **data overload** can result in the observer failing to notice significant events. Worse still, current monitors may flood clinicians with false alarms, providing further unnecessary distraction (Koski et al., 1990).

This can be compounded by the clinical environment itself, which provides many distractions which compete with monitored data for the clinician's attention. These include tasks other than monitoring which might need to be carried out at the same time, especially in situations like the emergency room, intensive care or in the delivery of anaesthesia. All of these sources of distraction reduce the cognitive effort that can be devoted to signal interpretation, and increase the likelihood of an error of interpretation or a failure to notice data events.

Varying expertise

It is also clear that the level of expertise that individuals bring to a task like the interpretation of signals varies enormously, and it is not always possible for such deficits to be remedied by consultation with more skilled colleagues. Consequently rare events may be missed or misinterpreted. Complexity is also introduced when more than one disease process is active in a patient. They may interact to alter the normal presentation of signals one expects. In the absence of previous experience, the only way such diagnoses can be made is to work back from first principles, often requiring a deep knowledge of the pathophysiological mechanisms involved.

Human error

Cognitive overload and inexperience are two of the major mechanisms that may lead to errors in diagnosis and selection of treatment. For example, the majority of complications associated with anaesthesia, in which clinicians are highly dependent on the use of monitoring equipment to assess patient status, result from inadequate training or insufficient experience of the anaesthetist (Cooper et al., 1984; Sykes, 1987).

There is, however, a wider literature on the causes and effects of human error (Reason, 1990). In particular, human reasoning is susceptible to certain biases that may result in incorrect conclusions being drawn, despite the evidence at hand (Ayton and Pascoe, 1995). The particular causes of error will vary significantly with the environment within which individuals are operating, as well as with the type of decision making problems that face them.

There are several ways in which computer based systems can assist in addressing such difficulties. Firstly, systems can be developed that issue alerts or alarms when clinically significant events are detected. There is now good evidence that such systems can have a positive effect on clinical outcomes, by either reducing the time between the event and it being detected, or by preventing events being completely missed (Shea, DuMouchel et al., 1996).

Computer systems do not only have value as automated safety nets for busy clinicians. It is also possible to design computer systems capable of diagnosing clinical conditions, to assist with rare or complex cases (Patil, 1988). Much of the research in medical artificial intelligence over the last two decades has been devoted to this area, and impressive diagnostic performances have been demonstrated in many specialised medical domains (Clancey and Shortliffe, 1984).

At the other end of the scale, the process of data validation can be automated. At present it is up to the clinician to ascertain whether a measurement accurately reflects a patient's status, or is in error. While in many situations, signal error is clear from the clinical context, it can also manifest itself as subtle changes in the shape of a waveform. Without quite specialised expertise, clinicians may misinterpret measured data as being clinically significant, when it in fact reflects an error in the measurement system. For example, changes in the height of a pressure transducer can significantly alter the measurements it produces.

21.2 System requirements

There are several basic requirements that must be met before a system for automatic interpretation or control can begin to provide clinical benefit.

Firstly, and most importantly, it is essential that any system developed actually fulfils a relevant clinical role. The long lag in the introduction of computerised decision support into medicine is more probably due to failure on this point than because of technological limitations (Shortliffe, 1987). Systems must be developed to fit in with the work practices of clinicians, and to support decision making processes that are clinically relevant (Coiera, 1993). There is little advantage in developing a complex system that mimics interpretative skills already possessed by all clinicians. Rather, it should attempt to provide support for cognitive functions that clinicians perform poorly. Thus the development of intelligent systems is as dependent on developing an understanding of the cognitive patterns of the clinicians who will work with them as it is on advances in technology.

To ensure that monitored parameters are interpreted in clinical context, one may also need access to clinical data other than the monitored signals themselves. This is because it may not be possible to come up with sufficiently useful interpretations without access to background information about a patient. This data may include the medical record, current medications, and values from other devices like the settings from an anaesthetic machine. Centralised patient record systems and clinical workstations seek to do just this.

21.3 Stages of development

Pragmatic considerations suggest that, because of the slow and uneven way in which the electronic patient record is coming into routine use, there needs to be a staged introduction of software capable of intelligent interpretation.

Current first generation systems are relatively simple, and require minimal interaction with the clinician, and minimal or no interaction with the patient record system. Most of these are likely to be found embedded within normal clinical devices. For example, programs exist within current generation patient monitoring devices that are capable of filtering out artefacts and suppressing false alarms.

The next level of system interpretation requires explicit interaction with clinicians, offering some form of active decision support. Such systems will come into their own as integrated electronic patient record systems appear and the medical profession becomes more accustomed to computer assistance. They will be able to assist in the selection of tests and the formulation of diagnoses, as well as the selection of optimal therapies. Interaction will be necessary because, although such systems are capable of drawing conclusions from patient data, they will not have access to the complete clinical picture. The clinician must supply vital clinical context and therapeutic goals unavailable to the system.

The third stage of system introduction could consist of autonomous intelligent systems, capable of independent activity. These are at present experimental, but could eventually form the heart of closed-loop systems. For example, drug delivery systems could automatically measure a drug's level and administer doses based upon that measurement (Blom, 1991; Packer, 1990). The development of such closed-loop systems is at present hampered as much by legal and ethical issues as it is by technological considerations.

21.4 Levels of interpretation

Signal interpretation can occur at a number of levels, starting from a low level assessment of the validity of a signal, through to a complex assessment of its clinical significance. The different levels of interpretation that a signal may pass through are illustrated in Figure 21.1.

A signal is first examined for evidence of artefact. Where possible, the signal is 'cleaned up' by removing the artefactual or noise components of the signal. Once it has been processed in this way, the modified signal is then presented to the next layer in the interpretative hierarchy.

Often a single measurement channel will contain sufficient information for a diagnosis to be made. In some circumstances, however, several alternative explanations might be possible, and a single channel does not contain enough information to disambiguate them. In such circumstances, an interpretative system can look for cross-signal correlations. In Figure 21.1, a flat portion of ECG trace is not diagnosed as an 'asystole' because examination of the corresponding arterial waveform reveals pulsatile behaviour consistent with normal cardiac function.

A higher level of interpretation is also possible, taking into account relevant contextual patient information where this is available. This level is concerned with making decisions based upon signal interpretations, and may include recommendations for further investigations or therapeutic actions. The tasks of artefact detection, single and cross-channel interpretation and decision support will be examined in more detail below.

Artefact detection

The first task in signal interpretation is to decide whether the values that are measured are physiologically valid. In other words, is the signal genuine or is it artefactual? An artefact is defined as any component of the measured signal that is unwanted. It may be caused by noise on the signal, or by distortions introduced through the measurement apparatus. Indeed, an artefact may be due to another physiological process that is not of interest in the current context, like a respiratory swing on an ECG trace. Thus 'one man's artefact is another's signal' (Rampil, 1987).

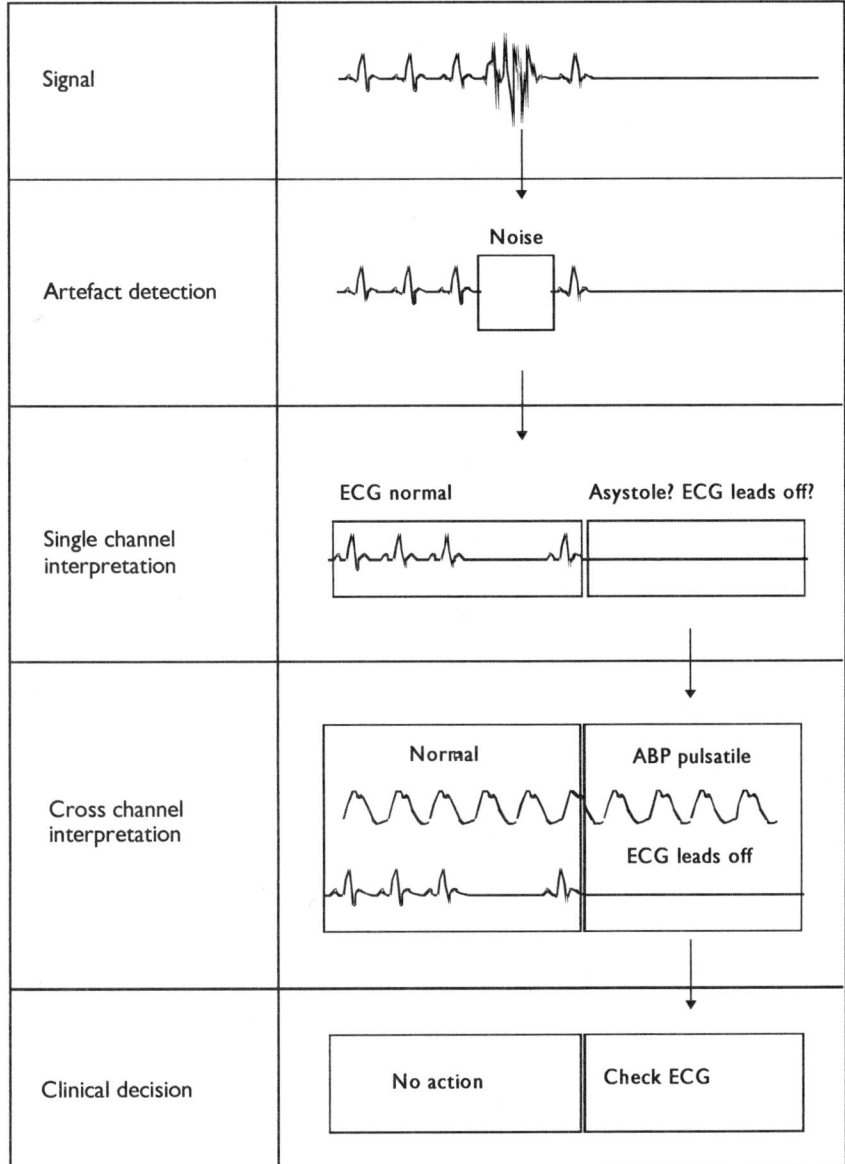

Figure 21.1: *Multiple levels of interpretation take a raw physiological signal and process it, with each level producing increasingly complex interpretations (adapted with permission of W B Saunders Co. Ltd., London, from Coiera, 1994).*

Artefact detection is important for several reasons. Firstly, an artefact may be misinterpreted as a genuine signal and lead to an erroneous therapeutic intervention. Next, invalid but abnormal values that are not filtered can cause alarm systems to register false alarms. Finally, artefact rejection improves the clarity of a signal when it is presented to a clinician for interpretation.

There are many sources of artefact in the clinical environment. False heart rate values can be generated by diathermy noise during surgery and by patient movement, and false high arterial blood pressure alarms are generated by flushing and sampling of arterial lines (Figure 21.2). These forms of artefact have contributed significantly to the generation of false alarms on patient monitoring equipment. Koski et al. (1990) found that only 10% of 1307 alarm events generated on cardiac postoperative patients were significant. Of these, 27% were due to artefacts, e.g. sampling of arterial blood. The net effect of the distraction caused by these high false alarm rates has been that alarms have often been turned off intraoperatively, despite the concomitant increase in risk to the patient.

While an artefact is best handled at its source through improvements in the design of the transducer system, or in low level signal processing, it is not always possible or practical to do so. The next best step is to filter out artefactual components of a signal or register their detection prior to using the signal for clinical interpretation. Many techniques have been developed to assist in this process and include Kalman filtering, rule-based expert systems, blackboard systems, and neural networks. It is in the nature of artefact that it cannot always be eliminated on the basis of a single signal, and cross-channel correlation may be needed, making artefact detection a feature at all levels of signal interpretation.

Single channel interpretation

Having established that a signal is probably artefact free, the next stage in its interpretation is to decide whether it defines a clinically significant condition. This may be done simply be comparing the value to a predefined patient or population normal range, but in most cases such simple thresholding is of limited value.

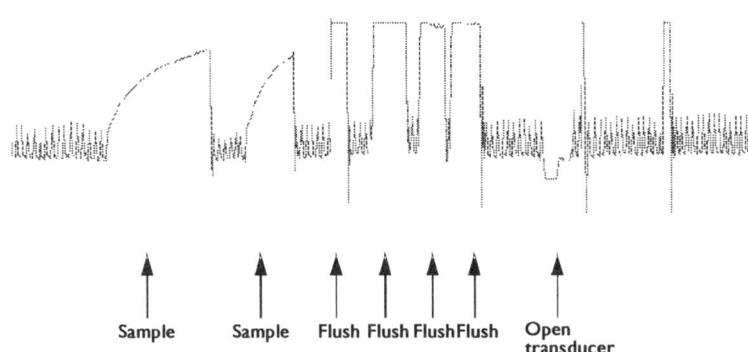

Sample　　Sample　　Flush Flush FlushFlush　　Open
transducer

Figure 21.2:
Examples of artefact
on the arterial blood
pressure channel.
(From Coiera, 1994,
with permission of W
B Saunders Co. Ltd.,
London).

Firstly, clinically appropriate ranges cannot always be defined because the notion of the acceptable range for a patient is highly context specific. One can in fact calculate statistically valid patient specific normal ranges (Harris, 1980, 1981) but these rely on a period of measurement stability which may not be attainable in a dynamic clinical context. Further, the notion of an acceptable range is often tied up with expectations defined by the patient's expected outcome and current therapeutic interventions.

Finally, even if one can decide upon an acceptable range for a specific parameter, the amount of information that a single out of range warning can convey is usually limited. Even wildly abnormal values may have several possible interpretations. These limitations of simple threshold based alarm techniques have spurred on the development of more complex techniques capable of delivering 'smart alarms' (Gravenstein et al., 1987).

Much more information can be obtained from the analysis of a single channel if is a time varying and continuous waveform, like arterial pressure. Specific pressure artefacts like sampling and flushing of the catheter line can be detected by their unique shape (Figure 21.2). Estimates of clinically useful measures like stroke volume can be derived by analysing the area under the curve of the wave (Figure 21.3). It is even possible to analyse the frequency components of the pressure waveform to obtain information about the fidelity of the measurement system itself (Figure 21.4).

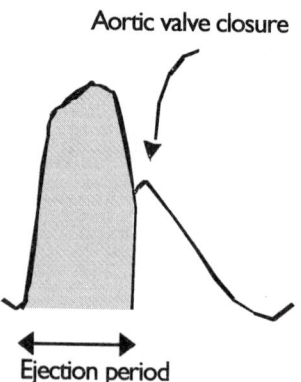

Aortic valve closure

Ejection period

Figure 21.3:
Derivation of information from a waveform's shape. The systolic ejection area beneath the arterial pressure waveform gives an indirect measure of stroke volume. It is demarcated by the beginning of systole and the dicrotic notch caused by the closure of the aortic valve. (From Coiera, 1994, with permission of W B Saunders Co. Ltd., London).

Alterations in the behaviour of a repetitive signal can also carry information. Changes in the ECG are a good example. Features such as the height of the QRS peak help to label individual components within beat complexes. The presence or absence of features like P waves, and the duration and regularity of intervals between waves and complexes can carry diagnostic information about cardiac rhythm. However, it is not always possible to unambiguously label events in an ECG strip, and sometimes one needs to use additional contextual information to assist in the labelling process (e.g. Greenwald et al., 1990).

Cross-channel interpretation

Often conditions can only be identified by examining the signals on several different channels. Such cross channel information is useful at several levels, starting with artefact detection and signal validation through to clinical diagnosis.

Cross-correlation for signal validation can be made with a number of sources, depending on the signal being measured. The alternatives for correlating a signal include the following methods.

Same Signal, different interpretation method. If, for example, an error is suspected when the heart rate is derived by a simple peak detection algorithm, one could attempt to validate the value by comparing it to one derived using a different method on the same data.

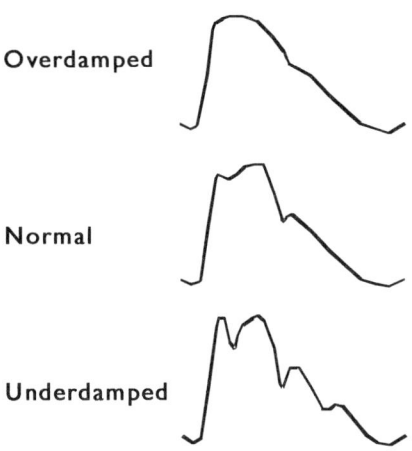

Overdamped

Normal

Underdamped

Figure 21.4: The shape of arterial pressure waves varies with the dynamic response of the catheter transducer. Analysis of the waveform frequency components following a fast flush can assist in detecting system damping and assist in optimising pressure measurements (adapted from Gardner, 1981).

Different physical source, but same signal. Comparing different ECG leads is a common technique for validating changes seen on one lead. Patterns across leads also have diagnostic importance.

Different signal. A flat ECG trace indicating asystole can be checked against the arterial pressure waveform or the plethysmograph, both of which should demonstrate pulsatile waves if the heart were contracting normally, and would loose their pulsatile characteristics if asystole was present.

Cross channel information can also be used to identify conditions not detectable with single channels alone. Many clinical conditions can be distinguished by the time ordering of events in their natural history (Coiera, 1990). For example, the cause of a hypotensive episode may be deducible from the order in which changes occurred across heart rate, blood pressure and CVP (Figure 21.5). In the presence of a vasodilator, the arterial blood pressure drop would precede the reflex tachycardia and CVP fall. In the presence of hypovolaemia, the first parameter to shift would be the heart rate followed by CVP and blood pressure.

Making clinical decisions

Once a computer system is able to diagnose complex disease patterns from measured signals and data stored in electronic patient records, it is in a position to assist clinicians in making therapeutic decisions. As noted earlier, intelligent interpretative systems will appear both as embedded systems hidden within instruments, and as explicit entities which can interact with a clinician.

The way in which an intelligent system is used affects its design. Systems that need to interact with humans may need to justify their decisions in a way that an embedded system does not. Equally, a system that acts as an advisor to a human is placed in a less critical position than one that acts independently to manage a patient's therapy. While embedded interpretative systems are already starting to appear, those that require explicit interaction have yet to make a significant impact.

Decision support systems

The classic model of computer based decision support requires a clinician to input details of a patient's clinical state, with the machine then suggesting one or more possible diagnoses. The MYCIN system is the archetype of this model, providing assistance with the selection of antibiotic therapy (Buchanan and Shortliffe 1984). Other examples include programs which assist in diagnosing abdominal pain (de Dombal, 1972) and chest pain (Goldman et al., 1988). In practice however, this model does not fit well with the realities of the clinical workplace.

Clinicians are often unable to spend the time required to use such systems, and if they do, the types of problems that they would like assistance with are often somewhat different. As a consequence, systems which offer different models of decision support have been developed. For example, to support the decision making that is characteristic of anaesthetists in the operating room, work is currently underway to develop intelligent patient monitors and anaesthetic workstations (e.g. Loeb et al., 1989).

Intelligent monitors will not only suppress spurious alarms generated by signal artefact, but will use cross-channel signal correlations to generate high level diagnostic alarms. They have a role in assisting with clinical vigilance of slowly evolving conditions, and of conditions which have been missed because of distraction.

When integrated with an anaesthetic machine, a monitor system can also warn of faults within the gas delivery system, and possibly suggest corrective actions. Research is also underway exploring

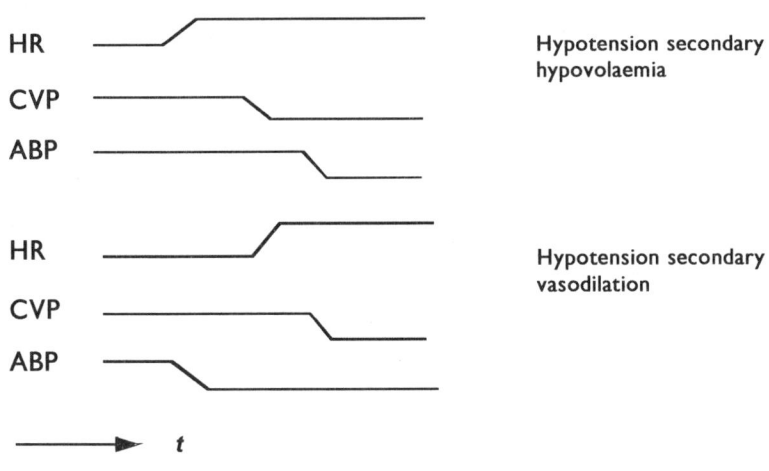

HR

CVP

ABP

Hypotension secondary to hypovolaemia

HR

CVP

ABP

Hypotension secondary to vasodilation

t

Figure 21.5: Time ordering of the onset of trends across different signals can help identify the onset of different clinical conditions. The cause of hypotension can be distinguished by the sequence of changes detected on heart rate (HR), central venous pressure (CVP) and arterial blood pressure (ABP). (From Coiera, 1994, with permission of W B Saunders Co. Ltd., London).

ways of integrating a predictive component into these systems. With such systems, a clinician could test changes to therapy before initiating them by simulating their effect on a mathematical model of the patient (Rutledge et al., 1993).

Other modes of decision support include therapy planning systems, which develop a treatment protocol based on a patient's clinical status (Hickman et al., 1985), and therapy critiquing systems which examine treatment plans generated by clinicians, and attempt to suggest improvements (Miller, 1983).

Autonomous therapeutic devices

In contrast to decision support systems, autonomous systems can operate independently of human interaction on complex tasks. Such systems are at the present moment purely vehicles for research. Perhaps the most studied application area is ventilator management.

Programs have been designed to adjust ventilator settings automatically in response to measurements of a patient's respiratory status. Early research into systems that could wean patients from ventilators (Fagan et al., 1984) has lead to more ambitious projects that seek to take control of most of the tasks associated with ventilator management (e.g. Hayes-Roth et al., 1992). While such projects may in the long term provide new classes of therapeutic devices, it is clear that their successful introduction will require continued advances in sensor design (e.g. implantable glucose sensors for insulin delivery systems), and in the technologies for signal interpretation.

21.5 Methods of interpretation

Intelligent signal interpretation can be divided into two tasks. Firstly, distinct events within a signal are identified using pattern recognition methods e.g. detecting individual peaks in an ECG signal. Secondly, a meaningful label is assigned to the detected events using pattern interpretation methods, e.g. picking a QRS complex from a T wave, and interpreting its clinical significance. There have been significant advances with techniques for performing both these tasks, and new methodologies have emerged, several specifically from research in AI.

Pattern recognition techniques are those that extract significant events from a signal. For example, they detect edges and curves in pictures, or letters, letter groups and words from speech. Pattern detection techniques vary in the way they model events within signals. For example they may be based on statistical models, in which the frequency of certain patterns is used in the recognition process. There are many classic recognition techniques that have clinical application - like blackboard systems (Nii, 1989) (initially developed for speech recognition) and Markov models. Neural networks are an alternative technique for pattern recognition, and they have become of increasing interest both to the biomedical research community in recent years.

Once patterns have been identified within a signal, they need to be interpreted. It is with this task that techniques from AI have made major contributions over the last two decades, especially through the introduction of expert systems. Rule based systems are more suited to cross-channel interpretation of signals than lower level signal processing.

Clinically deployed expert systems perform a variety of tasks from the interpretation of ECGs (Greenwald et al., 1990) to analysis of laboratory results such as thyroid hormone assays (Horn et al., 1985). Experimental expert systems have been developed with more ambitious goals in mind, including systems that can interpret respiratory parameters and automatically adjust ventilator settings during the process of weaning a patient off a ventilator (Fagan et al., 1984).

21.6 Conclusions

It is already the case that much monitoring technology is poorly understood by the clinicians who use it, and that clinicians are often unaware of how to use or interpret their output correctly. As more intelligence is added to the devices that populate the clinical workplace, there is an even greater need to understand their advantages and limitations.

There is no doubt that advances in AI will gradually change many of the ways clinicians handle day to day problems and that they will greatly improve many aspects of the clinical process. Of necessity, the high level at which these systems will perform, assisting both in diagnosis and therapy means that they have a direct impact on patient care.

It will often only be the clinician who will be in a position to assess the conclusions of these systems. Rather than accepting these as a given however, the onus remains on those who use them to do so correctly. While it will not always be necessary to understand the details of the technologies used, and indeed these will continue to evolve, it is necessary to understand their nature and in particular the types of mistake that they are prone to make.

Chapter summary

1. The automated interpretation of patient measurements is needed because of the difficulties clinicians face when they continuously monitor patient data. These human factors include the problems of cognitive overload, varying expertise, and human error.
2. Signal interpretation can occur at a number of levels, starting with artefact detection and removal, moving through to a complex assessment of its clinical significance.
3. Interpretations can be based on data within a single channel like arterial blood pressure, or look at multiple channels for cross-correlations and temporal patterns.
4. Once interpretations have been made, they can be presented for the consideration of a human, or can be used in closed-loop devices to autonomously control patient therapy, including ventilators and IV medication delivery.
5. Intelligent signal interpretation can be divided into two tasks. Firstly, distinct events within a signal are identified using pattern recognition methods e.g. detecting individual peaks in an ECG signal. Secondly, a meaningful label is assigned to the detected events using pattern interpretation methods e.g. picking a QRS complex from a T wave, and interpreting its clinical significance.
6. Neural networks are good at pattern recognition, but have limited ability to explain their conclusions. Expert systems are well suited to use in situations in which some form of explanation of reasoning is needed by the system's user.

Glossary

Abduction: A form of logical inference, commonly applied in the process of medical diagnosis. Given an observation, abduction generates all known causes. See also: Deduction, Induction, Inference.

Agent: Computer software constructed to operate with a degree of autonomy from its user, e.g. an agent may search the Internet for information based upon loose specifications provided by its user. See also: Artificial Intelligence.

Application: Synonym for a computer program that carries out a specific type of task. Word-processors or spreadsheets are common applications available on personal computers.

Arden syntax: A language created to encode actions within a clinical protocol into a set of situation-action rules, for computer interpretation, and also to facilitate exchange between different institutions.

ARPAnet: Advanced Research Projects network. A computer network developed by the United States Department of Defence in the late 1960s, and the forerunner of today's Internet.

Artificial intelligence (AI): Any artefact, whether embodied solely in computer software, or a physical structure like a robot, that exhibits behaviours associated with human intelligence. Also the study of the science and methods for constructing such artefacts. See also: Turing test.

Artificial intelligence in medicine: The application of artificial intelligence methods to solve problems in medicine e.g. developing expert systems to assist with diagnosis, or therapy planning. See also: Artificial Intelligence, Expert system.

Asynchronous communication: A mode of communication between two parties, when the exchange does not require both to be active participant in the conversation at the same time e.g. sending a letter. See also: Synchronous communication, E-mail.

ATM: Asynchronous Transfer Mode. A packet-based communication protocol that provides the high bandwidth transmission rates required for multimedia communication. See also: Packet-switched network, Circuit-switched network

Bandwidth: The amount of data that can be transmitted across a communication channel over a given period of time. See also, Bits per second, Channel.

Bayes' theorem: Theorem used to calculate the relative probability of an event given the probabilities of associated events. Used to calculate the probability of a disease given the frequencies of symptoms and signs within the disease and within the normal population.

B-ISDN: Broadband ISDN. A set of communication system standards for ATM systems. See: ATM, ISDN.

Bit: One binary digit, in base 2. The basic unit for electronically stored or transmitted data. See also: Byte.

Bits per second: A measure of data transmission rate. See also: Bit.

Broadband network: General term for a computer network capable of high-bandwidth transmission rated. See also: ATM.

Browser: A program used to view data e.g. examining the contents of a database or knowledge base, or viewing documents on the World Wide Web. See also: Mosaic, World Wide Web, Internet.

Byte: Eight bits. Bytes are usually counted in kilobytes (1024 bytes), megabytes, and gigabytes. See also: Bit.

Case-based reasoning: An approach to computer reasoning that uses knowledge from a library of similar cases, rather than by accessing a knowledge base containing more generalised knowledge, such as a set of rules. See also: Artificial intelligence, Expert system.

Causal reasoning: A form of reasoning based on following from cause to effect, in contrast to other methods in which the connection is weaker, such as probabilistic association.

CERN: Conseil Européan pour la Recherche Nucléaire. The European Particle Physics Laboratory. It was here that the initial set of standards were developed to create the World Wide Web. See: HTML, HTTP, WWW.

Channel: The connection between two parties that mediates their communication, such as a telephone or e-mail.

Circuit-switched network: A communication network that connects parties by establishing a dedicated circuit between them. See also: Packet-switched network.

Client: A computer connected to a network that does not store all the data or software it uses, but retrieves it across the network from another computer that acts as a server. See also: Client-server architecture, Server.

Client-server architecture: A computer network architecture that places commonly used resources on centrally accessible server computers, which can be retrieved as they are needed across the network by client computers on the network. See also: Client, Server.

Clinical guideline: An agreed set of steps to be taken in the management of a clinical condition.

Clinical pathway: See Clinical guideline.

Clinical protocol: See Clinical guideline.

Closed-loop control: Completely automated system control method in which no part of the control system need be given over to humans. See also: Open-loop control

Code: In medical terminological systems, the unique numerical identifier associated with a medical concept, which may be associated with a variety of terms, all with the same meaning. See also: Term.

Cognitive science: A multi-disciplinary field studying human cognitive processes, including their relationship to technologically embodied models of cognition. See also: Artificial Intelligence.

Computerised protocol: Clinical guideline or protocol stored on a computer system, so that it may be easily accessed or manipulated to support the delivery of care. See also: Clinical guideline.

CPR: Computer-based Patient Record. See: Electronic Medical Record.

Connectionism: The study of the theory and application if neural networks. See: Neural network.

CSCW: Computer supported co-operative work. The study of computer systems developed to support groups of individuals work together. See also: Groupware

Cybernetics: A name coined by Norbert Weiner in the 1950s to describe the study of feedback control systems and their application. Such systems were seen to exhibit properties associated with human intelligence and robotics, and so was an early contributory to the theory of artificial intelligence.

Cyberspace: Popular term now associated with the Internet, which describes the notional information 'space' that is created across computer networks. See also: Virtual reality.

Database: A structured repository for data, usually stored on a computer system. The existence of a regular and formal indexing structure permits rapid retrieval of individual elements of the database.

DECT: Digital European Cordless Telephony standard, which defines the architecture for wireless voice and data communication systems restricted to campus-size areas, rather than wide-area systems that would be publicly available.

Decision support system: General term for any computer application that enhances a human's ability to make decisions.

Decision Tree: A method of representing knowledge which makes structures decisions in a hierarchical tree-like fashion.

Deduction. A method of logical inference. Given a cause, deduction infers all logical effects that might arise as a consequence. See also: Inference, Abduction, Induction.

Distributed computing: Term for computer systems in which data and programs are distributed across different computers on a network, and shared.

DTMF: Dial Tone Multifrequency. The tones generated by punching in numbers on a telephone key-pad.

EDI: Electronic Data Interchange. General term describing the need for healthcare applications to be able to exchange data, requiring the adoption of agreed common standards for the form and content of the messages passing between applications. See also: HL7.

Electronic mail: See E-mail.

Electronic medical record: A general term describing computer-based patient record systems. It is sometimes extended to include other functions like order entry for medications and tests, amongst other common functions.

EMR: See: Electronic medical record

EPR: Electronic patient record. See: Electronic medical record

E-mail: Electronic mail. Messaging system available on computer networks, providing users with personal mail-boxes from which electronic messages can be sent and received.

Epistemology: The philosophical study of knowledge.

Evidence-based Medicine: A movement advocating the practice of medicine according to clinical guidelines, developed to reflect best-practice as captured from a meta-analysis of the clinical literature. See also: Clinical guideline, Protocol.

Expert system: A computer program that contains expert knowledge about a particular problem, often in the form of a set of if-then rules, that is able to solve problems at a level equivalent or greater than human experts. See also: Artificial intelligence.

FAQ: Frequently Asked Questions. Common term for information lists available on the Internet which have been compiled to newcomers to a particular subject, answering common questions that would otherwise often be asked by submitting e-mail requests to a Newsgroup.

Finite state machine: A knowledge representation that makes different states in a process explicit, and connects them with links which specify some transition condition that specifies how one traverses from one state to another.

Firewall: A security barrier erected between a public computer network like the Internet and a local private computer network.

FTP: File Transfer Protocol. A computer protocol that allows electronic files to be sent and received in a uniform fashion across a computer network.

Fuzzy logic: An Artificial intelligence method for representing and reasoning with imprecisely specified knowledge, for example defining loose boundaries to distinguish 'low' from 'high' values. See also: Qualitative reasoning, Artificial intelligence.

Group: A group collects together a number of different codes associated with medical events, that are considered to be sufficiently similar for some purpose e.g. the determination of an appropriate reimbursement for approximately similar clinical procedures or diseases. See also: Term, Code.

Groupware: A computer application that assists communication and shared working amongst groups of individuals with access to a common computer network, but who may be geographically or temporally separated. See also: CSCW.

GSM: The Global System of Mobility. A widely adopted international standard for the architecture and operation of digital cellular telephony systems that can carry voice and data circuits, as well as short packet-data messages.

GUI: Graphical User Interface. That part of a computer application seen and interacted with by its user. Specifically, that part of the interface that is based upon visual structures like icons, which act as metaphors for the different functions supported by the application e.g. deleting a file is enacted by dragging a visual symbol representing the file onto a trash can icon.

Hardware: For a computer system, all its physical components, as distinguished from the programs and data that are manipulated by the computer. See also: Software.

Heuristic: A rule of thumb that describes how things are commonly understood, without resorting to deeper or more formal knowledge. See also: Model-based reasoning.

HIS: Hospital information system. Typically used to describe hospital computer systems with functions like patient admission and discharge, order entry for laboratory tests or medications, and billing functions. See also: Electronic medical record.

HL7: Health Level 7. A healthcare specific communication standard for data exchange between computer appliactions.

Home page: A document on the World Wide Web that acts as a front page or point of welcome to a collection of documents that may introduce an individual, organisation, or point of interest.

HTML: Hypertext Mark-up Language. The description language used to create hypertext documents that can be viewed on the World Wide Web. See also: HTTP, World Wide Web.

HTTP: Hypertext Transfer Protocol. Communication protocol used on the Internet for the transfer of HTML documents. See also: HTML, World Wide Web.

Human-computer interaction: The study of the psychology and design principles associated with the way humans interact with computer systems.

Human-computer interface: The 'view' presented by a program to its user. Often literally a visual window that allows a program to be operated, an interface could just as easily be based on the recognition and synthesis of speech, or any other medium with which a human is able to sense or manipulate.

Hyperlink: A connection between hypertext documents, that allows a reader to trace concepts appearing in one document to related occurrence in other documents.

Hypertext: A method of presenting documents electronically that allows them to be read in a richly interconnected way. Rather than following a single document from beginning to end, sections of each document are connected to related occurrences in other documents via hyperlinks, permitting 'non-linear' reading following concepts of interest to the reader. See also: Hyperlink, HTML, World Wide Web.

ICD-9: The International Classification of Diseases, 9th edition. Published by World Health Organisation.

ICD-10: The International Classification of Diseases, 10th edition. Published by World Health Organisation.

Induction: A method of logical inference used to suggest relationships from observations. This is the process of generalisation we use to create models of the world. See also: Deduction, Abduction, Inference.

Inference: A logical conclusion drawn using one of several methods of reasoning, knowledge and data. See also: Abduction, Deduction, Induction.

Information superhighway: A popular term associated with the Internet, used to describe its role in the global mass transportation of information.

Information Theory: Initially developed by Claude Shannon, describes the amount of data that can be transmitted across a channel given specific encoding techniques and noise in the signal.

Internet: Technically, a network of computer networks. Today, associated with a specific global computer network which is publicly accessible, and upon which the World Wide Web is based. See also: ARPAnet, World Wide Web.

Intranet: A computer network, based upon World Wide Web and Internet technologies, but whose scope is limited to an organisation. An intranet may be connected to an Internet, so that there can be communication and flow of information between it and other intranets. See also: Internet, World Wide Web.

IP address: The address of a computer on the Internet, that permits it to send and receive messages from other computers on the Internet.

ISDN: Integrated Services Digital Network. A digital telephone network that is designed to provide channels for voice and data services.

Knowledge acquisition: Sub-speciality of artificial intelligence, usually associated with developing methods for capturing human knowledge and of converting it into a form that can be used by computer. See also: Machine learning, Wxpert system, Heuristic.

Knowledge-based system: See: Expert system.

LAN: Local Area Network. A computer network limited to servicing computers in a small locality. See also: Intranet.

Machine learning: Sub-speciality of artificial intelligence concerned with developing methods for software to learn from experience, or to extract knowledge from examples in a database. See also: Artificial intelligence, Knowledge acquisition.

Mailing List: A list of email addresses for individuals. Used to distribute information to small groups of individuals, who may, for example, have shared interests. See also: E-mail.

Megabyte: 1024 bytes. See: Byte.

Meta-analysis: Pooled statistical analysis of results from several individual statistical analyses of different experiments, searching for statistical significance which is not possible within the smaller sample sizes of individual studies.

Model: Any representation of a real object or phenomenon, or template for the creation of an object or phenomenon.

Model-based reasoning: Approach to the development of expert systems that uses formally defined models of systems, in contrast to more superficial rules of thumbs. See also Heuristic, Artificial intelligence.

Modem: Modulator-demodulator. Device used for converting a digital signal into tones that can be transmitted down a telephone wire.

Mosaic: The first commonly available World Wide Web browser for viewing hypertext documents, developed at CERN.

Multimedia: Computer systems or applications that are able to manipulate data in multiple forms, including still and video images, sound and text.

Network: Set of connected elements. For computers, any collection of computers connected together so that they are able to communicate, permitting the sharing of data or programs.

Neural computing: see Connectionism.

Neural network: Computer program or system designed to mimic some aspects of neurone connections, including summation of action potentials, refractory periods and firing thresholds.

Newsgroup: A bulletin board service provided on a computer network like the Internet, where messages can be sent by e-mail and be viewed by those who have an interest in the contents of a particular newsgroup. See also: E-mail, Internet.

Object-oriented programming: Computer languages and programming philosophy that emphasises modularity amongst the elements of a program and their sharing of properties and intercommunication.

Open-loop control: Partially automated control method in which a part of the control system is given over to humans.

Open system: Computer industry term for computer hardware and software that is built to common public standards, allowing purchasers to select components from a variety of vendors and use them together.

PABX: Public Area Branch Exchange. Telecommunication network switching station that connects telephones in an area with the wider telephone network.

Packet-switched network: Computer network which exchanges messages between different computers not by seizing a dedicated circuit, but by sending a message in a number of uniformly sized packets along common channels, shared with other computers. See also: Circuit-switched network

Physician's workstation: A computer system designed to support the clinical tasks of doctors. See also: Electronic medical record.

Postscript: Commercial language that describes a common format for electronic documents that can be understood by printing devices and converted to paper documents or images on a screen.

Practice parameter: See: Clinical guideline.

Protocol: See: Clinical guideline.

PSTN: Public Switched Telephone Network, providing ordinary voice-based telephone services.

Qualitative reasoning: A sub-speciality of artificial intelligence concerned with inference and knowledge representation when knowledge is not precisely defined, e.g. 'back of the envelope' calculations.

Read codes: Medical terminology system, developed initially for primary care medicine in the UK. Subsequently enlarged and developed to capture medical concepts in a wide variety of situations. See also: Terminology.

Reasoning: A method of thinking. See also: Inference.

Representation: The method chosen to model a process or object for example a building may be represented as a physical scale model, drawing or photograph. See also: Reasoning, Syntax.

Rule-based expert system: See: Expert system.

Search engine: Computer program capable of seeking information on the World Wide Web (or indeed any large data base) based upon search criteria specified by a user. See also: World Wide Web.

Semantics: The meaning associated with a set of symbols in a given language, which is determined by the syntactic structure of the symbols, as well as knowledge captured in an interpretative model. See also: Syntax.

Server: A computer on a network that stores commonly used resources such as data or programs, and makes these available on demand to clients on the network. See also: Client, Client-server architecture.

SGML: Standard General Mark-up Language. Document definition language used in printing, and used as the basis for the creation of HTML. See also: HTML.

SNOMED: The Systematised Nomenclature of Human and Veterinary Medicine. A commercially available general medical terminology, initially developed for the classification of pathological specimens. See also: Terminology.

Software: Synonym for computer program. See also: Application.

Synchronous communication: A mode of communication when two parties exchange messages across a communication channel at the same time, e.g. telephones. See also: Asynchronous communication.

Syntax: The rules of grammar that define the formal structure of a language. See also: Semantics.

Telco: Abbreviation for telecommunication company.

Telemedicine: The delivery of health care services between geographically separated individuals, using telecommunication systems e.g. video conferencing.

Teleconsultation: Clinical consultation carried out using a telemedical service. See also: Telemedicine.

Term: In medical terminologies an agreed name for a medical condition or treatment. See also: Code, Terminology.

Terminal: A screen and keyboard system that provides access to a shared computer system e.g. a mainframe or mini computer. In contrast to computers on a modern network, terminals are not computers in their own right.

Terminology: A set of standard terms used to describe clinical activities. See also: Term.

Turing test: Proposed by Alan Turing, the test suggests that an artefact can be considered intelligent if its behaviour cannot be distinguished by humans from other humans in controlled circumstances. See also: Artificial intelligence.

URL: Universal Resource Locator. The address for a document placed on the World Wide Web. See also: World Wide Web.

User interface: The view a user has of a computer program, usually understood to mean the visual look and feel of a program, but also extending to other modes of interaction, e.g. voice and touch.

Virtual Reality: Computer simulated environment within which humans are able to interact in some manner that approximates interactions in the physical world.

Vocabulary: See Terminology.

Voice mail: Computer based telephone messaging system, capable of recording and storing messages, for later review or other processing e.g. forwarding to other users. See also: E-mail.

WAN: Wide Area Network. Computer network extending beyond a local area such as a campus or office. See also: LAN.

World Wide Web: An easy-to-use hypertext document system developed for the Internet allowing users to access multimedia documents. See also: Internet, CERN, HTTP, HTML, URL.

WWW: See: World Wide Web.

W3: See: World Wide Web.

References

M. Ackerman, M. Ball, P. D. Clayton, M. E. Frisse, R. M Gardner, et al., Standards for medical identifiers, codes and messages needed to create an efficient computer-stored medical record, *JAMIA*,1,1-7, (1994).

K. P. Adlassnig, W. Horak, Hepaxpert I: Automatic interpretation of tests for Hepatitis A and B, *MD Computing*, 8(2), 118-119, (1991).

W. Ahn, D. L. Medin, A two-stage model of category construction, *Cognitive Science*, 16, 81-121, (1992).

S. Akelsen, S. Lillehaug, Teaching and learning aspects of remote medical consultation, *Telektronikk* ,89(1), 42-47, (1993).

S. Akelsen, G. Hartviksen, L. Vorland, Remote interpretation of microbiology specimens based on transmitted still images, *J Telemedicine and Telecare*, 1, 229-233, (1995).

A. Allen, L. Roman, R. Cox, B. Cardwell, Home health visits using a cable television network: user satisfaction, *J Telemedicine and Telecare*,2, Supplement 1, 92-4, (1996).

R. Anderson, NHS-wide networking and patient confidentiality, *BMJ*, 311, 5-6, (1995).

E. Antman, J. Lau, B. Kupelnick, F. Mosteller, T. Chalmers. A comparison of the results of meta-analysis of randomised controlled trials and recommendations of clinical experts. *JAMA*, 268, 240-8, (1992).

P. Ayton, E. Pascoe, Bias in human judgement under uncertainty? *Knowledge Engineering Review*, 10(1), 21-42, (1995).

C. Babbage, *On the Economy of Machinery and Manufactures*, Charles Knight, London, 3rd Edition, (1833).

G. O. Barnett, H. J. Sukenik, Hospital Information Systems, *in* Dickson and Brown (1969).

G. O. Barnett, J.J. Cimino, J.A. Huppa, et al., Dxplain: an evolving diagnostic decision-support system, *JAMA*, 258, 69-76, (1987).

R. C. Barrows, P. D. Clayton, Privacy, confidentiality, and electronic medical records, *JAMIA*, 3, 139-148, (1996).

N. Bean, Secrets of network success, *Physics World*, 30-34, Feb.,(1996).

T. Bereners-Lee, R. Calliau, A. Luotonen, H.F. Nielsen, A. Secret, The World Wide Web, *Communications of the ACM*, 37(8), 76-82, (1994).

A. Bhattacharyya, J. R. Davis, B. E. Halliday, A. R. Graham, S. A. Leavitt et al., Case triage model for the practice of telepathology, *Telemedicine J*, 1, 1, 9-17, (1995).

J. A. Blom, Expert control of the arterial blood pressure during surgery, *International Journal of Clinical Monitoring and Computing*, 8, 25-34, (1991).

Bolam v Friern Barnet, *HMC* 1 WRL 582, (1957).

D. Boden, *The business of talk - Organisations in Action*, Polity Press, (1994).

O. Bouhaddou, K. Cofrin, D. Larsen, H. Warner Jr., P. Huber, D. Sorenson et al., Implementation of practice guidelines in a clinical setting using a computerized knowledge base (Iliad), *Proceedings of 17th Symposium on Computer Applications in Medical Care*, 258-262, (1993).

H. Bourland, C. Wellekens, Links between markov models and multilayer perceptrons, *IEEE Transactions on Pattern Analysis and Machine Intelligence*, 12, 1167-1178, (1990).

H. Bower, Internet sees growth of unverified health claims, *BMJ*, 313, 381, (1996).

R. A. Bowles, R. Teale, Communications services in support of collaborative health care, *BT Technology Journal*,12(3), 29-44 (1994).

D. Brahams, The medicolegal implications of teleconsulting in the UK, *J Telemedicine and Telecare*, 1, 196-201, (1995).

P. J. Branger, J. C van der Wouden, B. R. Schudel, E. Verboog, et al., Electronic communication between providers of primary and secondary care, *BMJ*, 305,1068-1070, (1992).

I. Bratko, I. Mozetic, N.Lavrac, *KARDIO: A study in Deep and Qualitative Knowledge for Expert Systems*, MIT Press, Cambridge MA., (1989).

L. L. Bready, R. B. Smith, *Decision making in Anesthesiology*, B C Decker, Toronto, (1987).

F. Brennan, On the relevance of discipline in informatics, *JAMIA*,1, 200-201 (1994).

B.G.Buchanan, E.H.Shortliffe (eds.) *Rule-Based Expert Systems: the MYCIN experiments of the Stanford Heuristic Programming Project*, Addison-Wesley, Reading MA, (1984).

E. L. Buhle, J. W. Goldwein, I. Benjamin, OncoLink: A multimedia oncology information resource on the Internet, *JAMIA,* Symposium Supplement, 103-107, (1994).

J. E. Cabral Jr., Y. Kim, Multimedia systems for telemedicine and their communication requirements, *IEEE Communications Magazine*, 20-27, July (1996).

B. S. Caldwell, S. Uang, L. H. Taha, Appropriateness of communications media use in organizations: situation requirements and media characteristics, *Behaviour and Information Technology*, 14, 199-207, (1995).

J. R. Campbell, T. H. Payne, A comparison of four schemes for codification of problem lists, Proceedings of the Symposium on Computer Applications in Medicine, *JAMIA*, Symposium Supplement, 201-204, (1994).

CCC, A Guide to the use of tables of equivalence between ICD-9 and ICD-10, NHS Centre for Coding and Classification; Report F6110, (1995).

E. Charniak, D.V.McDermott, *Introduction to Artificial Intelligence*, Addison-Wesley, Reading MA, (1985).

J. J. Cimino, P. D. Clayton, Coping with changing controlled vocabularies, Proceedings of the Symposium on Computer Applications in Medicine, *JAMIA*, Symposium Supplement,135-139, (1994).

J. J. Cimino, Controlled medical vocabulary construction: Methods from the CANON group, *JAMIA*;1,296-297, (1994).

W.J. Clancey, E.H.Shortliffe (eds.), *Readings in Medical Artificial Intelligence - The First Decade,* Addison-Wesley, Reading MA, (1984).

W. J. Clancy, Notes on "Epistemology of a rule-based expert system", *Artificial Intelligence*, 59, 197-204, (1993a).

W. J. Clancy, Notes on "Heuristic Classification", *Artificial Intelligence*, 59, 191-196, (1993b).

H. Clarke, S. Brennan, Grounding in Communication, in L.B. Resnick J. Levine, and S. D. Behreno (Eds.), *Perspectives on socially shared cognition*, American Psychological Association, Washington, (1991).

B. Cohen, *The specification of complex systems*, Addison-Wesley, (1986).

E. Coiera, Monitoring diseases with empirical and model-generated histories, *Artificial Intelligence in Medicine*, 2, 135-147, (1990).

E. Coiera, Incorporating user and dialogue models into the interface design of an intelligent patient monitor, *Medical Informatics*, 16, 331-346, (1991).

E. Coiera, The qualitative representation of physical systems, *Knowledge Engineering Review*, 7,1, 55-77,(1992a).

E. Coiera, Intermediate depth representations, *Artificial Intelligence in Medicine*, 4, 431-445, (1992b).

E. Coiera, Editorial: Intelligent monitoring and control of dynamic physiological systems, *Artificial Intelligence in Medicine*, 5, 1-8, (1993).

E. Coiera, Automated signal interpretation, in P. Hutton, C. Prys-Roberts (eds.) *Monitoring in Anaesthesia and Intensive Care*, Bailliere Tindall Ltd., London, (1994).

E. Coiera, V. Tombs, G. Higgins, T. H. Clutton-Brock, Real-time clinical decision making, *HP Laboratories Technical Report*; HPL-94-79, (1994).

E. Coiera, Question the assumptions, in P. Barahona, J.P. Christensen (eds.), *Knowledge and Decisions in Health Telematics - The Next Decade*, IOS Press, Amsterdam, 61-66, (1994).

E. Coiera, S. C. R. Lewis, *Information Management System*, European patent application 94302119.6, 24th March, (1994); US patent application 08/409,444, 24th March, (1995).

E. Coiera, Medical Informatics, *BMJ*, 310, 1381-7, (1995).

E. Coiera, Editorial: The Internet's challenge to healthcare provision, *BMJ*, 311, 2-4, (1996a).

E. Coiera, Artificial intelligence in medicine - the challenges ahead, *JAMIA*, 3, 363-366, (1996b).

E. Coiera, Clinical communication - a new informatics paradigm, *Proc. 1996 AMIA Annual Fall symposium, JAMIA Symposium Supplement,* 17-21, (1996).

P. Compton, R. Jansen, A philosophical basis for knowledge acquisition, *Knowledge Acquisition*, 2, 241-257, (1990).

P. Compton, G. Edwards, B. Kang, L. Lazarus, R. Malor, et al., Ripple down rules: Turning knowledge acquisition into knowledge maintenance, *Artificial Intelligence in Medicine*, 4, 463-475, (1992).

J. Constable, Active Voice, *BJ Healthcare computing and Information management,* 11, 30-31, (1994).

J.B. Cooper, R. S. Newbower, R. J. Kitz, An analysis of major errors and equipment failures in anaesthesia management: considerations for prevention and detection, *Anesthesiology*, 60,1, 34-42,(1984).

R. A. Côté, D. J. Rothwell, J. L. Palotay, R. S. Beckett, L. Btochu, *The Systematised Nomenclature of Human and Veterinary Medicine - SNOMED International* (4 vols), College of American Pathologists (1993).

D. C. Cox, Wireless personal communications: What is it?, *IEEE Personal Communications*, April, 20-35, (1995).

P. Cutler, *Problem Solving in Clinical Medicine - from data to diagnosis*, Williams and Wilkins, Baltimore, (1979).

S. J. Darmoni, P. Massari, JM. Droy, E. Moirot, J. Le Roy. SETH: an expert system for the management on acute drug poisoning in adults. *Comput. Methods Programs Biomed.*; 43: 171-176 (1993).

R. Dawkins, *The Extended Phenotype*, Oxford University Press, Oxford, (1982).

R. S. Dick, E. B. Steen, (eds.), *The Computer-based Patient Record - An Essential Technology for Health Care*, National Academy Press, Washington, DC, (1991).

J. F. Dickson III, J. H. U. Brown (eds.)., *Future Goals of Engineering in Biology and Medicine*, Proceedings of an International Conference held at Washington DC, September 1967, Academic Press, New York, (1969).

F. T. de Dombal, D. J. Leaper, Computer-aided diagnosis of acute abdominal pain, *BMJ*,2, 9-13, (1972).

F. T. de Dombal, V. Dallos, W. A. F. McAdam, Can computer aided teaching packages improve clinical care in patients with acute abdominal pain?, *BMJ*, 302, 1495-1497, (1991).

T. Delamothe, Whose data are they anyway?, *BMJ*, 312, 1241-2, (1996).

V. Della Mea, S. Forti, F. Puglisi, P. Bellutta, N. Finato, et al., Telepathology using Internet multimedia electronic mail: remote consultation on gastrointestinal pathology, *J Telemedicine and Telecare*, 2, 28-34, (1996).

T. DeMarco, *Controlling Software Projects - Management, Measurement, Estimation*, Prentice-Hall, NJ, (1982).

M. Dojat , A. Harf , D. Touchard , M. Laforest , F. Lemaire and L. Brochard, Evaluation of a knowledge-based system providing ventilatory management and decision for extubation, *American Journal of Respiratory and Critical Care Medicine*, (1996).

G. C. Doolittle, A. Allen, From acute leukaemia to multiple myeloma: clarification of a diagnosis using tele-oncology, *J Telemedicine and Telecare*, 2, 119-121, (1996).

K. Doughty, K. Cameron, P. Garner, Three generations of telecare of the elderly, *J Telemedicine and Telecare*, 2, 71-80, (1996).

J. Durinck, E. Coiera, R. Baud et al, The role of knowledge based systems in clinical practice, in P. Barahona, J.P. Christensen (eds), *Knowledge and Decisions in Health Telematics - The Next Decade*, IOS Press, Amsterdam, 199-203, (1994).

T. D. East, A. H. Morris, T. Clemmer, J. F. Orme, C. J. Wallace, S. Henderson et al., Development of computerized critical care protocols - a strategy that really works!, *Proceedings of 14th Symposium on Computer Applications in Medical Care*, 564-568, (1990).

T. D. East, S. H. Bohm, C. J. Wallace, T. P. Clemmer, L. K. Weaver, J. F. Orme Jr., A H Morris, A successful computerized protocol for clinical management of pressure control inverse ratio ventilation in ARDS patients, *Chest*, 101(3), 697-710, (1992a).

T. D. East, A. H. Morris, C. J. Wallace, T. P. Clemmer, J. F. Orme Jr., L K Weaver et al., A strategy for development of computerized critical care decison support systems, *International Journal of Clinical Monitoring and Computing*, 8, 263-269, (1992b).

Economist, Doctors in the dock, *The Economist*, August 19, 23-4, (1995).

G. Edwards, P. Compton, R. Malor, A. Srinivasan, L. Lazarus. PEIRS: a pathologist maintained expert system for the interpretation of chemical pathology reports, *Pathology*, 25, 27-34, (1993).

A. S. Elstein, L. S. Shulman, S. A. Sprafka, *Medical Problem Solving - An Analysis of Clinical Reasoning*, Harvard University Press, Cambridge MA, (1978).

D. Evans, J. J. Cimino, W. R. Hersh, S. M. Huff, D. S. Bell, Toward a medical-concept representational language, *JAMIA*, 1, 207-217, (1994).

Evidence-Based Medicine Working Group, Evidence-based Medicine, *JAMA*, 268, 2420-5, (1992).

N. F. Ezquerra, R. Mullick, E. V. Garcia, C. D. Cooke, E. Kachouska, PERFEX: An Expert System for Interpreting 3D Myocardial Perfusion, *Expert Systems with Applications*, Pergamon Press, (1992).

D. Fafchamps, C.Y Young, P. C. Tang, Modeling work practices: Input to the design of a physician's workstation, *Proc. 15th SCAMC*, (1991).

L. Fagan, E. H. Shortliffe, B. Buchanan, Computer-based medical decision making: from MYCIN to VM, in J. Clancey, E. H. Shortliffe (eds), *Readings in Medical Artificial Intelligence - The First Decade*, 241-255, Addison-Wesley, Reading MA, (1984).

N. Fenton, G. Hill, *Systems Construction and Analysis: a Mathematical and Logical framework*, McGraw-Hill, London, (1993).

A. R. Feinstein, *Clinical Judgement*, Williams and Wilkins, Baltimore, (1967).

A. R. Feinstein, ICD, POR, and DRG: Unsolved scientific problems in the nosology of clinical medicine, *Arch Intern Med*, 148, 2269-2274, (1988).

M. J. Fisk, A comparison of personal response services in Canada and the UK, *J Telemedicine and Telecare*, 1, 145-156, (1995).

K. Fitzpatrick, E. Vineski, The role of cordless phones in improving patient care, *Physician Assistant*, June, 87-92, (1993).

G. H. Forman, J. Zahorjan, The challenges of mobile computing, *IEEE Computer*, 38-47, April, (1994).

J. Fox, N. Johns, A. Rahmanzadeh, R. Thomson, PROforma: a method and language for specifying clinical guidelines and protocols, *Proc. Medical Informatics Europe - MIE '96*, (1996).

E. A. Franken, K. S. Berbaum, W. L. Smith, P. J. Chang, D. A. Owen, G. R. Bergus, Teleradiology for rural hospitals: analysis of a field study, *J Telemedicine and Telecare*, 1, 202-208, (1995).

E. A. Franken Jr, K. S. Berbaum, Subspecialty radiology consultation by interactive telemedicine, *J Telemedicine and Telecare*, 2, 35-41, (1996).

D. B. Fridsma, P. Ford, R. Altman, A survey of patient access to electronic mail: attitudes, barriers and opportunities, Proceedings of the Symposium on Computer Applications in Medicine, *Journal of the American Medical Informatics Association*, Symposium Supplement, 15-19, (1994).

C. P. Freidman, J. C. Wyatt, *Evaluation Methods in Medical Informatics*, Springer-Verlag, New York, (1997).

J. K. French, B. F. Williams, H. H. Hart, S. Wyatt, J. E. Poole, et al., Prospective evaluation of eligibility for thrombolytic therapy in acute myocardial infarction, *BMJ*, 312, 1637-41, (1996).

C. Friedman, S. M. Huff, W. R. Hersh, E. Pattison-Gordon, J. J. Cimino, The CANON Group's Effort: Working toward a merged model, *JAMIA*, 2, 4-18, (1995).

R.M.Gardner, Direct blood pressure measurements - Dynamic Response Requirements, *Anesthesiology*, 54, 227-236, (1981).

M. R. Genesereth, N.J. Nilsson, *Logical Foundations of Artificial Intelligence*, Morgan Kauffman, Palo Alto CA, (1988).

M. Gersenovic, The ICD family of classifications, *Meth Info Med*, 34, 172-5, (1995).

L. Gierl, M. Feistle, H. Muller, K. Silva, D. Varnhlt, S. Villain, Task-specific authoring functions for end-users in a hospital information system, *Computer Methods and Programs in Biomedicine*, 48, 145-150, (1995).

N. S. Glance, B. A. Huberman, The Dynamics of Social Dilemmas, *Scientific American*, 58-63, March, (1994).

A. J. Glowinski, E. W. Coiera, M. J. O'Neil, the role of domain models in maintaining the consistency of large medical knowledge bases, Proceedings of the Third AIME, *Lecture Notes in Medical Informatics*, 44, 72-81, (1991).

A. J. Glowinski, Integrating guidelines and the clinical record: the role of semantically constrained terminologies, in *Health Telematics for clinical guidelines and protocols*, C. Gordon, J. P. Christensen (eds.), IOS Press: Amsterdam, (1994).

C. A. Goble, A. J. Glowinski, K. G. Jeffery, Semantic constraints in a medical information system, *Proc. 11th BNCOD*, B. Worbuys, A. F. Grundy, (eds.), Lecture Notes in Computer Science 696, 40-57, (1993a).

C. A. Goble, A. J. Glowinski, A. Nowlan, A. Rector, A descriptive semantic formalism for medicine, *Proc 9th IEEE Intl Conf Data Enginnering*, IEEE Computer Society Press, 624-632, (1993b).

F. Goodlee, The Cochrane Collaboration, *BMJ*, 309, 969-70, (1994).

L. Goldman, E. F. Cook, et al., A computer protocol to predict myocardial infarction in emergency department patients with chest pain, *NEJM*, 318, 797-803, (1988).

P. Gorman, Does the medical literature contain the evidence to answer the questions of primary care physicians? Preliminary findings of a study, *Proc. 17th Annual Symposium on Computer Applications in Medical Care,* 571-575, (1993).

J. Gravenstein, R. Newbower, A. Ream, N. Smith, (eds.), *The Automated Anaesthesia Record and Alarm Systems,* Butterworths, Boston, (1987).

D. Greatbatch, P. Luff, C. Heath, P. Campion, Interpersonal communication and human-computer interaction: an examination of the use of computers in medical consultations, *Interacting with Computers,* 5(2),193-216, (1993).

S. Greenwald, R. Patil, R. Mark, Improved detection and classification of arrhythmias in noise-corrupted electrocardiograms using contextual information, *Computers in Cardiology,* (1990).

J. Gregory, J. E. Mattison, C. Linde, Naming Notes: Transitions from free text to structured entry, *Meth Inform Med*, 34, 57-67, (1995).

R. L. Gregory (ed.), *The Oxford Companion to the Mind*, Oxford University Press, Oxford, (1987).

P. A. Halvorsen, I. S. Kristiansen, Radiology services for remote communities: cost minimisation study of telemedicine, *BMJ*, 312, 1333-6, (1996).

C. Ham, Health care rationing, *BMJ*, 310, 1483-4, (1995).

R. Handel, M. Huber, *Integrated Broadband Networks - An introduction to ATM-based networks*, Addison-Wesley, (1991).

D. Hau, E. Coiera, Learning Qualitative models of dynamic systems, *Machine Learning*, 26, 177-211, (1997).

E. K. Harris, On the use of statistical models of within-person variation in long term studies of healthy individuals, *Clinical Chemistry*, 26, 383-391, (1980).

E. K. Harris, Use of statistical models to detect subject specific changes, in *Progress in Health Monitoring - Proceedings of The International Conference on Automated Multiphasic Health Testing and Services*, T. Yasaka (ed), Excerpta Medica, Amsterdam (1981).

A. Hart, J. Wyatt, Connectionist models in medicine: an investigation of their potential, in J. Hunter, J. Vookson, J. Wyatt (eds), *Lecture Notes in Medical Informatics,* volume 38, 115-124, Springer-Verlag, (1989).

B. Hayes-Roth, R. Washington, D. Ash, et al., Guardian: A prototype intelligent agent for intensive care monitoring, *Artificial Intelligence in Medicine*, 4, 165-185, (1992).

H. A. Heathfield, J. Wyatt, Medical informatics: hiding our light under a bushel, or the emperor's new clothes ? *Meth Inf Med*, 32,181-2, (1993).

H. A. Heathfield, J. Kirby, N. R. Hardiker, Data entry in computer-based care planning, *Computer Methods and Programs in Biomedicine*, 48, 103-107, (1995).

J. Heinsohn, D. Kudenko, B. Nobel, H. Profitlich, An empirical analysis of terminological representation systems, *Artificial Intelligence*,68,367-397, (1994).

Henderson, R. O. Crapo, C. J. Wallace, T. D. East, A. H. Morris, R. M. Gardner, Performance of computerised protocols for the management of arterial oxygenation in an intensive care unit, *International Journal of Clinical Monitoring and Computing*, 8, 271-280, (1992).

S. Henry, K. Campbell, W. Holzemer, Representation of nursing terms for the description of patient problems using SNOMED III, *Proceedings of the Symposium on Computer Applications in Medicine*, McGraw Hill: New York; 700-704, (1993).

D. H. Hickam, E. H. Shortliffe, et al., A study of the treatment advice of a computer-based cancer chemotherapy protocol advisor, *Ann. Intern. Med.*, 101, 928, (1985).

D. F. Hochstrasser, R. D. Appel, O. Golaz, Ch. Pasquali, J. C. Sanchez, A. Bairoch, Sharing of worldwide spread knowledge using hypermedia facilities and fast communnication protocols (Mosaic and World Wide Web): The example of ExPASy, *Meth Inform Med*, 34, 75-8, (1995).

R. M. Hogarth, Generalisation in decision research: The role of formal models, *IEEE Trans. Syst. Man. Cybernet*; 16(3), 439-449, (1986).

J. H. Hohnloser, F. Pürner, P. Kadlec, Coding medical concepts: A controlled experiment with a computerised coding tool, *Int J Clin Monit Comput*, 12, 141-145, (1995).

J. H. Hohnloser, F. Pürner, H. Soltanian, Improving coded data entry by an electronic patient record system, *Methods of Information in Medicine*, 35, 108-11, (1996).

K.Horn, P. Compton, et al., An expert system for the interpretation of thyroid assays in a clinical laboratory, *Australian Computer Journal*, 17, 7-11, (1985).

B. Hydo, Designing an effective clinical pathway for stroke, *Am. J.Nursing Continuing Education Series*, (1995), http://www.ajn.org/ajn/5.3/a503044e.1t

L. Hunter (ed.), *Artificial Intelligence and Molecular Biology*, AAAI Press/ The MIT Press, Menlo Park, CA, (1993).

ICD-9, *Manual of the International Statistical Classification of Diseases, Injuries and Causes of Death*, World Health Organisation, Geneva , (1977).

ICD-10, *International Statistical Classification of Diseases and Related Health Problems - 10th Revision*, World Health Organisation, Geneva, (1993).

L. Ironi, M. Stefannelli, G.Lanzola, Qualitative models in medical diagnosis, *Artificial Intelligence in Medicine*, 2, 85-101, (1990).

R. Johansen et al., *Leading business teams*, Addison Wesley, (1991).

D. H. Jones, C. Crichton, A. Macdonald, S. Potts, D. Sime et al., Teledermatology in the Highlands of Scotland, *J Telemedicine and Telecare*,2, Supplement 1, 7-9, (1996).

M. G. Kahn, S. A. Steib, V. J. Fraser, W. C. Dunagan. An expert system for culture-based infection control surveillance, *Proceedings Symposium on Computer Applications in Medical Care*. New York, NY: McGraw Hill,:171-5, (1993).

C. E. Kahn Jr., Validation, clinical trial and evaluation of a radiology expert system, *Methods of Information in Medicine*, 30, 268-274, (1991).

D. Kahneman, P. Slovic, A. Tversky (eds), *Judgment Under Uncertainty: Heuristics and Biases*, Cambridge University Press, NY (1982).

S. Kay, I. N. Purves, Medical records and other stories: a narratological framework, *Methods of Information in Medicine*, 35, 72-87, (1996).

E. Keravnou (ed.), *Deep models for medical knowledge engineering*, Elsevier Science Publishers B.V.:Amsterdam, (1992).

R. D. King, S. Muggleton, R. A. Lewis, M.J.E. Sternberg, Drug design by machine learning: the use of inductive logic programming to model the structure-activity relationship of trimethoprim analogues binding to dihydrofolate reductase, *Proc. Nat. Acad. Sci., USA*, 89, 11322-11326, (1992).

G. A. Klein, R. Calderwood, Decision models: some lessons from the field, *IEEE Transactions on Systems, Man and Cybernetics*, 21 (5), 1018-1026, (1991).

R. Klein, Priorities and rationing:pragmatism or principles? *BMJ*, 311, 761-2, (1995).

T. J. Kline, T. S. Kline, Radiologists, communication and resolution 5: A medicolegal issue, *Radiology*,184,131-134,(1992).

J. Klir, M. Valach, *Cybernetic Modelling*, Iliffe Books, London, 1967.

T. Kohonen, An Introduction to neural computing, *Neural Networks*, 1, 3-16, (1988).

E. Koski, A. Makivirta, T. Sukuvaara, A. Kari, Frequency and reliability of alarms in the monitoring of cardiac postoperative patients, *International Journal of Clinical Monitoring and Computing*, 7, 129-133, (1990).

L. P. Krall, R. S. Beaser, *Joslin Diabetes Manual*, 12th Edn., Lea and Febiger, Philadelphia, (1989).

B.J. Kuipers, J.P. Kassirer, Causal reasoning in medicine: analysis of a protocol, *Cognitive Science*, 8, 363-385, (1984).

G. J. Kuperman, R. M. Gardner, The impact of the HELP computer system on the LDS Hospital paper medical record, *Proc. SCAMC*, 673-7, (1990).

G. J. Kuperman, R. M. Gardner, T. A. Pryor, *The HELP System*, Springer-Verlag New York, (1991).

S. E. Labkoff, S. Shah, R. A. Greenes, Patterns of information resource access in patient care: a study of the use of portable computers to support the clinical encounter, *Capturing the Clinical Encounter, Proc AMIA Spring Congress*, 33, (1995).

R. E. LaPorte, E. Marler, S. Akazawa, F. Sauer, C. Gamboa, C. Shenton et al, The death of biomedical journals, *BMJ*,310,1387-9, (1995).

R. E LaPorte, Patterns of disease: diabetes mellitus and the rest, *BMJ*, 310, 545-6, (1995a).

R. E. LaPorte, Global public health and the information superhighway, *BMJ*, 308, 1651-2, (1995b).

L. S. Lawton, *Integrated Digital Networks*, Sigma, Wilmslow, England (1993).

R. S. Ledley, L. B. Lusted, Reasoning foundations of medical diagnosis, *Science*, 130, 9-21, (1959).

V. O. Leirer, D. G. Morrow, E. D. Tanke, G. M. Pariante, Elders' nonadherence: Its assessment and medication reminding by voice mail, *The Gerontologist*, 31(4), 514-520, (1991).

N. G. Leveson, C. S. Turner, An investigation of the Therac-25 accidents, *IEEE Computer*, 18-41, July, (1993).

R. C. Lewontin, *The Doctrine of DNA - Biology as Ideology*, Penguin, (1993).

A. D. Little, *Telecommunications: Can it help solve America's health care problems?* Little, Cambridge, MA (1992).

B. Littlewood (ed), *Software Reliability - Achievement and Assessment*, Blackwell Scientific Publications, Oxford, (1987).

D. F. Lobach, W. E Hammond, Development and evaluation of a computer-assisted management protocol (CAMP): Improved compliance with care guidelines for diabetes mellitus, *Proc. 18th Annual Symposium on Computer Applications in Medical Care, Journal of the American Medical Informatics Association*, Symposium Supplement, 787-791, (1994).

C. Lock, What value do computers provide to NHS hospitals?, *BMJ*, 312, 1407-10, (1996).

R. Loeb, J. Brunner, D. Westenskow et al., The Utah Anaesthesia Workstation, *Anesthesiology*, 70, 999- 1007, (1989).

H. J. Lowe, E. C. Lomax, S. E. Polonkey. The World Wide Web: A Review of an emerging Internet-based technology for the distribution of biomedical information, *JAMIA,* 3,1-14, (1996).

H. Ma, Mapping clause of Arden syntax with the HL7 and ASTM E 1238-88 standard, *Int J Bio-Med Comp*, 38, 9-21 (1995).

D. MacNeill, V. Huang, Pen Computers in Healthcare, *Pen Computing Magazine*, 18-25, April, (1996).

F. Majidi, J. P. Enterline, M. S. B. Ashley, M. E. Fowler, L. L. Ogorzalek, J. D. R. Gaudette et al., Chemotherapy and treatment scheduling: The Johns Hopkins Oncology Center Outpatient Department, *Proc. 17th Annual Symposium on Computer Applications in Medical Care,* 154-158, (1993).

J. Martel, M. D Jimenez, F. J Martin-Santos, A. Lopez-Alonso, Accuracy of teleradiology in skeletal disorders: solitary bone lesions and fractures, *J Telemedicine and Telecare*, 1, 13-18, (1995).

J. Martin, *The Great Transition - using the seven disciplines of enterprise engineering to align people, technology, and strategy*, AMACOM, American Management Association, New York, (1995).

N. Mays, C. Pope (eds), *Qualitative Research in Health Care*, BMJ Publishing Group, London, (1996).

J. C. McCarthy, A. F. Monk, Channels, conversation, co-operation and relevance: all you wanted to know about communication but were afraid to ask, *Collaborative Computing*, 1, 35-60, (1994).

P. McLaren, Telepsychiatry in the USA, *J Telemedicine and Telecare*, 1, 121, (1995).

S. Miksch , M. Dobner , W. Horn , C. Popow, VIE-PNN: An Expert System for Parenteral Nutrition of Neonates, *Ninth IEEE Conference on Artificial Intelligence for Applications (CAIA-93)*, Orlando, Florida, March 1-5, 285-91, (1993).

P. L. Miller, Critiquing anesthetic management: the ATTENDING computer system, *Anesthesiology*, 58, 362-369, (1983).

P. L. Miller, *Selected Topics in Medical Artificial Intelligence*, Springer-Verlag, New York, (1988).

R. A. Miller, Medical Diagnostic Decision Support Systems - Past, Present, and Future: A threaded bibliography and brief commentary, *JAMIA*, 1, 8-27, (1994).

R. Monk, *Ludwig Wittgenstein - The Duty of Genius*, Jonathan Cape, (1990).

R. M. Morrell, B. L. Wasilauskas, R. M. Winslow. Personal computer-based expert system for quality assurance of antimicrobial therapy. *Am J Hosp Pharm.*, 50, 2067-73, (1993).

A. Morris, C. Wallace, R. Menlove, T. Clemmer, J. Orme, L. Weaver et al., A randomised clinical trial of pressure-controlled inverse ratio ventilation and extracorporeal CO_2 removal from ARDS, *Am J Respir Crit Care Med*, 149(2), 295-305, (1994).

A. Morris, T. East, C. Wallace, J. Orme, T. Clemmer, L. Weaver et al., Ethical implications of standardization of ICU care with computerized protocols, *Proceedings of the Symposium on Computer Applications in Medicine*, *JAMIA* Symposium Supplement, 501-505, (1994).

M. A. Musen, S. W. Tu, A. K. Das, Y. Shahar, A Component-based architecture for automation of protocol-directed care, in Lecture Notes in Artificial Intelligence 934 - *Proc. 5th Conference on Artificial Intelligence in Medicine Europe - AIME-95*, Springer, Berlin, 1-13, (1995).

C. D. Mulrow, Rationale for systematic reviews *BMJ*, 309, 597-9, (1994).

S. M Murphy-Muth, *Medical Records - Management in a changing environment*, Aspen, Rockville MA , (1987).

N. Negroponte, *Being Digital*, Knopf, NY, (1995).

T. H. Nelson, A file structure for the complex, the changing and the indeterminate, *Proc. 20th National ACM Conf.*, 84-100, (1965).

H. P. Nii, Blackboard Systems, in A. Barr, P. Cohen, E. A. Feigenbaum (eds), *The Handbook of Artificial Intelligence* Vol. IV, Addison-Wesley, Reading, MA , 1-82, (1989).

M. Nikoonahad, D.C. Liu, Medical ultrasound imaging using neural networks, *Electronic Letters*, 26, 545-546, (1990).

R. E. Nisbett and T. D. Wilson. Telling more than we can know: Verbal reports on mental processes. *Psychological Review*, 84, 231–259, (1977).

D. A. Norman, Cognition in the Head and in the World: An introduction to the special issue on situated action, *Cognitive Science*, 17(1), 1-6, (1993).

J. Nymo, Telemedicine, *Telektronikk*, 89(1), 4-11, (1993).

M O'Neil, C Payne, J Read, Read Codes Version 3: A user led terminology, *Meth Info Med*, 34, 187-92, (1995).

F. Oesterlen, *Medical Logic*, (English Translation), Sydenham Society, London, (1855).

J. S. Packer, Patient care using closed-loop computer control, *Computing and Control Engineering Journal*, 1,1, 23-28, (1990).

J. E. Padgett, C. G. Gunther, T. Hattori, Overview of Wireless Personal Communications, *IEEE Communications Magazine*, January, 28-41, (1995).

S. Paterson-Brown, J. Wyatt, N. Fisk. Are clinicians interested in up-to-date reviews of effective care ? *BMJ*, 307, 1464, (1993).

S. Paterson-Brown, N. M. Fisk, J. C. Wyatt. Uptake of meta-analytical overviews of effective care in English obstetric units. *BJOG*, 102, 297-301, (1995).

R. S. Patil, Artificial Intelligence Techniques for Diagnostic Reasoning in Medicine, in H. Shrobe (ed), *Exploring Artificial Intelligence*: Survey Talks from the National Conferences on Artificial Intelligence, 347-380, Morgan Kaufmann, San Mateo, (1988).

D. Pendleton, T. Schofield, P. Tate, P Havelock, *The Consultation - an approach to learning and teaching*, Oxford University Press, Oxford, (1984).

P. Phaal, *LAN traffic management*, Prentice Hall International, Hemel Hempstead, (1994).

E. Pietka, Neural nets for ECG classification, in *Images of the 21st century: IEEE Engineering in Medicine and Biology 11th annual Conference*, 2021-2022, (1989).

H. Pince, R. Verberckmoes , J. L. Willems , Computer aided interpretation of acid-base disorders, *Int. J. Biomed. Comp.*, 25, 177-192, (1990).

D. J. Protti. The synergism of health/medical informatics revisited, *Methods of Information in Medicine*, 34, 441-5, (1995).

K. Popper, *Unended Quest*, Fontana, (1976).

J. R. Quinlan, Induction of Decision Trees, *Machine Learning*, 1, 81-106, (1986).

D. Raggett, J. Lam, I. Alexander, *HTML 3: Electronic Publishing on the World Wide Web*, Addison-Wesley, Harlow, (1996).

I. J. Rampil, Intelligent Detection of Artifact, in *The Automated Anaesthesia Record and Alarm Systems*, J. Gravenstein, R. Newbower, A. Ream, N. Ty Smith (eds.), 175-190, Butterworths, Boston, (1987).

J. Ramsay, A. Barabesi, J. Preece, Informal communication is about sharing objects and media, *Interacting with Computers*, 8 (3), 277-283, (1996).

J. N. Rao, Follow up by telephone, *BMJ*, 309,1527-1528, (1994).

J. Reason, *Human Error*, Cambridge University Press, Cambridge, (1990).

A. L. Rector, W. A. Nolan, A. Glowinski, Goals for concept representation in the GALEN project, *Proc. 17th SCAMC*, 414-418, (1993).

A. L. Rector, W. D. Solomon, W. A. Nolan, T. W. Rush, P. E. Zanstra, W. M. A. Claassen, A terminology server for medical language and medical information systems, *Meth Info Med*, 34, 147-57, (1995).

J. L. Renaud-Salis, Distributed Clinical Management-Information Systems: An enabling technology for future health care programmes, in P. Barahona, J. P. Christensen (eds.), *Knowledge and Decisions in Health Telematics - The Next Decade*, IOS Press: Amsterdam, 139-146, (1994).

R. E. Rice, Task analyzability, use of new media, and effectiveness: a multi-site exploration of media richness, *Organizational Science*, 3, 475-500, (1992).

R. J. Richardson, M. A. Goldberg, H. S. Sharif, D. Matthew, Implementing global telemedicine: experience with 1097 cases from the Middle East to the USA, *J Telemedicine and Telecare*,2, Supplement 1, 79-82, (1996).

M. J. Rodriquez, M. T. Arredono, F. del Pozo, E. J. Gomez , A. Martinez, A. Dopico, A home telecare management system, *J Telemedicine and Telecare*, 1, 86-94, (1995).

W. L. Roper, W. Winkenwerder, G. H. Hackbarth, H. Krakauer, Effectiveness in Health Care - an initiative to evaluate and improve medical practice, *New England Journal of Medicine*, 319 (18), 1197-1202, (1988).

E. Rosch, Principles of Categorization, in E. Rosch, B. B. Lloyd (eds.), *Readings in Cognitive Science*, Morgan Kaufmann:Los Altos, CA; 312-322, (1988).

D. J. Rothwell, SNOMED-based knowledge representation, *Meth Info Med*, 34, 209-13, (1995).

G. Rutledge, G. Thomsen, B. Farr et al., The design and implementation of a ventilator-management advisor, *Artificial Intelligence in Medicine*, 5, 67-82, (1993).

M. J.Sawar, T. G. Brennan, A. J. Cole and J. Stewart, An Expert System for PostOperative Care (POEMS), in *Proceedings of MEDINFO-92*, Geneva, Switzerland, Sept (1992).

E. A. Schafer, G. D. Thane, *Quain's Elements of Anatomy*, Vol 1 - Part III, Longmans, Green and Co., London, (1891).

A. Sebald, Use of neural networks for detection of artifacts in arterial pressure waveforms, in *Images of the 21st Century* - IEEE Engineering in Medicine and Biology 11th Annual Conference, 2034-35,(1989).

D. Shanit, A. Cheng, R. A. Greenbaum, Telecardiology: supporting the decision-making process in general practice, *J Telemedicine and Telecare*, 2, 7-13, (1996).

S. Shea, R. V. Sidell, W. DuMouchel, G. Pulver, R. R. Arsons, P. D. Clayton, Computer-generated information messages directed to physicians: effect on length of hospital stay, *JAMIA*, 2, 58-64, (1995).

S. Shea, R., W. DuMouchel, L. Bahamonde, A meta-analysis of 16 randomized controlled trials to evaluate computer-based clinical reminder systems for preventative care in the ambulatory setting, JAMIA, 3, 399-409, (1996).

R. N. Shiffman, Towards effective implementation of a pediatric asthma guideline: Integration of decision support and clinical workflow support, *Proceedings of 18th Symposium on Computer Applications in Medical Care*, 797-801, (1994).

E. H. Shortliffe, Computer Programs to Support Clinical Decision Making, *JAMA*, 258, 61-66, (1987).

I. Sim, M. A. Hlatky, Growing pains of meta-analysis, *BMJ*, 313, 702-3, (1996).

D. Slepian (Ed.), *Key papers in the Development of Information Theory*, IEEE Press, New York, (1974).

B. H. Smith; N. T. James; D. L. Sackett, W. M. C. Rosenberg, J. A Muir Gray, R. B. Haines, Correspondence: Evidence Based Medicine, *BMJ*, 313, 169-171 (1996).

H. T. Smith, P. A. Hennessy, G.A. Lunt, An object-oriented framework for modelling organisational communication, *Studies in computer supported cooperative work*, J. M. Bowers, S. D. Benford (eds.), Elsevier Science (North-Holland),145-157, (1991).

M. F. Smith, Telemedicine Safety, *J Telemedicine and Telecare*, 2, Supplement 1, 33-36, (1996).

R. Smith, The greatest breakthrough since fire or just more technology?, *BMJ* 312, ii, (1996a).

R. Smith, What clinical information do doctors need?, *BMJ*, 313(7064), 1062-67, (1996b).

M. G. Snow, R. J. Fallat, W. R. Tyler, S. P. Hsu,. Pulmonary consult: concept to application of an expert system, *Journal of Clinical Engineering*, 13(3), 201-205, (1988).

S. Staender, J. M. Davies, R. L. Helmreich, B. Sexton, M. Kaufmann, Anesthesia critical incident reporting system: an experience database, *Proc. Mednet '96 - European Congress of the Internet in Medicne*, 44-5, (1996).

L. Steels, R. Brooks (Eds.), *The Artificial Life route to Artificial Intelligence*, Lawrence Erlbaum, NJ, (1995).

M. Stefik, *Introduction to Knowledge Systems*, Morgan Kauffman, San Francisco, (1995).

M. Stinchombe, H. White, Multilayer Feedforward Networks are Universal Approximators, *Neural Networks*, 2, 359-366, (1989).

R. Stoupa, J. Campbell, Documentation of ambulatory care rendered by telephone: Use of a computerized nursing module, *Proceedings of the Symposium on Computer Applications in Medicine*, IEEE Computer Society Press:Los Alamitos, CA, 890-893, (1990).

M..K. Sykes, Essential Monitoring, *Br. J. Anaesth.*, 59, 901-912, (1987).

P. Szolovits, , *Artificial Intelligence in Medicine*, AAAS Selected Symposia Series, Westview Press, Colorado, (1982).

A. S. Tanenbaum, *Computer Networks*, Third Ed., Prentice Hall, NJ, (1996).

P.C. Tang, D. Fafchamps, E. H. Shortliffe, Traditional Hospital Records as a Source of Clinical Data in the Outpatient Setting, *Proc. SCAMC*, 575-9, (1994).

H.J. Tange, The paper-based patient record: Is it really so bad?, *Computer Methods and Programs in Biomedicine*, 48, 127-131, (1995).

H. Tange, How to approach the structuring of the medical record? Towards a model for flexible access to free text medical data, *International Journal of Bio-medical computing*, 42, 27-34, (1996).

E. Tenner, *Why Things Bite Back - Technology and the Revenge Effect*, (1996).

G. E. Thomsen, D. Pope, T. East, A Morris, A. Tupper Kinder, D. Carlsom et al., Clinical Performance of a rule-based decision support system for mechanical ventilation of ARDS patients, *Proceedings of the Symposium on Computer Applications in Medicine*, McGraw Hill, New York, 339-343, (1993).

L. A. Thompson, W. C. Ogden, Visible speech improves human language understanding: implications for speech processing systems, *Artificial Intelligence Review*, 9, 347-358, (1995).

C. Trendelenburg: Interpretation of special findings in laboratory medicine and medical responsibility. *Lab. Med.*,18, 545-582, (1994).

S. W. Tu, M. G. Kahn, M. A. Musen, J. Ferguson, E. H. Shortliffe, L.M. Fagan, Episodic skeletal-plan refinement based upon temporal data, *Communications of the ACM*, 32 (12), 1439-1455, (1989).

H. M. Tufo, J. J. Speidel, Problems with Medical Records, *Medical Care*, 9, 509-517, (1971).

M.G. Turnin, R. H. Beddok, J. P. Clottes, P. F. Martini, R. G. Abadie et al., Telematic Expert System Diabeto, *Diabetes Care*, 15, 204-12, (1992)

M. S. Tuttle, The position of the CANON group: A reality check, *JAMIA*, 1, 298-299, (1994).

M. S. Tuttle, S. J. Nelson, The role of the UMLS in 'storing' and 'sharing' across systems, *Int J Bio-Med Comp*, 34, 207-237, (1994).

M. S. Tuttle, W. G. Cole, D. D. Sherertz, S. J. Nelson, Navigation to Knowledge, *Meth Inform Med*, 34, 214-31, (1995).

M. C. Vissers, J. Biert, C. J. v.d. Linden, A. Hasman, Effects of a supportive protocol processing system (protoVIEW) on clinical behaviour of residents in the accident and emergency department, *Computer Methods and Programs in Biomedicine*, 49, 177-184, (1996).

S. Uckun, Model-Based Reasoning in Biomedicine, *Critical Reviews in Biomedical Engineering*, 19(4), 261-292, (1992).

S. Uckun, B. Dawant, D. Lindstrom, Model-based diagnosis in intensive care monitoring: the YAQ approach, *Artificial Intelligence in Medicine*, 31-48, (1993).

J. M. Utterback, *Mastering the Dynamics of Innovation*, Harvard Business School Press, Boston, (1994).

R. P. van der Loo, E. M. van Gennip, A. R. Bakker, A. Hasman, F. F. Rutten, Evaluation of automated information systems in health care: an approach to classifying evaluative studies, Computer Methods and Programs in Biomedicine, 48, 45-52, (1995).

H. R. Warner, P. Haug, O. Bouhaddou, M. Lincoln, H. R. Warner Jr, D. Sorenson, J. W. Williamson, C. Fan. Iliad: An Expert Consultant to Teach Differential Diagnosis, *Proc. SCAMC*, 371, (1988).

M. B. Weigner, C. E. Englund, Ergonomic and human factors affecting anesthetic vigilance and monitoring performance in the operating room environment, *Anesthesiology*, 73, 5, 995-1021,(1990).

S. Whittaker, Rethinking video as a technology for interpersonal communications: theory and design implications, *Int. J. Human-Computer Studies*, 42, 501-529, (1995).

C. D. Wickens, *Engineering Psychology and Human Performance*, Harper Collins, New York, (1992).

A. W. Wicker, Attitudes v. Actions: the Relationship of Verbal and Overt Responses to Attitude Objects, in *Attitudes*, N. Warren, M. Jahoda (eds), 2nd. Ed. Penguin Books Ltd., Middlesex, (1976).

L. E. Widman, A model-based approach to the diagnosis of cardiac arrhythmias, *Artificial Intelligence in Medicine*, 4, 1-19, (1992).

E. Williams, Experimental comparisons of face-to-face and mediated communication: a review, *Psychological Bulletin*, 84, 963-976, (1977).

P.H. Winston, *Artificial Intelligence*, Addison-Wesley MA , (1984).

E. J. Wisniewski, D. L. Medin, On the interaction of theory and data in concept learning, *Cognitive Science*, 18, 221-281, (1994)

C.B. Withers. Electronic voicemail: one hospital's experience, *Computers in Healthcare*, 28-30, (1988).

L. Wittgenstein, *Philosophical Investigations*, Macmillan, New York, (1953).

J. Wyatt, The evaluation of clinical decision support systems: a discussion of the methodology used in the ACORN project, *Proceedings of AIME 87, Lecture Notes in Medical Informatics,* Springer-Verlag, Berlin, 33, 15-24, (1987).

J. Wyatt, Lessons learned from the field trial of ACORN, an expert system to advise on chest pain. In: B. Barber, D. Cao, D. Qin, eds. *Proc. Sixth World Conference on Medical Informatics*, Singapore, North Holland, Amsterdam, 111-115, (1989).

J. Wyatt, Use and sources of medical knowledge, *The Lancet*, 338,1368-1373, (1991).

J. Wyatt, Evidence-based decision support. - Is it feasible? *Workshop on Decision support in primary and secondary care - priorities for implementation*, NTRHA, 20 December, (1995).

Index

Page numbers appearing in **bold** refer to figures and page numbers appearing in *italic* refer to tables